Fabulous Females and Peerless Pīrs

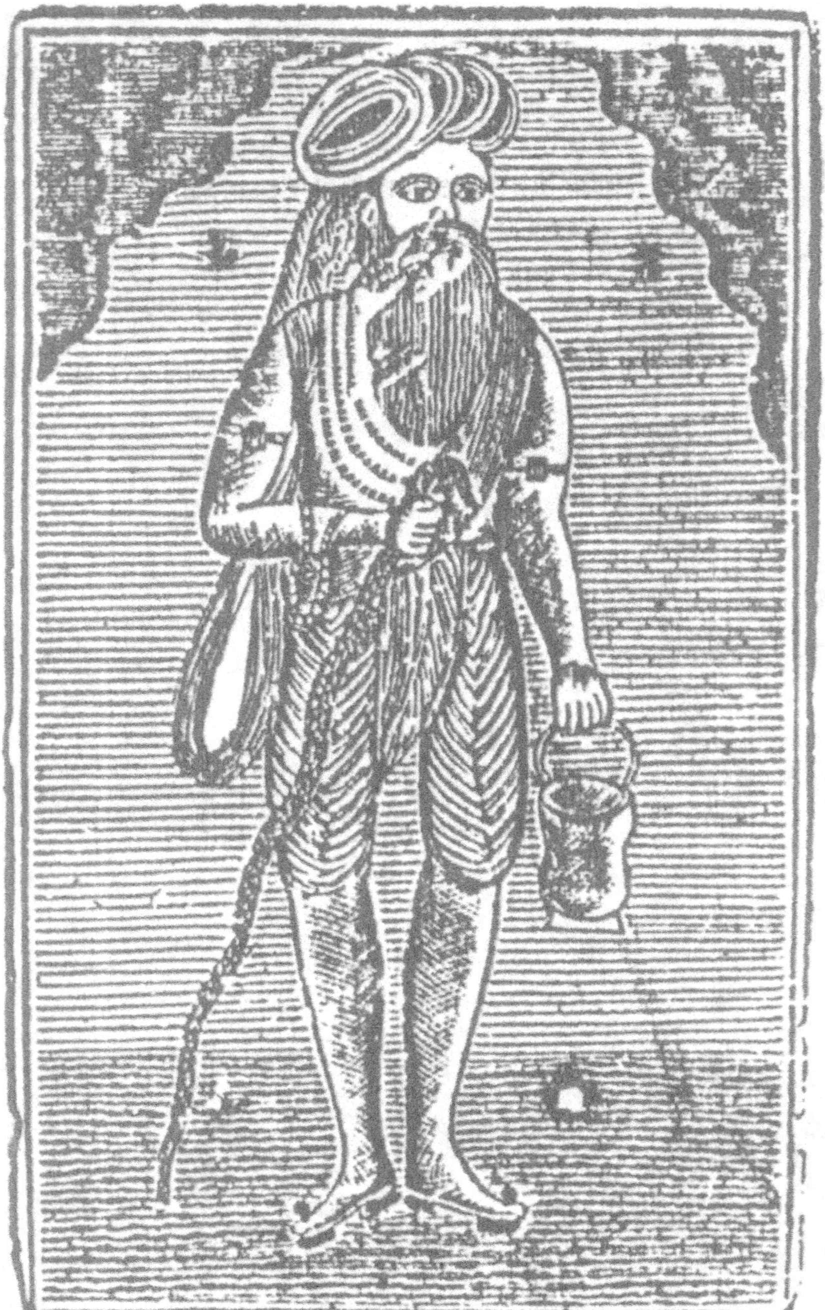

Fabulous Females and Peerless Pīrs

Tales of Mad Adventure in Old Bengal

TRANSLATED BY

Tony K. Stewart

OXFORD
UNIVERSITY PRESS
2004

OXFORD
UNIVERSITY PRESS

Oxford New York
Auckland Bangkok Buenos Aires Cape Town Chennai
Dar es Salaam Delhi Hong Kong Istanbul Karachi Kolkata
Kuala Lumpur Madrid Melbourne Mexico City Mumbai
Nairobi São Paulo Shanghai Taipei Tokyo Toronto

Published by Oxford University Press, Inc.
198 Madison Avenue, New York, New York 10016

www.oup.com

Library of Congress Cataloging-in-Publication Data
Fabulous females and peerless pīrs: tales of mad adventure in old bengal / translated by Tony K. Stewart.
p. cm.
Includes bibliographical references and index.
Translated from Bengali.
ISBN 0-19-516529-2; 0-19-516530-6 (pbk.)
1. Short stories, Bengali—Translations into English. 2. Bengal (India)—Social life and customs. 3. Bangladesh—Social life and customs. 4. Religious pluralism. I. Stewart, Tony K., 1954–
PK1716.5.Faa 2003
891.4'430108—dc21 2003000165

1 3 5 7 9 8 6 4 2

Printed in the United States of America
on acid-free paper

for Joan R.

whose story,

if it isn't already here,

should be

PREFACE

This is a book I never set out to write, but after years of working in this literature I found the need to do so. It began as curiosity about the figure of Satya Pīr, who seemed to be a syncretistic figure, an odd mixture of Hindu and Muslim, packaged in tales that were not easily classified according to any standard genres I knew. These seemingly insignificant tales turned out to be anything but—in intellectual content, in style and range, in geographic distribution, and in number—even though, when pressed, few scholars seemed to know anything about them. I have located more than 750 handwritten manuscripts and more than 160 printed works by at least one hundred different authors, writing mainly in Bangla (Bengali), but even some in Sanskrit—texts that were composed in every region within Bengal. It was in the long period of wrestling with Asim Roy's important characterization of syncretism in this and related literatures of precolonial Islam that I rejected his classification nearly completely and formulated an alternative model to conceptualize this figure—and I thank Asim dearly for that stimulation.[1] Satya Pīr is a generic holy man and as such is a locus of power to whom anyone can turn when they have the need. It is the orientation of this practical use—not some ideological standard that measures according to pristine and exclusive categories of Hindu and Muslim—that dictates how he is depicted and understood. The eight tales I have chosen to translate bear this out as well as any, for they defy classification along sectarian lines—for reasons I have outlined in the introduction—and exercise a kind of situation creativity that invites the reader or listener to grapple with morally ambiguous situations apart from the dictates of some religious injunction.

The origins of this book are a little obscure, but date back to materials on Satya Pīr that I began to gather somewhat casually in 1978–79 while in search of representative reading materials when I was studying Bengali in Calcutta (now Kolkata) in the intensive language program run by the American Institute of Indian Studies. When I returned to Kolkata in 1981–82 to do dissertation research on the topic of Gauḍīya Vaiṣṇava hagiography, under the auspices of the Fulbright-Hays Doctoral Dissertation Research Abroad program run by the U.S. Department of Education, I discovered many more references to Satya Pīr and Satya Nārāyaṇa and their connections to that Vaiṣṇava world. The bookstalls of College Street were very generous in starting to fill my shelves with this popular literature; my good friend and colleague Robert Evans helped me in that endeavor to collect materials in Kolkata, and subsequently provided copies of print materials from his extensive private collection of Vaiṣṇava and popular literature. When I returned to the University of Chicago, Regenstein Library yielded another small cache of printed materials (to which I added), and I thank both Maureen Patterson and James Nye for their help in locating these. In 1989, during a highly successful but all-too-short fishing expedition to the Oriental and India Office Collections (OIOC) of the British Library located in the old building on Blackfriars I discovered a trove. I returned in 1991, courtesy of the National Endowment for the Humanities "travel to collections" grant to mine the OIOC's vast holdings, picking up copies and references to numerous nineteenth-century editions, as well as a few mold spores from the same period that continue to plague me every time I enter their collections. Then Deputy Director Graham Shaw was very generous with his time and staff, and Bengali bibliographer Dipali Ghosh went out of her way to raid the stacks and introduce me to the secret handwritten "blue cards" of uncataloged materials that yielded three of the stories in this collection.

Until that point, most of my research on Satya Pīr had been as invisible as the literature itself, but in 1991–92, I was awarded a fellowship by the Fulbright-Hays Faculty Reseach Abroad program specifically to investigate the manuscript literature of Satya Pīr in Bangladesh. At the same time I was granted a fellowship from the American Institute of Bangladesh Studies for a dovetailed project on Satya Pīr that focused more on print materials. That dual support enabled me to extend my stay in Dhaka, where I worked largely in the manuscript collection of Dhaka University Library, and the libraries of the Asiatic Society of Bangladesh and the Bangla Academy. Unfortunately, because of the political unrest during that year, which culminated in December when the Babri Masjid was razed in Ayodhya, India, work was often cut short. Dhaka University itself was closed for more than one hundred days that year, with sixteen student political assassinations on campus; and scheduled trips to Kumilla, Rajshahi, and Rangpur were variously canceled. But intellectual life in Dhaka does not stop because of politics and strikes, so I benefited from long relaxed evenings with the late Professor M. R. Tarafdar, Dhaka University, whose knowledge of Bengali history was without peer—and whose study on the Awadhi romance literatures as they traveled to Bengal helped me perhaps more than any other to see the importance of that source of inspiration to these tales. Many hours were spent with other scholars whose ideas and resources contributed directly, including Dhaka University professors Anisuzzaman and the late Ahmad Sharif, and, toward the end of that stay, A.K.M. Zakariah, who shared a unique manuscript of the text of *Baḍa satya pīr o sandhyāvatī kaṇyār punthi,* previously known to me only in printed form—a manuscript not found in any public collection. At the urging of Professor Tarafdar, Professor Shah Jahan Miya of the Bengali Department, Dhaka University, worked with me in 1992 to transcribe five previously unnoticed manuscripts of Satya Pīr; two of those tales are included in the current volume, and it is our hope that the edited Bengali texts will soon, although belatedly, be published.

In 1992 I gave my first public presentation of these materials to a combined meeting of the Itihas Parisad, Dhaka, and the Department of Islamic Civilization and History, Dhaka University. I offered a more extended survey to the Carolina Seminar on Comparative Islamic Societies in 1994, and two workshops at the University of Pennsylvania, one in 1995, and the other, a substantially expanded and revised form, in 1997. In 1995 Carl W. Ernst, University of North Carolina–Chapel Hill, and I ran a National Endowment for the Humanities Summer Seminar for College Teachers under the title "Rethinking Religious Boundaries in South Asia," where a very appreciative group laughed their way through lengthy synopses of many of the tales in this volume, with special scepticism being directed at the thirteen-cubit cucumber in the *Bāghāmbara pālā* (translated here as "The Disconsolate Yogī Who Turned the Merchant's Wife into a Dog"), a translation to which I steadfastly hold. Out of that group I am especially grateful to suggestions by Robin C. Rinehart, Lafayette College, and Lakhi Sabaratnam, Davidson College. Since that time patient audiences have contributed substantially at the American Historical Association annual meeting (1996—in the middle of a very distracting snowstorm), twice at the Triangle South Asia Consortium's colloquium (1996, 1998), and at the Conference on Religion in South India (1999). I was slated to deliver a survey of the literature to the Rockefeller Residency Institute for the Study of South Asian Islam at Duke University in 1996, but was foiled by yet another lingering respiratory infection engendered at the British Library some two months earlier, but that article was subsequently published in the volume *Beyond Turk and Hindu: Rethinking Religious Identities in Islamicate South Asia*, edited by David Gilmartin and Bruce B. Lawrence. The College of Humanities and Social Sciences, North Carolina State University, partially subsidized several subsequent trips to Dhaka (2000, 2002) and London (2000, 2001), where I tidied up some loose ends.

Along the way I bored many a colleague and friend with talk of these tales and insistent requests to read them and respond. Most willing and always able to press the limits of my knowledge was David Gilmartin, North Carolina State University, a colleague of inestimable value. The late Edward C. Dimock, Jr., of the University of Chicago discussed with me, among many other issues related to Bengali culture and literature, how to present these tales in a way that would make them accessible to English-speaking audiences—and I trust that those who knew him will detect some of his presence in the wit and humor of these translations. Bruce B. Lawrence and Katherine P. Ewing, both of Duke University, Carl W. Ernst of the University of North Carolina-Chapel Hill, David Ludden and Guy Welbon, both of the University of Pennsylvania, Dick Eaton of the University of Arizona, Fran Pritchett of Columbia University, Barbara Metcalf of the University of California-Davis, and Ralph W. Nicholas of the University of Chicago all gave me ideas that were incorporated here and elsewhere in my approach to Satya Pīr. Ms. Hena Basu of Kolkata, my longtime friend and research assistant, provided much-needed help in surveying the literature in the early stages of the project, including hand-copying the Bengali original story of *Bāghāmbara* and *Manohara phāsarā* when photocopying was not available. Ms. Bharati Roy, also of Kolkata, worked closely with Hena and hand-copied the story of *Motilāl*. This book would never have come to light in its present form without their help, and for that I am deeply grateful.

On a more personal note, Jamal and Tuli Ahmed have over the years opened their home in Dhaka with a hospitality that has made this and other works truly possible; it was while sitting in their guest bedroom in July 2000 that I commited finally to preparing these translations as a separate volume, and in that same room in March 2002 that I edited the manuscript for the last time before submitting it for press review. In Kolkata, A. P. "Kaka" Roy and his wife, Anna, and Jaweed "Miyan" Moiz and his wife, Rukhsana, have made me a part of their familes with a love and affection and an honest incredulity at my study of Bengali culture that no one else can ever understand. For nearly a quarter century Kaka's and Miyan's fondness for bourbon and jazz has bound us tighter than brothers ever could be; and it was the third member of this troika, Jayanta Sengupta, of Kolkata and sometimes Mumbai, whose zest for storytelling convinced me that even in the urban metropolis the art of the tale was far from dead (an impromptu drunken recitation from memory of a ten-page section of *The Hitchhiker's Guide to the Galaxy* cinched it). In 1993 and 1994, Alice and Jeffrey Barr gave me carte blanche to use their Dhaka home as my base, an act of kindness that freed me from mundane logistical concerns in my frequent trips. My Canadian friends in Dhaka, Christine Spoerel and the late Ron Audette, and honorary Canadian Sara Bennett, looked after my living arrangements in 1992, making work time more productive and my personal life much enriched. Both Liz Sherwood of Chapel Hill and Mary Vilas of Raleigh pressed me to tell these stories and in that process made me realize more of their general appeal, and for that I am grateful. Carolyn Hall's keen editorial eye transformed the uneven typescript into a manuscript worthy of submission, a tedious and time-consuming task that greatly eased my burden. Oxford University Press ushered this book through the process of production much more easily than I had imagined possible. Special thanks goes to Cynthia Read, Theo Calderara, Margaret Case, and Rebecca Johns-Danes. And to Mary Beth Coffman-Heston I am deeply indebted for support during the final stages of production, as she turned over her own study to my extended use and provided personal encouragement and helpful feedback along the way. There are of course others unnamed who have lent a helping hand, to all of whom I can only say thanks.

In all of these venues and with all of these willing and unwilling collaborators, what has become glaringly clear is that few know anything at all about these tales, even though collectively these stories make for one of the largest blocks of a very rich Bengali literary corpus. So, bowing to the inevitable, I finally decided to translate the primary material I was attempting to analyze. I hope this little volume will convey a brighter side of the wonderfully complex world that is Bengal.

As the book neared its end, the I. A. Blumenthal Foundation offered me much-needed support to spend three weeks in the writer's cabin at the Wildacres Retreat in the mountains near Little Switzerland, North Carolina, in the summer of 2001. The solitude afforded by cabin life made possible the retranslation of the last of the eight tales. To Wildacres Director Mike House and his wife, Kathy, to Annie Bixler, who runs the Owl's Nest program and her husband, Joe, to the entire staff at Wildacres, and to Philip Blumenthal, I owe a debt of gratitude for creating a relaxed, indeed inspired, environment that allows creative work to take precedence over all else. As these last words are written, is it surprising that outside the cabin window, the mountain forests are shrouded in mist, with the dark creeping in, and I am reminded of Śaśīdhara on the isle of Laṅka, as the cry of a she-owl echoes through the mountains.

CONTENTS

The Bloodthirsty Ogress Who Would Be Queen
Kiṅkara Dāsa's *Śaśīdhara Pālā*
172

The Princess Who Nursed Her Own Husband
Gayārāma Dāsa's *Madanamañjarī Pālā*

Fabulous Females and Peerless Pīrs

Introduction

During one of my first trips to the South Asian subcontinent, I visited a village outside Delhi with a group of other Fulbright scholars and their spouses as part of an official effort to introduce us to "rural India." As we toured the village, we stopped at one small house where we were introduced to the oldest member of the community, a great-great-grandmother, who received us outside on the stoop. The organizers of the visit provided translations since few of us knew Hindi, and we were encouraged to ask questions, any question on any topic. At some point—and in retrospect one can only surmise that this was rehearsed—a young woman in our group was prompted to ask this aging toothless matriarch how the roles of men and women differed in her village.

The old woman laughed with a certain amount of embarrassment, pulled the end of her sari across her face, rubbed her hands together, and with everyone now duly attentive, very quietly but with a little gleam in her eye said something along the lines of: "Oh, the differences are very clear and very easy, Memsaheb. Men do all of the important things in life. Women do everything else." At the opening to this old saw, the other women in her family could barely restrain themselves, giggling and exchanging knowing glances. The old woman continued. "Men decide elections, direct foreign policy, and prognosticate the weather and our cricket matches. Women just do what's left. We manage the money, do the marketing, cook for the family, bear and raise the children, see to their education, repair the house, arrange marriages, act as doctor and midwife, and make sure that in times of need we always have a little pittance to tide us over." Then pausing for dramatic effect, she concluded, "Yes, women do all the unimportant things. Men do what is important."

And with this dry commentary on gender responsibilities—amid a widespread vocal affirmation from other women present—we were left to interpret for ourselves. As I was preparing this book, I realized that the eight tales in this volume function in much the same way: they explore the unusual while explaining the obvious. The stories celebrate Satya Pīr, a figure of religious power who is nominally both Muslim and Hindu; they vault women or their offspring into heroic roles as the men flounder in uncertainty and helplessness, they traffic freely in the symbolic capital of gender distinctions, all in an effort to comment, critique, and even stretch the traditional values reaffirmed in the conclusions of each tale. Not suprisingly, these tales are often wickedly humorous as they play out stock situations that challenge the listeners' expectations, much as the old woman's tale did for our little group of Fulbrighters—and our different interpretations can be just as instructive.

The initial response of the individuals in our group, myself included, was to reduce the old woman's critique to a stereotype of gender roles, relying on such basic analytical distinctions as public/private, communal/domestic, and so forth, and their neat analogues of male/female and a host of other binary distinctions to which we had grown accustomed in the study of South Asia. Stereotyping is of course a highly condensed shorthand for encapsulating in essentialist terms a fixed anecdotal image. In this case we arrived at a notion of "traditional" Indic culture that would play to our students and other consumers of our experience. The anti-Orientalist critique could and should make an easy target of our group's willingness to accept this offering in such simplistic and reductionist terms. But it fails to explain what that old woman was doing when she told us that story.

Since that wonderfully choreographed moment several decades ago, I have heard friends and acquaintances all over India and Bangladesh recite the same story in a multitude of languages and with equal relish, differing in only the slightest detail. The tale's ubiquity and the inevitable laughter it elicits suggest that it is part of a larger common "cultural narrative," in this case one shared by women and, seemingly ironically, almost never denied by men. Narratives of this sort inevitably help to make sense of one's place in a given culture by laying out the parameters within which action can be contemplated and certain types of identity imagined. Such stories are neither essentialized or schematic depictions of worldly experience nor idealized statements of perfect identities; rather they acknowledge the range of possibilities, setting the parameters within which one can envision a life. Within a playground of possibilities come opportunities to exercise individual initiative. Participating in playful narratives allows the individual to appropriate those parts that resonate. Narrative allows for exploration with a kind of protection and impunity not granted to the impetuous real-life actor. And yet avid participation in such narratives can give shape to eventual courses of action, help explain why things are, or why decisions are made the way they are, and even justify who we are. Because they test cultural limits, such narratives are much fun for their tellers and listeners. They say what cannot be said, poke fun at those in authority, play off of sexual tensions, and in many small ways challenge what passes as standard. These types of narratives are vitally important to any culture.

Enacting Gender, Enacting Religion

To live in any society is to participate willy-nilly in the perpetuation of cultural narratives, but how they are created and circulated is not always transparent or completely accessible to the casual visitor or even the professional student. Part of this is due to the oral nature of their circulation, their sharing as a social event, and any reconstruction misses the immediacy and inevitably of much of the complexity of interplay, because reconstrutions nearly always reflect the concerns, interests, and sophistication of awareness of the individual observer. Cultural anthropologists and folklorists are trained to try to capture the myriad threads that make up these complex interactions, and recent scholarship such as that of Kirin Narayan,[1] Margaret Mills,[2] and Joyce Flueckiger[3] has given us glimpses of a lived environment previously unknown to those not present. But what about historical reconstructions for those of us who do not work in the contemporary period? How can we read tales from earlier periods? Or, put another way, what kind of historical understanding is possible from narratives that are largely devoid of context?[4] It is perhaps one of the most important features of literature—especially what we lump together as "folk literature"—to crystallize moments of cultural narration, ossifying them in some standardized way that is delivered in an acceptable genre. These crystallized moments are not an index to what was—or even to what was considered—ideal, although there is probably a certain amount of that. Rather I would argue that these literatures reveal the range of the imagination of earlier times, mapping constraints on what could be thought, what might be contemplated, and testing the limits of the work's discursive space.[5] Much of the literature that has survived from historical periods has inevitably been a court literature, produced by professional literati and patronized by kings and the wealthy, and, by the late nineteenth century in this region of the subcontinent, religious institutions. The written record favors a privileged few, and will of necessity reflect that perspective, as the subaltern and other postcolonial readings have reminded us. But the tales in this volume are not the currency of courts and literati but of a more common sort of Bangla-speaking audience.

Bangla is spoken in the northeastern regions of the South Asian subcontinent, the areas that today constitute the nation-state of Bangladesh and the Indian state of West Bengal. The literature dates back easily to the fourteenth century, although some would push it several centuries earlier. Commissioned court works translated and mimicked the epics of classical India and Persia, although with increasingly local perspectives; by the sixteenth century a distinctively Bengali voice began to emerge. Few topics were off limits, including India's greatest heroes. Rāma was taken to task repeatedly in Kṛtttibāsa's *Rāmāyaṇa*,[6] and Saiyad Sultān's *Nabī Vaṃśa* turned Muhammad and Abraham into *avatāras* and Kṛṣṇa and Rāma into prophets.[7] New goddesses were fêted in semi-epic poems called *maṅgala kāvya*,[8] and Sufi poets composed abstruse instructions for yoga in such texts as the *Yoga Kalandar* and *Jñānasāgar*.[9]

But within this vast literature I never encountered anything approaching the bald challenge to gender roles I heard in the old woman's anecdote, and certainly nothing that seemed to champion women or present the upper classes from the perspective of the lower—that is, until I stumbled across the story of Lālmon, the *Lālmoner kecchā* (or *Lālmoner kāhini*) translated here as "The Wazir's Daughter Who Married a Sacrificial Goat."[10] Lālmon did everything I had come to expect of men in these traditional tales and at the same time managed to discharge all of her duties as a traditional woman as well. Through Lālmon I was introduced to a genre of tales wherein women assume the commanding position to order and set right the world. These heroines don armor to fight *dacoits*, slay raging rhinos (and naturally cut off their horns in wonderfully Freudian fashion), harness flying horses to rescue their lovers, transform ignorant men into billy goats to serve as breeding stock for their passions, weave magic garlands that ensorcell the men while in other contexts proving their own fidelity, and generally instruct the kings and princes of the world in the ways of statecraft. These are independent, politically savvy women, who step outside the confines of the home to tame a world that according to tradition is known but to men. These are women who seem to turn the old woman's anecdote on its head, or perhaps more accurately, confirm it to be truer than her public pronouncements, however sarcastic, could admit—and it is just these stories that I have chosen to translate for this volume.

There are of course many active heroines of all sorts in the long history of Indian letters; one need only look at the great mythological traditions so lovingly enumerated in their complexity by Wendy Doniger[11] and others, and of course a host of literary works as Somadeva's "Ocean of Story," the *Kathāsaritsāgara.*[12] In the regions of the Bangla vernacular, the well-known story of Behulā is a prime local example of a woman in a "take-charge" mode; her love and devotion to the goddess of serpents, Manasā, give her the strength to cradle her dead husband's body on her lap until she floats down the river to heaven itself and receives the boon of his life.[13] In many respects, the narrative of Lālmon and the others in the cycle confirm an independence similar to Behulā's, and perhaps more important, demonstrate that the power of the women is not only formidable but, not surprisingly to these uniformly male authors, ambiguous. Their power, like Behulā's, is directed toward the end of preserving the lives and welfare of their husbands and families at all costs. That same power has a strange, magical side that—perhaps leaping ahead somewhat in anticipation of the argument to come—can in its extreme forms invoke the dark mysteries of Tantra, powers granted through esoteric rituals that strive to defeat mortality itself by mastering the elements of the earth and the body, often by manipulating the messy, polluting world of blood and other bodily substances. In this sense, then, these are the powers that historians of religion generally associate with the goddess, with Śāktas who worship her, and with Nāthas and a host of related practitioners who seek immortality through yogic mastery. But what is different here—and very unlike Behulā—is that the heroines of these tales have no direct connection to the arcane arts of Tāntrikas or Śāktas. In fact they are generally opposed to such figures and practices, for their foes frequently are cast in such roles: self-indulgent yogīs, spell-inducing witches, and so forth.

These eight stories tell of women such as Lālmon, Rambhāvatī,[14] Madanamañjarī,[15] and others who must violate any number of cultural mores, stretching and breaking the limit of what is socially acceptable, in order to establish or reestablish a morality that only they seem fit to instantiate. Their world is a pragmatic one, where the need to maintain a proper order requires unusual remedies for equally unusual situations. If there is one common thread in the complicated plots of these tales, it is the response of resourceful women who find themselves plunged into situations that compromise them at every turn; they must find their way out of what is socially awkward if not truly unacceptable. These are women who, we are led to believe, as a rule are not allowed to make major decisions about their lives until fate deals them a different hand, and in these tales invariably that fate comes in the form of an insensitive, naïve, or just plain stupid decision made by the men who are somehow responsible for them. That bungling engenders radical action that falls outside the standards of expectation and flies into the realm of the fabulous.

All of the tales of Satya Pīr, but most especially the nonsectarian fabulous tales, can be understood as "folk literature." These are not officially sanctioned or commissioned pieces like the great semi-epics and epics of the Mughal and Sultanate courts. The authors are not famous even when we know who they are, nor are they always particularly gifted as poets, although some are accomplished raconteurs who manage to make the written word as lively as its oral counterpart—and this should be reflected in the style of the translations. But in many instances the written version is perfunctory in its diction and narrative structure, and of course on occasion repetitive (such as the story of Motilāl). It is a "popular" literature, but like the term "folk" literature, that label serves at best as a vague classification that usually lumps together all types of literature that are in form and function different from courtly or high literary works, a kind of non- or less-literary class, generally understood to be oral in composition and transmission. Inevitably this classification invites comparison with the well-known and often fuzzy genres of "folk tales," "fairy tales," and "legends"; yet the narratives of Satya Pīr do not comfortably fall into any of those categories—not that those labels themselves manage to be clearly defined.[16] Although the issues in many of the fabulous tales are reminiscent of the ambiguities one encounters in fairy tales, especially in their function as described by Bruno Bettelheim, these are for the most part adult tales that describe uniquely adult kinds of moral dilemmas.[17]

These tales tend to be longer and more complex than what is generally circulated as a fairy tale, and the Bangla-speaking community has many such collections of the latter. Perhaps the most famous collections started with Dakṣiṇārañjana Mitra Majumdār's *Ṭhākurmār Jhuli* at the turn of the twentieth century; a host of similarly titled volumes remain in print today, a handful of whose tales have been translated into English and other European languages, but none of which includes the tales in this volume.[18] Not surprisingly, a limited number of motifs are recycled from these and related tales, such as the two magical sticks of silver and gold that are used to put to sleep and awaken the unsuspecting woman, utilized in both "The Story of the Rakshasas" and "The Origin of Rubies," in the Reverend Lal Behari Day's *Folk-Tales of Bengal*,[19] in "A Stick of Gold, a Stick of Silver," in F. B. Bradley-Birt's *Bengal Fairy Tales*,[20] and resurface in the translation below of the tale of Bāghāmbara[21] or "The Disconsolate Yogī Who Turned the Merchant's Wife into a Dog." In other instances, entire plots or substantial portions of them seem to be interchangeable, for example in Kabir Chowdhury's *Folktales of Bangladesh*, "The Story of Koonch Baran Kanya" tells of a boy who magically hides inside a bel fruit or wood apple.[22] He then drops into the waters of a lake, only to be eaten by a bottom-feeding sheatfish from whose stomach the young boy is soon to be released to do further battle with ogresses or *rākṣasīs*, who in turn are forced to regurgitate all of the animals and humans they have devoured. Nearly that entire tale can be found imbedded within the tale of Śaśīdhara, translated below as "The Bloodthirsty Ogress Who Would Be Queen."[23] It would be easy to multiply the examples, which would serve only to confirm what is already well known about the often formulaic nature of these types of literatures as described by Stith Thompson in his motif index[24] and by Vladimir Propp in *The Morphology of the Folktale*.[25] Where they differ is in the compositional skill required to string together these motifs into a tale of somewhat greater complexity than the average fairy tale or folk tale; these stories verge on more contemporary notions of fiction, a genre that developed in Bangla in the late nineteenth century. It is in those vignettes that we see the transitional nature of the literature as it moves from genres devoted to public performance to the more purely chirographic.

Three performance genres engender these tales: *pālā* or *pālāgāna*, *pāñcālī*, and *kecchā* or *kissā*. Each of these names can be translated simply as "story" or "tale," but the first two classifications indicate the primary material for public performances by professional troupes who stage these minidramas to audiences all over Bengal. The designation by the authors and publishers as *pālā* or *pāñcālī* indicates clearly that the stories had been or are meant to be orally transmitted, even though they are on occasion recorded by hand or printed. Orality depends for its success on an immediate social concern, or the audience will not respond; that is, the authors must explore themes relevant to their audiences to incite a response. In form, however, it is the Urdu *qissa* (from the Persian *qiṣṣah*, Bangla *kecchā* or *kissā*) that shares most with these narratives: fixed tales that were printed in popular editions, widely circulated, but performed by raconteurs in coffee houses throughout northern India. As Frances Pritchett has documented, *qissa* popularity soared in the nineteenth century, roughly parallel to the rise in popularity of the tales in this volume. *Qissa* primarily circulated in print, although they were narrated publicly.[26] Only the first tale in the current volume carries the marker of *kecchā* (or, in one of its Bengali substitutions, *kāhini*), but the features of the genre are replicated throughout the set. All of the tales are framed by the narrator, indicated by the intermittent signature lines or *bhaṇitās*. The author (or sometimes the publication editor, taking liberties) breaks the tale into parts, interjecting occasional comments about the complications of the plot, the motives of the characters, and the role of Satya Pīr. The implied narrator's voice (which is almost always taken to be the author himself because of the signature line, *bhaṇitā*), functions as a framing device that, following Gerard Genette, qualifies as paratextual, part of the threshold of the text whose discursive practices mediate the narrative proper.[27] Most of the narrative (and the paratext) is delivered in the fourteen-syllable, end-rhymed couplet called *payār*, while moments laden with emotion and the direct addressing of God or Satya Pīr will slip into the more complex three-footed meter called *tripadi*. *Tripadi* is rhymed in a variety of ways, but usually in the form of *a-a-b c-c-b*, with the feet varying in length from 6-6-8 to 8-8-10, and so forth. The lengths of all of these tales are equivalent, the Madanamañjarī tale the real exception. And like the *qissa*, the printed versions tend to be in chapbook size.

The tales also mimic their *qissa* cousins in their subject matter, and in the abundance of fairies, demons, flying horses, talking birds, and corrupt yogīs who work a black kind of magic. It is a world we have conveniently labeled "fabulous," a fictional world quite apart from that depicted in the more sectarian tales of Satya Pīr noted below. Although the sectarian tales do display some of the fabulae, they are generally attributed to God, either Allah Khodā or Kṛṣṇa-Nārāyaṇa, or to the Pīr, whose power derives from God. The sectarian tales always have overtly religious explanations for the powers that be; the fabulous tales, however, allow for a much wider range of extraordinary or supernatural display by all manner of characters. Many of these characters are familiar to classical Indic literary traditions, and in that sense they are not unusual at all, so the divisions should not be understood as absolute (as any genre classification inevitably breaks down or blurs in the face of its examplars). Characters act well outside the range of any accepted normalcy, and challenges to gender are essential to nearly every plot. Unlike their sectarian counterparts, the treatment of religion and the religious life itself is sidelined in the fabulous tales of Satya Pīr. In short, the unlikely, the unexpected, and the fabulous reign. But the presence of the fabulous—or features of the related genres of the "marvelous" and the "fantastic" as outlined by Todorov—fail to address the real issue of the imagination, which ultimately sets these tales apart as fictions.[28]

The incorporation of the fabulous into these tales signals that the action occurs in fictional worlds that are automatically set apart from ordinary experience. In these not-altogether-familiar worlds, the listener encounters possibilities that may otherwise remain unimagined, exploring alternate realities that produce a sense of marvel, entertaining while they occasionally offer new ways of conceiving traditional roles. As I have already intimated, gender forms in these worlds seem to be challenged directly by the actions of both men, who are frequently wimpy and obtuse, and women, who are nearly always either heroic or the opposite, bewitchingly malevolent.[29] Many of the narratives hinge on apparent confusions and inversions of traditional gender roles, and by the nature of that action one cannot but be reminded of Judith Butler's argument that gender is neither ascribed by cultural environment or the concretization of something biologically innate, but is "enacted."[30] She proposes that gender is not a matter of adherence to prescribed social roles but of habitual enactment, shifting the emphasis from ideology to action. By stepping out of their normal activities, the women in these tales clarify what these forms have been or might become. Following Butler, we can also argue that it is not surprising or coincidental that these women demonstrate two of her focal strategies for articulating gender: cross-dressing and parody, both of which find wide play in these eight stories. It is not necessary to rehearse all of the implications except to note that when read in this way, these tales come alive as much more than the wild adventures that drive their plots; they suggest ways of exploring gender, the relationship between the sexes, the expectations for young and old and for common and royal blood.

As we contemplate the range of possibilities offered by these tales, especially regarding the women in them, we must remember that as far as can be determined from the authors' names, the tales were written exclusively by men. Before we get bogged down in the prospect that these tales might really do little more than portray men's perspectives on what is permissible in the enactment of gender, we might complicate the picture further by looking to the other major issue that dances around the periphery of these eight tales, but which seldom intrudes directly: what it means to be religious. As will become apparent, this issue curiously mimics the gender challenges. All religions in the subcontinent are united in asking central ethical questions, and, in these cases especially, how one makes moral decisions when all of the options are vexed with unhappy implications. Today it is often unreflectively accepted that to be religious means to participate in a specific religious community, to be committed to a doctrine or general religious ideology that is in turn somehow constituitive of identity. In greater Bengal this usually means one of two communities (and identities): Hindu or Muslim. It is true that since the late nineteenth century, perhaps most conveniently located in the census of 1871, the affiliation of Hindu and Muslim became an indicator or mark of political identity; but the labeling did not quite as conveniently create a concomitant religious identity that was dependent on ideological or doctrinal commitment.[31]

If we might oversimplify as a starting point for this argument, religion in South Asia is as much about right action (orthopraxy) as belief (orthodoxy), and action is not just formal ritual action associated with an icon or a place of worship, but habitual action and the observed morality that informs those habits. Habitual enactment constitutes religious identity in much the same way as Butler argues that it constitutes gender. The parallel is not only striking but also integral to the structure of the narratives. Where the gender issues cluster around the actions of women in men's roles, the issues of religious morality cluster around the actions of holy men and their devotees. Like the gender complications, religious and moral issues are most eloquently adjudicated in parody, in this case of the generic holy man—the Muslim *pīr* or fakir and the Hindu yogī or renunciant *saṃnyāsī*—in the figure of Satya Pīr. Appropriately, Satya Pīr effects a religious cross-dressing that includes a brahmin's sacred thread, the Sufi beard and wooden sandals, the chain belt and dagger of the *gāzi* or warrior-defender of God, and the simple loincloth of the renunciant or occasionally the *dhoti* of a brahmin. As a figure of local power, this holy man extracts promises of devotion in exchange for material aid in his devotees' lives. Depending on the teller of the story, Satya Pīr is either guided by the light and power of the Prophet Muhammad, or is none other than God, Kṛṣṇa himself, come to earth—and sometimes both. Their parodic structure, however, suggests that these eight tales are not immediately and overtly theological in their impulse, for then they would cease to be the exploratory fictions they are. In fact, Satya Pīr appears in them only sporadically, either to provide a crucial helping hand as the invisible deus ex machina, or more often as the instigator of the trouble that allows the protagonists to discover solutions to their unexpected events—although the effects of Satya Pīr's intervention do become proof positive of his miracle-working power, his *karamāt*. None of the stories is particularly didactic, although there are occasional digressions in that direction. Rather, these tales seem to depend for their theology and didacticism on the other Satya Pīr literature, and for the object of their parody and political commentary on the sectarian literature of both Hindus and Muslims. Just how these tales relate should offer some insight into the complexity of their fiction.

The Sectarian Literatures of Satya Pīr: Muslim and Hindu

To those accustomed to the politics of contemporary religious conflict in South Asia, the popular mythic figure of Satya Pīr presents something more than an anomaly. His name combines the Sanskrit word for truth, *satya*, and the appellation of a Muslim spiritual guide, "*pīr*." He dresses in a distinctive garb that signals allegiance to both Muslim and Hindu religious sensibilities, reflecting the religious interests of the two communities that populate the Bangla-speaking world. The Bengali authors who began to write about this mythic figure as early as the late sixteenth century uniformly agree that Hindus and Muslims should and do come together in his worship, because the gods extolled in the sacred Hindu *purāṇas* and the God of Islam praised in the Qur'ān are in reality not different. One nineteenth-century author, in the opening lines of his story of Motilāl, celebrates him this way, calling him both Satya Pīr and Satya Nārāyaṇa:

In an act of contrition,
cross both arms over your chest and
  bow to pay your respects to Satya Nārāyaṇa,
the one imagined in the calculus of the Veda,
the *avatāra* of the Kali Age here on earth as
  the Lord God Khodā, Nirañjana the Stainless One.
Rāma and Rahim—these two are but one;
they are distinct neither in the heavens,
  nor in their qualities rehearsed in the Qur'ān and the Purāṇa.
To navigate this vast ocean of sin
may Satya Pīr be your helmsman—
  allow no other thought to enter your heart.[32]

Hindus, Muslims, and other people in the region worship Satya Pīr for the most basic reasons of instinct and survival: the generation of wealth and provision for the family. The foundational truism of this worship provides a constant in support of the plots: the exigencies of abject penury undercut the most basic morality, so the first step to a religiously productive life is to gain wealth sufficient to allay the nagging demands of providing food and shelter for the general weal of the family. Seen this way, the worship of Satya Pīr is a recipe for success in the world, and when the protagonists of his tales meet with success—and many of the stories tell of people from the highly successful and socially dominant classes, that is merchants and royal families—they become witness if not proof of his efficacy. But the tales are about more than simply generating wealth, for they tell of Satya Pīr's guidance in matters of personal fortitude, in helping the protagonists through situations that are socially, politically, and theologically fraught with ambiguity. Even today the environment of Bengal can be harsh, the political landscape treacherous for the unwary and socially inept. In these trying circumstances, Satya Pīr can provide for the health of families and the general welfare of the household—in short, for any issue that qualifies as domestic. For this reason—and we must be careful of the generalizations here—it is primarily women who perform the worship of Satya Pīr in today's world, for the domestic has traditionally been their domain, even in the expansive version suggested by the old woman's anecdote. At least since the late eighteenth century, Hindu women have incorporated this worship directly in the monthly cycle of domestic rituals called *vrata*, sometimes translated as "vow," and many continue to do so today.[33] One worships Satya Pīr to get rich, to live well.

Historically, and certainly in the stories about Satya Pīr, men too have undertaken worship to great effect, usually connected with larger public ventures such as trading journeys or royal pursuits. No matter who does it, the worship of Satya Pīr is easy, so easy that all one needs is a clear determination and promise, accompanied by a small food offering. Traditionally this food offering is called *śirṇi*, a familiar concoction of rice flower, banana, milk, sugar, and spices, although the forms can be elaborated in excess by those better situated to finance the transactions.[34] If possible, a small space is demarcated with sticks, banana stalks, or arrows placed on the four corners, and a golden platform seat or *āstānā* installed, that seat becoming the aniconic focal point of the worship. Anyone can proffer this worship, regardless of social standing. During the performance, whether undertaken by urbane brahmins of high standing and their kings, or less sophisticated countrymen and women of no particular religious persuasion, Satya Pīr's tales are recited. Following that recitation comes a great feast, as nearly all of the tales attest in their closing verses. Some say Satya Pīr magically conjures himself from his home in Mecca, flying to the spot at a moment's notice to acknowledge his devotees' prestations; others imagine an invisible formless presence, not automatically perceived by the normal senses. Regardless of how the *pīr* is believed to manifest himself, all of the authors agree that Hindus and Muslims, and any other religious peoples for that matter, are bound together in this common worship, commited to upholding a basic moral order that guarantees a lasting peace and productivity in the world. Overt religious divisions dissolve in the face of a palpable localized power dedicated to social good. When formal worship with offerings is not possible, the stories can be and still are told, propagating Satya Pīr's fame and with it the teller's and listeners' fortunes.

Since Independence in 1947, Satya Pīr stories seem to have slowed in their print circulation, which suggests that the tales have lost some of their immediacy—not surpising given the dramatic and all-too-often bloody division of Hindus from Muslims at the time and, unfortunately, since. Today in Bangladesh I have detected some anecdotal evidence of a renewed interest in Satya Pīr as an example of popular solutions to official doctrinal enmities between the communities, but it would be overstating it to say that his literature is enjoying a comeback. During the height of their circulation in the late eighteenth and the nineteenth centuries, the narratives of Satya Pīr enjoyed a popularity very nearly without a second, judging from the formidable number of manuscripts preserved in the repositories of Dhaka, Kolkata, and Kumilla, among others in the Bangla-speaking region. Historically, only the Vaiṣṇava literature, devoted to the charismatic figure of Kṛṣṇa Caitanya (1486–1533), has exceeded the scope of Satya Pīr's corpus. There are extant today more than 750 manuscripts and more than 150 printed texts, composed by no fewer than one hundred different authors. Some of the stories translated in this volume come from editions that by the early twentieth century had reached their twelfth printing. Within the vast range of tales, there seem to be three distinct trajectories: two doctrinally driven narratives, one Islamic, the other Vaiṣṇava, as opposed to the fabulous narratives that are primarily fictional, with only a hint of doctrinal motivation. Common to all is the message that the worship of Satya Pīr knows no boundaries and is open to everyone.

This theme of religion without barriers, which pirates and undermines the symbol systems that differentiate groups, is echoed throughout the literatures, yet, as will become obvious, each author articulates it somewhat differently. Those who favor an orientation toward the overt tenets of Islam have developed tales that can be easily laced into a cycle that takes on the features of *malfuẓat* or hagiography, generally taking the form of conversations with the saint.[35] Perhaps best known and most extensive among these is the tale told by Kṛṣṇahari Dāsa in his *Baḍa satya pīr o sandhyāvati kaṇyāra punthi,* where he creates a comprehensive life narrative replete with all the triumphs and miracles worthy of the genre.[36] These episodes, assembled sometime in the nineteenth century, follow a trajectory that is discernibly Islamic in orientation, and that orientation is generally Sufi. Most traditional South Asian Sufi hagiographies extol the triumphs of the saint among both Hindu and Muslim populations. The tales celebrate power over the physical world, animate and inanimate, as well as power over the lives of individuals, both followers and opponents. In the latter instance, the target of persuasion is usually an individual of prominence, regardless of his or her religious affiliation, and is generally a king or a learned *paṇḍita.* But wealthy landowners and even highly successful farmers can likewise bear the brunt of Satya Pīr's ire when they are guilty of the basic "sin" of not paying proper respect, which is a manifestation of the underlying hubris that the Pīr must crack to effect their moral salvation. In these encounters the value of brahmins is measured in their actions, by the virtue of their personal qualities, not by some mysterious status conferred by birth, and of course many are lacking. Kings, too, are held to an idealized standard that demands support for all members of society regardless of religious orientation and social status; they are not valued for upholding a particular sectarian ideal that favors one community over another. It is up to Satya Pīr to set these people straight and, as these tales powerfully predict, so he does with overwhelming displays of saintly power, the focused *karamāt* directed at antagonists. The antagonists in these tales of Satya Pīr-as-saint tend as a rule to be men, and the stories that are primarily about men more often than not exhibit a corresponding tendency to moralize in ways that suggest the impetus if not the imprimatur of an organized religion. Put another way, most of the stories about Satya Pīr and his interaction with men can be classified as nominally doctrinally driven, and in this they move away from fiction to something motivated by a world outside the book; that is, the stories are in the service of a religious ideal. Predictably, then, parallel to the Muslim-oriented narratives we find overtly Hindu versions of Satya Pīr's tales.

Those authors who favor a Hindu interpretation of Satya Pīr are exclusively Vaiṣṇava in orientation; Śaivas, Śāktas, Nāthas, and members of other Hindu sects are often vilified in opposition to Vaiṣṇavas and Muslims in the tales. These Vaiṣṇava authors bring a simple form of theology to bear on Satya Pīr's image and, like their Muslim counterparts, tell the tales in decidedly masculine terms with masculine protagonists and masculine triumphs. Compared with their Muslim counterparts, these tales tend to be even more overtly sectarian, for Satya Pīr is revealed to be Satya

Nārāyaṇa, a descent of Lord Kṛṣṇ in this the last and most degenerate of ages, the Kali. Satya Pīr is God who has taken the form of Muslim holy man, a *pīr*, to teach basic right and wrong. It is a rather unsophisticated but systematically articulated version of basic puranic *avatāra* theory, the theological assertion that harks back to that ancient dictum of the *Bhagavad Gītā* (4.7–8) that whenever the constraining moral order of the universe, *dharma*, begins to languish, it is incumbent upon Viṣṇu or Kṛṣṇa to descend and set humans back onto the path of righteousness. Śaṅkarācārya and Rāmeśvara, whose tales are the most popular and widely disseminated of these Vaiṣṇava offerings, eloquently argue that Satya Pīr is this long-awaited *avatāra* of the age who accommodates the presence of Muslims and domesticates the land for proper Hindu habitation.[37] This strategy of accommodation appears to be a telling recognition of the realities of the land of Bengal, where for the last several centuries two out of three Bengalis have been Muslim, and where Hindus who live outside the pale of the traditional Hindu heartland of the *madhyadeśa* must account for their minority status. Proper Hindu conduct is rare in this unruly place, say the tales, and the exigencies of the environment make it all the more difficult, perhaps contributing to Vaiṣṇava alliance with Muslims, who find themselves opposed to many of the same religious groups. The worship of the goddess, with her blood rituals, and the *tantrika* activities of less centrally organized but widely spread groups seem to be anathema to both Gauḍīya Vaiṣṇavas and Bengali Sufis, hence obvious factors for their alliance in the figure of Satya Pīr. Yet this accommodation also signals an ideal, if not historical, reality where Muslims and Hindus of various persuasions were not locked in mortal combat; it is a scenario that flies in the face of contemporary expectations, where such enmity is assumed to have been an eternal norm. The tales themselves offer up new ways to impute social and religious value to individuals based on a common acceptance of the figure of Satya Pīr, producing a religious outlook that is regional, uniquely Bengali.[38]

In their seemingly endless iterations, these Hindu-oriented stories tend to fall into three basic thematic modes: the stories of the poor brahmin and his wife who finally acquiesce to Satya Pīr's demand that they worship Kṛṣṇa in the form of the *pīr* and, as promised, do get rich; the woodcutters who learn from the brahmin the secret of his new-found wealth and follow it to success; and the more dynamic and often lengthy sagas of the merchant who sets off across the waters to parts unknown and meets obstacles surmountable only by the aid of Satya Pīr, or by the intervention of the wife or daughter of the merchant who worships Satya Pīr on his behalf. Generally these Vaiṣṇava sectarian tales have been composed and circulated in manuscript or printed form as a set, although the merchant's tale can and often does stand alone.[39] Very rarely a fourth tale will be inserted between the woodcutter's and merchant's stories, the tale of a king who is hunting in the wilds, loses his way, and, as he sits exhausted, is accosted by a cowherd who invites him to worship Satya Pīr, which he declines to his family's peril. Once the king realizes his mistake, Satya Pīr restores him and his family.[40] The plots of the merchant's tale and the king's adventure in the forest blur into the the last class of Satya Pīr literature, a class that as we have already intimated eliminates the sectarian bent, depends on folk motifs, and features the well-considered actions of women over the general ineptitude of men. Although the tropes may blur the line, the Vaiṣṇava literature, like the Muslim hagiographical literature, is motivated by theology and concerns that lie outside the fictional world.

The Fiction of the Fabulous: Framing the Tale and Parody of Roles

The motif of a king or prince losing his way after giving chase to a stag is a predictable one and a common mark of folk narratives, legends, and fairy tales. So too are parts of the merchant's adventure, where all manner of strange events occur when the trader slips out of sight of land and enters the realm of the unknown, usually making landfall in south India, which for ancient Bengal is the stereotypical "Other." The third and final class of Satya Pīr tales—and nearly all of the ones found in this volume—often depend on some permutation of these basic tropes to initiate or complicate the action. Unlike the two doctrinally driven sets of stories, the fabulous tales address situations created by the general ineptitude of men or of men in power under the sway of women, that is, not "real men." This shift in the locus of heroism undermines the normally accepted solutions to worldly problems: radical situations require radical action. It is left to those normally not in charge to set the world straight. Kings, merchants, and courtiers relinquish control of their own destinies as well as those of their women, and it is the mothers, wives, and daughters of these men—or in a few cases preadolescent boys with the help of their mothers and lovers—who have to make things right. For instance, in the story of the adolescent Madanamañjarī, her father the king gives her in marriage to a six-month-old baby boy, son of the minister, an unthinkable compromise of her position in a society that traditionally holds that men must marry women considerably younger in order to have the fortitude and experience necessary to keep the woman under control.[41] As we have already noted in the tale of Lālmon, the daughter of the *wazir* runs away with the prince and lives as a man, a warrior who eventually wins the kingdom. In other tales the women are active antagonists, usually in the form of witches or demons who pit the men against the righteous and worthy women of the kingdom. In all instances the world is eventually reordered, the wrongs avenged, the protagonists restored to their rightful places, often with accumulations of wealth and social standing far above where they began. Satya Pīr in these tales seems to be but a device to ensure the action at critical moments, sometimes capriciously, at other times in direct response to the request of his devotees. After order is restored, Satya Pīr graciously accepts their worship, but his absence during most of the narrative sets these tales apart from their more sectarian counterparts. That absence requires comment because it hinges on the difference between doctrinally driven and fictional genres.

The two central issues of gender and religious commitment bring to a head the fundamental difference of this cycle from its sectarian counterparts. Pierre Macherey (who follows Althusser) argues that fiction, if it is really fiction, cannot refer ultimately to anything outside itself, that is, the world that is created by the words of the work constitute a self-contained reality, a position not altogether unfamiliar to contemporary literary critical circles. He continues, however, to argue that ideology—and we can extend that to religious doctrine—likewise must lie outside the realm of fiction. Ideology can and does inform the fiction, but ideology proper must be pushed aside lest the fiction become propaganda and lose its fictional quality, because the fiction of propaganda and the ideology that drives it are rooted in some kind of social reality that lies outside the text. The language of the text constitutes its own reality and does not concern itself with the distinctions of truth and falsity, "in so far as it establishes—reflexively but not speculatively—its own truth: the illusion that it produces is its own peculiar norm. This language does not express the existence of an order independent of itself, to which it claims to conform; it suggests itself the category of truth to which it is to be referred. Language does not designate; it begets, in a new form of expression."[42] He goes on to argue that the writer creates "both an object and the standards by which it is to be judged," which means that any intimations of ideology or doctrine that may be detected within the fictional narrative can only be parodies of the political reality.[43] The literary work mimics theoretical discourse and functions as "an analogy of knowledge and a caricature of customary ideology."[44] The implication for this last set of tales is clear enough: as literary (or oral) fictions, they are not concerned directly with the doctrinal and religiously ideological positions of the other two strands of literature, which also make their function different. If these tales are not directly addressing the religious life, then what are we to make of the many clear references to things ostensibly religious, to Allah and Nārāyaṇa, to the offering of *śirṇi*, and so forth? What does it mean that the doctrinal dimension is parodied—or is it? There are two tendencies we can observe to clarify the stakes: the rhetorical strategy of framing the narrative and the inverse relationship of demonstrable power displayed by the heroines (and two heroes) and Satya Pīr himself.

The author inserts himself into and around the narrative through the use of asides and section-closing signature lines that often include an embedded commentary on the action, part of the paratext noted above—a discourse that falls outside of but mediates the narrative proper. Following a traditional formula in old Bangla literature, the author inserts salutations to Satya Pīr and to God, often asserting that the identity of Allah and Kṛṣṇa Nārāyaṇa is not different. The author will exhort the reader or listener to live the good life, to honor religious activity, and to be compassionate, and describes the glories that await those who heed the moral of the tale about to be told. At the end of the story, there is always complete resolution, with each character fully restored to socially sanctioned propriety and place, followed by a description of the offering of *śirṇi* to be made to Satya Pīr in response to his graciousness. But between these two framing devices we have a story that is essentially free of exhortation, save a mock deference to the powers of the *pīr*. Let us look at one example in some detail, an example that proves that the fictional narrative is itself basically doctrine-free.

There is a story not included here that goes by three diffferent names, depending on the name chosen for the hero: The tale or *pālā* of Madana-Sundara, or Madanasundara. This hero discovers that his sisters are witches, and, after turning himself into a white fly, secretes himself in the magical trees by which they fly around the country in endless search of pleasure and debauchery. That in turn results in the young man's transformation into a bird possessed by a beautiful young princess; eventually he is transformed back again and wins everyone's favor, not least that of the princess.[45] The three versions of the text respective to their hero's names noted above are Vallabha,[46] Wazed (Oyājed) Āli Sāheb,[47] and Kavikarṇa.[48] Each wrote in a different region of Bengal and place his hero variously around the countryside—in the Sunderban, in Hugli, and in Murshidabad, respectively. But for those minor variations, and the unmistakable facility with language that marks both Vallabha's and Wazed Āli's texts, the tale is essentially the same. Two of the stories seek to position the audience to interpret the tale along doctrinal lines in their openings and in their insertion of similes that draw overt comparisons with religious mythology; the oldest text, Vallabha's, does not. Just what a profoundly different tone this creates is worth examining. Kavikarṇa's tale begins this way:

> May all kinsmen listen carefully to the tale of the Pīr, for it includes the unparalleled tale of a truly extraordinary trader. Sānanda and Binanda were the names of two merchants, and their youngest brother was Madanasundara. Their home was in Saptagrāma on the banks of the Bhāgīrathī, and all three brothers lived together in a single compound. Their interactions were not dissimilar to those of Śrī Rāma and Lakṣmaṇa, for they were accustomed to a happy leisure with each other.
>
> In that region Rājā Ratnākara was the king and lord, and every human and beast within his protection was able to savor life to the fullest. When the king held court, he sat among them in a way that seemed as if a celestial *gandharva* had magically appeared as the ruler himself. In his court were maintained accomplished poets who were equal to Vālmikī in skill. These learned *paṇḍitas* publicly recited various of the Purāṇas and the epic *[Mahā]bhārata*. To the music of *vīṇā* and flute did performers dance and sing, acting out the exploits of Kṛṣṇa to the wonder and amazement of the king. Each and every day did the king perform the ritual worship of Hari and Hara, but, he began to realize, "My stores of black sandalwood and aloe have been gradually depleted. . . ."

And just at the time the two merchant brothers Sānanda and Binanda arrived to pay their respects to the king. . . . [49]

The royal world constructed here is ideal and the ideal is Hindu: learned brahmins chanting the sacred texts, daily worship to Śiva and Viṣṇu, the tales of Lord Kṛṣṇa extolled to the joy of the king, who inhabits a paradise on earth, so that it would appear to the unwary to be nothing less than the court of a celestial being, a *gandharva*. These overt statements are reinforced by the narrator, who inserts numerous allusions to Hindu mythology for the edification of his listeners.

Wazed Āli Sāheb, not surprisingly, takes a completely different tack. He does not feel compelled to punctuate the narrative itself with so many allusions and textual or mythological references, but instead steps forward and frames the story proper with a eulogy and a mildly didactic introduction to ensure the tale's proper reception and the benefits to the reader that are sure to ensue. He begins:

> It was for the sake of all, however shameless and depraved, that Khodā, the Lord God, created this manifest world in which we live. After he had populated it with all manner of animals and sentient creatures, he also thought to provide proper sustenance for them as well. Among the myriad sentient creatures in this world, none was overlooked. But the Lord kept some of these provisions aside as exceptions and he proscribed the eating and drinking of these to all concerned. Following jealously the dictates provided by Lord God, let us praise and honor the apostle of God, the epitome of these beings, the Messenger and Last Prophet. And how does this declaration serve as an introduction? In the end these dictates, if properly followed, determine your progeny and general weal. I make salaam to all those firmly fixed in their practice.
>
> May everyone in the assembly repeat the name of God: "Allah, Allah." May you, Allah, who are stainless, save and protect all present.
>
> I make obeisance to your feet, O Satya Pīr. May you come and be merciful to everyone within my ken. I make a thousand salaams, bowing over and again. Grant us your grace, Satya Pīr, in this horrific time of the Kali Age, as you would view benevolently the innocent children who manage to survive to the eighth day of life. It is through the power and majesty of the Pīr that riches are made and destroyed—that becomes certain upon reflection. One who has been steadfast and true will gain the blessings of the Pīr, just as [the author] Āli, devout of God, became a rich man of hard-earned wealth. What can I know to say about the full majesty and glory of the Pīr? I can only bow my head to honor those holy tombs favored by Allah and entreat you to listen with rapt attention to the tale of the merchant.[50]

The remainder of Wazed Āli's version is only occasionally punctuated with references to Islamic concerns.

That Vallabha, the author who wrote first (although the dating is not altogether certain), composed his version of the story with little hint of sectarian frame makes clear that the content of the story, the basic narrative structure, is not concerned with doctrinal or ideological issues except obliquely, that is, it is informed by them and plays off of them. Doctrine tends to remain limited to the paratextual apparatus. This is repeated throughout the cycle of tales when identical episodes are played out in different venues: for example, Husain, who, under the spell of a flower vendor, leaves a coded message on the wall of the mosque for Lālmon, which ultimately leads to his rescue; this is mirrored by Vidyādhara, who does the same on the wall of a Hindu temple in the story of Manohar the cutthroat.[51] And this absence of ideological import is confirmed repeatedly in the cycle in the way that Satya Pīr's role is delineated vis-à-vis the heroine's.

We have noted that Satya Pīr seems to sit largely on the periphery of these fabulous tales, whereas he is the subject of the stories in the Muslim sectarian versions and is the object of devotion and the instigator of all action, although not the primary subject, in the Vaiṣṇava versions. The reasons for this deemphasis are probably several, but it is telling that the centrality of Satya Pīr is generally inversely symmetrical to the role of the female heroine. The more active the heroine, the less active and more invisible Satya Pīr and his religious ideology; conversely, the more assertive the male heroes, the more intrusive Satya Pīr and doctrine. It is as if the violations of norms are embodied in either the heroines or in Satya Pīr, but seldom both; the former is a challenge to social sensibilities, the latter is a challenge to the overtly religious but is powered by God. Put another way, when Satya Pīr plays the primary role, we enter the realm of doctrine delivered in a narrative form, but in the more fictional narratives of the heroines such as Lālmon, the doctrinal dimension is implied as a condition of possibility, undergirding a differently created world than is the norm. Either God through Satya Pīr intervenes in the affairs of men, or women act out of place and intervene in the affairs of men; to have both in the same narrative overloads the plot and destabilizes the action. One confirms the world and its stability, the other seems to challenge it only to be resolved in the end to the former's position of acceptable roles for men and women. Six of the tales in this anthology are clearly about women, displacing Satya Pīr's centrality, but two of the tales are less clear, and in that ambiguity confirm the proposed distinction between doctrinal and fictional. In the story of Ākhoṭi, the fowler and the stupid prince, the fabled *beṅgamā* bird advises the king and his court about matters pertaining to the religion of Lord Kṛṣṇa—in overt doctrinal statements—and male figures come to dominate the action.[52] To a lesser extent we see the same in Motilāl's tale and the tale of Bāghāmbara, although in both of those cases it is a youth (not a man) who shares the lead with his mother or aunt, and the intrusion of overt doctrine is likewise diffused but more present than in other tales. In short, the corpus of Satya Pīr literature seems to say that when men do what they are supposed to do (the sectarian tales), God and Satya Pīr occupy the liminal space that crowds and impinges on normalcy; when men cannot (the fabulous tales), the gods and Satya Pīr are effectively displaced, and women step in to fill the liminal space outside the bounds of the normal. But the keen observer will see that the women who have to right the crazy world created by men do so with the discreet aid of Satya Pīr, who lurks in the background as the foundation of stability, his occasional overt intervention testament to his miracle-working power, his *karamāt*. Somehow the tales end up at the same point, to restore an order in which men can again act and the world can become "normal," but how they get there depends on dramatic inversions of roles. Satya Pīr and religion are thus parodied by the flagrant acts of women, empowered by the Pīr, who, like their male counterparts, ultimately seek a stable and frutiful moral existence. With this in mind, perhaps the tales you are about to read can elicit some of that same glee that energized our small band of scholars who set out that day to discover something of India.

ABOUT THE TRANSLATIONS

The art of translation is mysterious at best and of little import to most readers who simply—and rightly—want a story. Collections of folk tales, however, present special problems for translators because, more often than not, the stories are delivered orally and orality requires the translator first to become a storyteller who hears the story before retelling it, albeit in a different language. That process places the translator directly in the tradition itself, because the emphasis is on the tale, with value placed on the virtuosity of the teller. It not only invites, it requires the storyteller to step forward and reinvent the story in the target language, giving much license to edit. In the bibliographies that are appended to this volume, retelling is the norm, and most especially among those books that have proved most popular and widespread, such as Lal Behari Day's *Folk-Tales of Bengal* and F. B. Bradley-Birt's *Bengal Fairy Tales*; much the same holds for other regional and pan-South Asian traditions. It is clear that some of the editors of the current narratives intruded as storytellers when the tale moved from manuscript to printed form. But in this anthology, I have taken a slightly different tack: the translations are not retellings, but faithful renderings of the handwritten and printed originals, with many of the qualities of Bangla retained, including some that might qualify as quirks and oddities in English. Consequently, the stories will inevitably be somewhat uneven, because some of the authors are, quite frankly, better than others in telling a tale; the reader can decide their relative merits. I have chosen not to even out the translations to give the impression of a single voice, although that inevitably happens when one person is responsible for translating different authors in the same volume. At the same time, I have chosen to include stories that duplicate episodes or motifs, sometimes in nearly identical language, a choice that, as noted in the introduction, allows the reader to see the stock-in-trade of the storyteller on full display.

These translations are different from any of the Bangla folk collections I have seen, and they differ in three significant ways: the mode of composition and circulation of the texts, the size of the texts, and the style of the translations themselves.

These are tales that appear to have been composed and circulated in writing as much as they were told, aligning them more with the rich literary traditions of Bangla. I was unable to locate manuscripts for all of the tales, but many of them clearly circulated in handwritten form before printing. But in most instances, the time between writing and printing was no more than a century, and in some cases only a few years. Catching these tales on the cusp of transition from an orally dominated mode of production (represented by the solitary or occasional manuscript) to a transmission through mass circulation (represented by printed text) gives us an opportunity to understand something more of both processes—their limitations and opportunities. For instance, in those texts published by Nihar Press, the authors or perhaps the editors seem to have "padded" the text with numerous cross-references to classical mythology, in itself not unusual, but in a repetitive manner, with the same anecdotes referenced in the same way by different authors in different tales, clearly the work of a redactor. This is arguably a case of Sanskritization or some other form of legitimation extraneous to the tale—and uniformly those tales are Hindu in orientation, even though the same tale often exists in other orientations, as has been pointed out in the introduction. In one case, the *Manohara phāsarā*, a tale found in manuscript by an author named Rasamaya, seems to have been copied and made anonymous, with a series of changes primarily to the framing of the text, and the insertion of more didactic material and references of the type noted in the introduction.

Major textual divisions are here replicated from the original. In manuscripts these are often signaled by special marks or in some cases numbering. In printed editions, editors routinely append short titles to these sections, which I have never seen in any manuscript. Following Gerard Genette (1977), I have removed those titles that I have determined are paratextual because they are obviously not intended by the original author but, more important, because they break dramatically the flow of the narrative. They appear, in most instances, to serve as a kind of plot index; none of these printed texts carried an index and few had tables of contents. The narrator, however, usually in the persona of the author, will make various asides, at the end of each section, and sometimes at the beginning. Those asides—which usually take the form of an admonition to the audience or as a signature line of the poet—are rendered in italics throughout, even when they appear in the middle of a narrative section. Ellipsis points, however, *do not* indicate the absence of material or editing, but signal an unfinished conversation the audience is expected to fill in, or some dramatic pause in the telling.

The length of these tales also sets them apart from other types of Bangla tales. Most of the fairy tales and folk tales collected and translated into English, as well as those that are compiled in Bangla, such Dakṣiṇārañjana Mitra Majumdāra's *Ṭhākurmār Jhuli* (1907) or Upendra Kishore Raychaudhuri's *Tuntunir Bāi* (1910), tend to be short, as few as two and seldom more than fifteen pages, and are generally in prose in their original creation or transcription, often replete with line drawings or simple black-and-white illustrations. Only on rare occasions do any of the tales from those and similar collections run to greater length. The tales translated here, however, routinely run fifteen to twenty folios in traditional manuscript form, which means handwritten text with no word divisions, couplets and triplets marked, written front and back with approximately ten to twelve lines per page, each folio measuring about 4½" × 14". That works out to somewhere between 450 and 600 couplets, or thirty to forty pages in translation. This makes the Satya Pīr stories somewhat smaller than the classic *maṅgala kāvya*, Hindu panegyrics to the Goddess and accompanying tales of the trials of her devotees, or the romance literature migrating to Bangla from Persian and Urdu, and yet considerably larger than fairy tales or other humorous narratives, such as the Gopāl Bhāḍ cycle. The tales probably come closest in length and tone to the Urdu *qissa*, which, as noted in the introduction, Frances Pritchett has shown to have flourished with the advent of printing in the nineteenth century.

Finally, the style of translation here is of necessity different from that in most collections precisely because these are translations of fixed texts. The translations in this volume are never paraphrastic or summary, but try to recreate in English the tenor of the original, while retaining narrative order. The rhymed fourteen-syllable couplet or *payār* has been translated as prose; the more metrically sophisticated triplet or *tripadī* has been variously translated as prose or blank verse, with little attempt to make it any more poetic (at least in a formalist sense), but rather as a signal that the original author has shifted into the more elaborate meter at moments of great emotional impact. For those with the wherewithal to read the original texts, it should be noted that when in my estimation that emotional impact did not carry weight in English, I ignored the shift and continued with prose.

Explanatory notes are whenever possible incorporated directly into the text, usually involving a reference to a piece of classical mythology, where I have added a qualifying phrase to help make the allusion clear without resorting to footnotes. If the reference is generally well known, such as a comparison of a king to Rāma, the paragon of kingship in the *Rāmāyaṇa* epic, I have not interrupted the flow of the narrative to point out the reference; but when even well-known references make a specific, often minor allusion, I have chosen to provide explanations and, in a few cases, specific textual references. I have often paired a technical term, such as *pakṣirāja*, with its translation "king of birds" or "flying horse." These are often connected by the phrase, "which means." Epithets are likewise often translated, but never eliminated from the text. These epithets not only signal the role of the character, for instance a king who, when describing his general rule, may be styled *nṛpavara* or "chief among men," but when angry and meting out punishments may be called *daṇḍapati*, "lord of justice" or "dispenser of punishment." These epithets often appear as vocatives, which remind the reader that these texts have their origins in the oral traditions; vocatives alert the listener to the direction of the action and conversation, conventions of speech not generally deemed necessary when a text is exclusively chirographic. Likewise stock phrases, such as *kaṇyā bale*, literally "the young woman said," will always be translated contextually; for example, the woman said, spoke, continued, asked, queried, exclaimed, asserted, and so forth. Only in instances where vocatives or stock phrases are used in excess have they been trimmed to make the narrative flow better for an English reader. It should be noted, however, that when read aloud, some of these passages derive their humor from the exchanges that are marked in these simple ways—"he said, . . ." "she said, . . ."—sometimes running as many as dozen alternating lines. In those instances, I have tried to leave the repetition intact to convey something of that humor, a style not altogether lost in English. Similarly, repeated passages are retained, for example in the story of Motilāl, where the lament of the woman's misfortune, how she was wrongly banished from her house by her mother-in-law, then had her baby stolen, is repeated in each new episode. Many translators will eliminate these repetitions, but I have chosen to leave them intact, for the tension mounts with each telling, and with each telling the story reveals an often subtle shift, although by the end of the tale even the author has tired of it, as will become apparent. With perhaps no more than six or seven lines in the entire set of texts, all direct speech has been translated as direct speech, rather than as reported speech or material supplied by the narrative voice.

The names of gods present special problems. I have always left the name as it appears in the text, occasionally appending the more common name. It is not unusual to find Kṛṣṇa referred to by the names Hari, Nārāyaṇa, Gopāla, Govinda, Ghanaśyāma, and Viṣṇu in a two- or three-couplet stretch. Unlike their use in more theologically nuanced texts, these names tend to be used indiscriminately, more for meter and rhyme than theological orientation. The names of flora often have no equivalent in English; they are translated whenever possible, sometimes with a short explanation in the form of an adjective, or with the generic name (e.g., jasmine) prefaced by the type (e.g., *jui-*). Some flowers and fruits used repeatedly in similes (e.g., *bimba* fruit) have been included in the glossary; botanical designations have not.

For those few linguists who are interested in the grammatical features of the text, it should be noted that it is not unusual for the simple past tense (e.g., *dekhile*, "he saw or met") to be used for the desiderative ("he hoped to see or meet") and occasionally for the simple future ("he will see or meet"). Vowel shifts are not at all uncommon, nor are the usual confusions of spelling often seen in handwritten Bangla literature. As is often the case in manuscript materials, there are numerous instances of haplology, vowel epenthesis, and a not unusual form of scribal spelling error that breaks apart conjunct consonants in what Rich Salomon has called in a personal communication "graphic epenthesis," for example *śāsatere*, which is the locative of the more familiar *śāstra*. One unusual construction is *dhiyāne*—which can be construed as the instrumental of *dhyāna* ("meditation"), or as a past active participle ("having meditated")—when used with another past active participle, such as, *jāniyā* ("knowing or having known"), functions in the manner of the finite third person singular present tense coupled with an infinitve (so "knows by his meditation" becomes "meditates to realize"). There are of course many words that are Urdu or Persian in their origin, and I have attempted to capture as much of the etymological sense of those terms as possible. In every case, however, I have exercised judgment about the best contextual reading, while minding the patience of the English reader.

The Fabulous Tales of Satya Pīr

The Wazir's Daughter Who Married a Sacrificial Goat

Kavi Ārif's *Lālmon Kecchā*

Say Allah, Allah, brother. Speak to the memory of Allah.
How can you err to take the name of Allah with every breath?
Never neglect to recite the name of Allah,
for your every utterance will become salutary and your mind stayed.
Everything you see in this world is without solid base,
a conjured trick; this play in the dust of earth does not endure.
I can sing my encomia ceaselessly and forever,
but listen closely for a while
to the saga of Lālmon.
Through Satya Pīr's manipulations
the winsome young maiden Lālmon
managed to elope to a faraway land
with the crown prince Hosen Shāh.

In the city of Korava lived the emperor's wife Hosenā, who bore a son named Hosen. How can I portray this emperor? He was renowned in all ways, he looked after his subjects as if they were his own offspring. But alas no issue of his own—male or female—was to be seen. Every day without fail he prostrated himself in salutation, a continuous praise of Allah. When in his advanced age the salutations and praise eventually proved fruitful, the emperor finally fathered the son Hosen, who in due time was formally remanded to the custody of the traditional *muktab*, the primary school.

There lived in that same city a sayyid named Jāmāl, and born to his house was a daughter he called Lālmon. Replete with all good qualities and the beauty of a celestial nymph, it was as if Bidhātā, the god of fate, had cast a new mold for girls with this little one. Since this sonless father had no other, he raised his only daughter, Lālmon, with the love and affection generally reserved for boys. Jāmāl felt deep in his heart that she was in truth a male in disguise, and so he committed her to the regimen of the local *muktab*. Each day the young lady Lālmon headed to school, toting a copy of the Qur'ān under her arm. For her first official action each day, she recited the *Bismillah* to commence work, and then took to the study of the Qur'ān.[1] After that the young lady studied the Farsi or Persian tongue. After completing the oral recitation of her Persian, she would at last turn to the study of Arabic. And so did the two young students come to sit together as one, for Lāl faithfully attended, never missing a day of school. In this routine did many days manage to pass without event. But pay attention to how God, Khodā, can create mischief!

One day Lālmon began to feel a little light-headed, so she hurried to take her bath. When she finished bathing, the young lady returned to her private chambers. To better dry her hair, this precious girl climbed to the second-floor balcony. Bending over, she twisted the water from her hair and shook it dry; her chest arched forward, causing her simple shift to slip down from her breast. As this beauty stood there—naked from the waist up—the crown prince Hosen Shāh chanced to look up. With but a glimpse, this heir to the throne sputtered with the excitement of the first-smitten. As the day passed he could neither eat nor drink.

The crown prince arose early the next morning and went to the school, to the study area known as the *darasa*. Once there the prince tried to study—if study is the word for it.

So has written the Poet Ārif about his friend and companion Satya Pīr.

That morning the crown prince sat down and opened his book to read, when Lālmon arrived at the school as usual. The crown prince was in a daze, indeed enchanted, staring at Lālmon, who came in and took her place with a light heart. The book in which she had begun to write her lessons was soon filled with the giddy joys that ran rampant in her heart, and for some little time more she was able to continue this charade. But watch the mischief of which God alone is capable of stirring.

As she wrote, Lāl's hand slipped to the left and her half-finished page fell directly in front of the crown prince. Watching it slip away, Lāl called out to the prince, "I've dropped my paper. Please pick it up and hand it to me."

Paying heed to Lāl's request, he timidly replied to her, "I feel constrained, indeed I do not have the courage, to speak to you directly." Lāl listened and then told the son of the emperor, "First fetch me my paper, then speak your mind."

"I am haunted without respite by thoughts of you. Gloom grips my heart when I cannot see you. Be merciful, my dear, and save my pitiful life! I crave the intimacy of eating betel, Lāl, directly from your hand."[2]

When she heard his words, Lāl was flabbergasted. "You want to eat betel from me, a woman, a lowly being devoid of any good qualities? As soon as your father the emperor hears of this he will slit both our throats with his own hand! Put these crazy thoughts out of your mind and let me back to my quill, for I must strive to compose my lyrics without further disruption."

Hearing her rebuke, the crown prince wailed, "Hāya, hāya!" in despair. "I will give up my kingdom to be with you! I shall abandon this world for your sake alone. I shall become a wandering fakir, wrapping my neck in their distinctive patchwork rags."

As the daughter of the wazir listened, she chided the crown prince, "Why would you become a fakir on account of a worthless woman? You are the only son of the emperor and darling to all. You need but command and countless female servants come running. I have already told you, good Prince, that you cannot have me. Don't even dream about me!" And of course upon hearing this, the young prince wailed all the more loudly and could do little else.

Distressed, he pressed his case again to Lāl, this time more solicitously, "Listen to the timbre of my voice that it may better convey my appeal!" The crown prince continued, "Listen, my dear girl, you who are so beautiful. You alone will I make the prince consort! Elephants, horses, jewels, and land—all will be yours. I shall speak to the emperor and get full sanction and approval of the court for the two of us. Otherwise, your mother and father will marry you off to someone who is not even a local. How could you stand that, Lāl? How could you continue to live having to forget everyone here? Love is an object difficult to obtain, the most prized experience of this world. You must be extremely cautious to nurture this fragile love. My life, my wealth—everything have I offered you, O beautiful one! After I ascend the throne as emperor, it is you, Lāl, who will give the commands! If you pay no heed and ignore what I say, Lāl, I shall commit suicide by impaling myself on my scimitar. You and you alone shall bear full and complete responsibility for my death all the days of your life. You shall suffer miserably throughout this life and the afterlife as well. All the wealth you can see about you is yours. Listen, protect too this treasure that is my paltry life, my dearly beloved Lālmon!"

By the end of his declarations, Lālmon was completely distraught. Exasperated and desperate she replied, "Love is indeed the cool and creamy essence of experience in this world of honorable men, but for those of questionable motives, O Prince, it is like a searing fire. You have spoken freely of what is in your heart. I recognize your love as true, so please extend your right right hand to me. Love and protect me, O Prince, for as long as you live! Should you abandon me any time in the future, you will bear the burden of this heinous evil. Because we are alone, this is our private vow to each other and before no one else. The only witness present before us is the Master himself, Satya Pīr."

Listening carefully to the conditions set forth, the crown prince proffered his right hand. The daughter of the wazir stood up and acknowledged him with a formal salaam. Grasping the prince's hand, she guided it to her head and solemnly declared, "This body is now yours, O Prince among princes, I have entrusted it entirely to you and your safekeeping." Leading the prince by the hand, she sat on the bed. Opening a box of gold, she fed him betel with her own hand. The king's son and Lālmon were transfixed. Kissing gently they stretched out and lay on the bed together as a couple. There on that bed the couple surrendered themselves to unmitigated joy. Lālmon's extraordinary beauty glowed even brighter, if that were possible.

While the two savor their love play, extended and intense, on that nuptial bed, may Satya Pīr be merciful and save our hero! May everyone recite Allah, Allah, and take refuge in the Prophet. Serving his murśid, the poet Ārif sings.

The couple was absorbed in their mutual pleasures, whispering sweet nothings, and playing as only new lovers do, when magically Satya Pīr materialized in their midst. The Pīr interrupted them, "Lāl, you called me as witness to your betrothal. Out of mercy I have come. Now stretch out your hands to make offering to me." Slowly and deliberately Satya Pīr slid away and suddenly floated above the doorway. Extending his magical power over the physical world, he called out to Lāl, "I have come to your chambers to receive alms!"

The son of the emperor grew belligerent in his pride and arrogance as he listened to the Pīr's words. He picked up a pen—the only item close at hand—and hurled it with all his might at Satya Pīr. "I worked long and hard to win Lāl, so be off with you!" cried out the heir apparent. But when the eminent Satya Pīr registered the vitriol spewing from the prince's mouth, he calmly observed, "You who have cast aspersions on me do not merit the likes of Lāl." The prince unsheathed his scimitar and lunged to strike, but Satya Pīr prudently and deftly sidestepped just beyond his reach. The Pīr retorted, "O son of the emperor, you have failed utterly to recognize me. You struck me with a pen from your own hand." Anger rising unchecked, Satya Pīr let fly a retaliatory curse, "Suffer greatly you will on account of Lāl. You came at me to hack me to pieces with your sword, but it is you who will be felled by the hand of a witch, one possessed, in a land far away." Having had his say, the Pīr suddenly vanished as quickly as he had come, while the crown prince and the wazir's daughter remained frozen on the bed.

They returned to their respective abodes only to eat. The couple tried to resume their normal studies, attending school every day. The days began to slip by, one just like the other—but just watch and see what mischief God can stir up.

Sinful acts always will out, and so they did. One day Lāl, the minister's daughter, was caught giving a meaningful look at the crown prince. Even though that daughter of a wazir gave but a single look and said nothing whatsoever, from that solitary act Lāl's demise was plotted by those who saw: "When the emperor hears the whole story, he will take his own son's life, hurling him into a lime pit, be sure of it." Nearly instantly a servant was assigned as a chaperone there in the ornate gazebo in which they studied—and to him fell the order to murder Lāl.

It happened that a maidservant, a wet nurse named Hīra—the embodiment of clarity and strength, as her name, "Diamond," suggests—was in that very same place and heard with her own ears everything that was plotted. Now Hīra was Lāl's favorite servant and she was very partial to Lāl, so she rushed to the school under the pretext of going to the bazaar. Presenting herself with the utmost formality and courtesy, she stood firm and placed her hand over her heart as a sign of sincerity. "O my prince, O daughter of the minister! Listen carefully to my words: Your sins of the flesh, the fact that you are illicit lovers, has been discovered. When you return home, your throat is to be slit."

The wazir's daughter listened and the pleaded with the crown prince, "Hear me, lord of my life, what can we do? The news is out, so everyone now must know. Come, let us escape the kingdom and flee for our lives!"

The prince gave heed and immediately ordered Lāl, "Go back and slip quietly through the back door into your private chambers. Put on the clothes of a man and wrap your torso with a broad cummerbund to disguise yourself. Take some gold coins—*moharas* of value—to cover travel expenses. We shall saddle two of the finest horses and under the cloak of night make good our escape." When they had worked out the details of their plan, each returned home surreptitiously, entering their private ward through the back, while the ministers sat in ambush outside. Through secret back passageways and alleys they wended their way through the confines and equipped themselves quickly as they arrived in their chambers. They wound compact turbans around their heads in the Mongolian style, and Lāl, who was such a beauty, chose outer garments that matched the prince's. They slipped into pajamas of finest muslin, called *mulmul*, and around their waists they strapped dagger, sword, and shield. Over these they slipped their matching red jackets and leather helmets. Finally they packed a change of clean clothes and picked well-tempered Kharasani scimitars, renowned for their icy-edged sharpness. After fixing handkerchiefs in their tightly bound cummerbunds, they at last set off. From the palace they fled, dressed as soldiers of fortune. From the stable each picked a handsome steed, bridled and saddled it. They carefully tucked an extra gold *mohara* into an inner pocket and then leaped upon their mounts. With a magical twinkling the high-strung horses were off, and the couple abandoned everything to this sorry world, speeding onto the open greenway. They paused only when they reached a distant stand of flowering *kadamba* trees.

The poet Ārif serves the feet of his spiritual preceptor by singing.

As Lāl despaired, openly wallowing in her misery, she spoke abjectly to the prince. "I have abandoned my home, everything for which I hoped and held dear. And here I sit crying, alone at the foot of the orange-flowering *kadamba* tree. By what ill fate was I destined to become a woman of ill repute, tarnished goods? I have become guideless, my lord and master Satya Pīr has completely forsaken me."

Standing beneath the *kadamba* tree
Lālmon spoke through her tears.
   "Get up my prince, wake up!
The night is fast becoming dawn.
How and where shall we go?"
   Lālmon cried out in anguish.
"When we were in the school,
what power compelled us to love
   once your real feelings were made known?
I was a defenseless girl
saddled with the guilt of your destruction
   when you declared your love for me.
Before you I was everyone's darling.
I went to school to study,
   carefully raised by my mother and father.
Not realizing the consequences
I committed immoral sins of the flesh—
   to you I surrendered my body completely.
Your heart was hard,
when forgetting all else you took me,
   now a few short days later your fortune has turned sour. . . ."
But the crown prince had been asleep
and was only gradually waking to consciousness.
   He stood up and looked around to get his bearings.
He called out to Lāl,
"Stay here under the *kadamba* tree.
   Please forgive my mistakes and bad qualities,
pardon my faults.
The palace still sleeps.
   Let us get dressed. Be quick!"
Lāl nodded her assent
and began to pull on her garments.
   Carefully did she clothe and disguise her body.
On her lithe form went fine muslin pajama,
decorated with delicate beads of pearls.
   Then she emerged from beneath the shelter of the tree.
She held in her hand a shield and scimitar.
The liveliest stallion from the stable

she mounted on the spot.
The trials of love are severe.
Abandoning her mother, father, and wet nurse,
Lāl stepped onto the roadway and joined the prince.
He who never knows love
lives peacefully and in happiness.
If one is lucky, he stays that way.
Lāl spoke forcefully,
"We cannot stay here any longer,
lest someone catch sight of us."
Love suffers no shame.
Abandoning royal convention and propriety
the two lovers bolted.
Ārif the poet lives,
his mind focused on the feet of truth,
serving the feet of the Pīr.

The couple turned and headed north. They passed through the city without anyone recognizing them. Tensions eased and they conversed lightheartedly. The stallions never relented, gallantly carrying them forward. They made good time, covering about twenty-five miles in three hours, just as the sun came up. When they had distanced themselves by those twenty-five miles, they decided to veer off the path and make for the border. The two lovers seemed to fly effortlessly over hundreds and hundreds of miles.

On her right, in the distance, Lālmon noticed a town slip by. Then they reached the city of Magāna. Off to the left they saw seven women and quickly turned their horses away. When they reached Cherāpa, they left the road and skirted around the town. Riding back into the middle of the main road, the son of the emperor spoke, "We can certainly lay over in the city of Ājama." And saying that, the prince rode on ahead . . . but he had blundered and was nowhere near the road to Ājama. As it dawned on him, the prince grew worried and pulled up to a stop. "I don't understand. When are we ever going to reach Ājama?" cried the prince to Lālmon. "Hear me! My body trembles for food, and it has made my head ache."

Lāl parried this august son of the emperor, "Listen, lord of my life. How am I to prepare food in the middle of this foreign jungly wasteland?" And with this short, somewhat pointed exchange, the two pressed forward, when they suddenly found themselves unwittingly at the house of some *phāsarās*, particularly bloodthirsty highwaymen, a merciless brand of brigands. The entire group of *phāsarās* was out hunting, but an old crone was sitting on the threshold of the house. Lāl addressed her politely and with respect, "Listen, Grandmother, could you please give me a pot to cook some food for us to eat?"

When she heard this plaintive voice, that mean old woman was nearly ecstatic. She instantly handed Lāl some wood, but it was wet, wood stacked in standing water, and a cracked pot that would hold nothing at all. While the crown prince announced that he was going to lie down on the veranda and nap, Lāl went off alone to cook. Filling her leaky pot with water, she began to sift the rice for cooking. This sweet young girl then sat down to cook it. Water seeped out of the pot's cracks, adding its deluge to the already wet wood of her smoky fire. It was only then that Lāl realized what the old crone had been up to. She had feigned affection when she had spoken to Lālmon, with an obvious bounce in her step as she stole occasional glances at the young and healthy Lālmon. When the old crone lavished just a bit too much attention on Lāl—but tricked her with the delaying tactic of the leaky pot and wet wood—it was then and only then that Lāl realized they had stumbled onto the homestead of a band of *phāsarās*. Carrying on and fussing about, the old woman finally went inside, and just as suddenly as she had disappeared a very young girl—the *phāsarā* household's newest bride—was standing there. Gesturing for attention, the girl quietly confided to Lāl, "Be warned. Get away as quickly as you can! But first, listen carefully. Ask the old hag for a little bit of ghee to prepare your food." Hearing her out, the young Lāl began to see her strategy, so she called the old lady plaintively, "Please give me some ghee to prepare my food!" Immediately the old woman ordered the child-bride, "Little Mother, give a little ghee for our honored guests' use!" As soon as she heard the order, the young girl was gleeful and ran off to collect a small cup of ghee, which she handed over to Lāl. She instructed her, "Pour this directly onto the wood in the embers of your small stove. You will see that the heat will cook the rice in no time at all, even though the wood be wet."

Heeding her instruction, Lālmon poured the ghee on the flames, which instantly roared to life, cooking the rice. Then the young Lāl called out, "Prince, O my prince! Wake up quickly. Listen, treasure of my life, the Fates have guided us to the house of a *phāsarā*." When this finally registered with the groggy emperor's heir apparent, he woke with a start. The couple wolfed down their food and made ready to flee. They jumped on their horses and rode hard and fast, slipping away from the *phāsarās*' house. Lāl urged them on, "O Prince, drive the horses harder, harder!" while following hard behind the old hag screamed the alarm.

Gaining on them, the crone tried to cut them off at a pass, but the prince and the wazir's daughter spurred their horses onward. Unable to stop them, the old hag could only watch mournfully as they rode away. In her anguish at having failed she flung herself hard to the ground, weeping and rolling in the dirt, but soon collected herself and began to scream at the top of her voice. With the alarm she sounded, more than seven hundred *phāsarās* responded by returning to the estate compound. Finding the old woman in such a state, they questioned her closely, "Why are you rolling around on the ground in such a frenzy? Why are you weeping?" The crone spoke, "A stranger came here from Chephāi. The young man had the wealth of seven kings on his person. I finagled to hold them here as long as possible, but the couple mounted up and rode off hard." The chief *phāsarā* listened attentively and then spoke, "Listen, Old Mother, you must tell us everything you know, for they may already have gotten away." The old woman responded, "Listen to what I tell you, Khelārām, my boy. I figure that they could not have covered more than about four miles by now." The old woman then showed the men the horses' hoofprints and all seven hundred *phāsarā*s took off after them in a mad rush. Anger welled in their hearts—for they were an innately malevolent breed—and they urged themselves forward with screams of "Kill! Kill!" Meanwhile, the crown prince and the wazir's daughter had paused to rest under a small stand of *kadamba* trees. Then Lālmon saw the *phāsarā*s and panic was upon her.

May the Stainless One protect them, mutters the poet Ārif. Who can fathom the complex magic of the Pīr's compassion? May you be enveloped in the aura of Satya Pīr's grace.

Lāl cried out, "Listen, O Prince, lord of my life! The hand of this wicked *phāsarā* has put us into a desperate state. O my lord, you must mount your horse and ride to freedom, while I stay behind and give battle to the *phāsarā*s!" Lālmon was emotionally overwrought and she clipped her words. "Why should you be struck down by the hand of the *phāsarā*s? You are male, you are the touchstone. Wherever you go untold numbers of beautiful women will happily run with your summons. I am but a terribly unfortunate woman who is little more than a dark blot on her family and lineage. You will find many loving women who are gold compared to my dross. Give up this crazy infatuation you have for me and turn your attention to someone else. Save yourself! Do not delay, O my prince, ride like the wind!"

After hearing her out, the son of the emperor rejoined, "If I give up you, what will I do? Where will I go? With whom shall I run? I have extended my right hand to you for love's sake. How can I survive, Lāl, if I abandon you? You are the treasure of my life, the very ring on my finger. It was only for you, Lāl, that I have become a fugitive, a refugee from my own land."

The couple stood there, absorbed in their argument, until suddenly they were surrounded by the full contingent of seven hundred *phāsarā*s. Lālmon vented her passion with a deafening roar and every single *phāsarā* without exception involuntarily recoiled. The brave Gopāla Jagāi was the man at the point, but he called on someone else to take the lead, "Hey, listen, brother! . . ." Dāmodara then tried, "Hey, Roghu, my good brother, why not order Hari to lead the charge! . . ." Listening to their spineless chatter, Hari flew into a rage and advanced. Lāl met him on her horse and quickly thrust her sword deep into his belly. Hard on her heels the emperor's son spurred his horse, and with a swing of his scimitar he separated head from body. The *phāsarā*s quickly blocked the road forward and backward, for they outnumbered the couple. Forced into a corner, the two began to hack their way forward. The *phāsarā*s proved no match against them, falling one by one to their incessant rain of blows until only one was left standing, a small boy. Lāl was with the emperor's son every step of the way, fighting back to back.

As this delicate daughter of the wazir was about to let fly one final blow, the prince called out to her, "Lāl, do not strike. Don't kill this one!" Lāl replied, "My prince, you do not understand. It will never do to save this child, for he is a black snake, the serpent of death!"

"Why would you behead this lovely child? This tiny child of such delicate constitution and tender age can hardly know anything at all." The prince continued, saying, "Listen, Lālmon, I plan to raise this child as if it were my own. I shall pick it up and take it with me to sate its hunger." Lāl argued, "O son of the emperor, I am at a loss! It is not meet that we have slain these many people, but now that it is done, you must finish the job, sever the lotus's stalk and deprive it of its life-giving water. Listen, O lord of my life, should you try to rear that child, you are certain to suffer, for it will bite the hand that feeds it. Listen, let us not procrastinate over what must be done. Pull yourself together and let us go. I will then cook some food."

Unable to agree, the pair rode slowly away from the scene, taking the boy. Deep within the jungle they came upon a lake. They pulled up beside it and loosed their gear. The prince instructed the child *phāsarā*, "Take yourself to the market and be quick about it! Fetch some rice, lentils, flour, and ghee and bring them back here at once!" The *phāsarā* did as told and headed for the local bazaar. He later presented the lentils, rice, etc., exactly according to the instructions of the crown prince. As usual the prince spread out some bedding and promptly lay down, dozing off, while the daughter of the wazir jumped to the labor of cooking. When the food was prepared, they sat down and ate and drank together. As their stomachs filled, the pair began to exchange the humorous nonsense of those in love. Lāl fashioned a betel quid and slipped it into the prince's mouth, while the young *phāsarā* sat silently and watched their increasingly amorous play. Their two bodies quickly joined as one; nothing could have pried them apart. And for seven straight days did they vent their passions, making this humble place their home.

One morning when Lālmon had gone out for her toilet, the prince's new child lay beside him all alone. The prince was in the unconscious bliss of a deep sleep. Gazing intently at the face of this crown prince, the young child saw only his family's death. With the idea gradually taking shape in his *phāsarā* mind, he concluded that he would decapitate this monster, then retrieve Lāl and carry her off to his former home. He quickly raised the prince's scimitar and swung, neatly separating the prince's head from his body in a single stroke. Examining the severed head he grew drunk with pleasure.

The severed head screamed, "Lālmon, where are you?" Rolling around in the dust it screeched between its final grunts and groans. "Where are you, love of my life? Show yourself to me! Befitting this worldly life you can go home. In this birth we two have been torn asunder, but, my beautiful Lāl, we shall meet in the next life, I swear it." As the head prattled on, the *phāsarā* quickly exchanged his tattered clothes for those elegant ones worn by the decapitated prince. He put them on with great glee. He strapped the scimitar to his side, picked up a shield, a dagger, and a stubby machete for close-in fighting. He then mounted the prince's gallant steed and waited for Lālmon. When she returned from her bath, the *phāsarā* eyed her lecherously and said, "See for yourself, my dear, I have hacked your husband to death. Come, let us go, my lovely, for you are mine and I'm taking you to my home."

When everything registered, Lāl broke into wails of agony and grief. It was as if the vault of the heavens had shattered and rained down on her head. "Where has my treasure gone, leaving me in this world without a guide?"

Ārif replies, "My girl, the Fates have veered dangerously off course."

As she gazed at the severed head lying on the ground,
her eyes blurred with the upsurge of tears,
casting her adrift on an ocean of sorrow
barely able to cling to life itself.
Weeping, Lāl reckoned it was the circumstance of birth
that occasioned this vile and black death.
"Get up, get up!" she screamed,
"I shall pour water in your mouth and make you live.
Apart from you, who else is there
by whom I can stand?"
When he heard Lāl's pathetic mourning,
the *phāsarā* spoke unsympathetically.
"Now who is your man? Who is in charge?
You must come with me now! Quick!"
She contemplated her options and quickly cast her lot
and answered, "I will come with you.
You go on a little ahead,
while I follow behind as is proper."
And so the *phāsarā* foolishly led the way
While Lālmon came after in a quiet rage.
Quietly did she raise high her scimitar
and let it fall at the crown of the *phāsarā*.
His head flew, bouncing to the ground
while Lāl pulled up on the reins to stop the horse.
Lāl had slain the *phāsar* without remorse.
She pulled hard on the reins, wheeled her horse around,
and headed back to that dreadful place
where she had dallied amorously,
but where her husband's corpse now lay.

Ārif the poet composes
while serving the feet of Truth, Satya Pīr.

Lāl picked up the prince's head and cradled it in her lap. Striking her own head in grief, she cried bitterly, lost in her delirium. "Where have you gone, O lord of my life, casting me adrift in this fathomless ocean of existence? I have no one else save you! Who else can I possibly have in this world? Save you, the lord of my life, on whom shall I lean? With whom shall I play and indulge each day, for when I lost your side there was none left on whom to lavish my affections. We rolled the dice together, but no longer."[3] She cradled the severed head in her lap and traced its features with her fingers. "Through this mouth would you eat betel, my life's lord. You have abandoned me, O my lord, where have you gone? How can I forget you and continue to live? I have no friends, male or female, in this sea of life. It is as if I float hither and yon on the surface of the water like a rootless water hyacinth. Did I steal away someone else's husband in a previous birth? Perhaps that would explain why my lord has now parted. Float me across this ocean of existence and make me your mate. We two shall become one as we are consumed with our love. Listen, my lord, half of the day has already passed. Too long have you slept without food; wake up and eat some rice. Apart from you I have no other in this river of life."

Just as waters without swans have lost their true beauty, her body, which had once glowed golden from her love play, now lost all luster and turned dark. A flood of tears soaked her shirt. As she relinquished her grief, the tears began to flow, increasing until they drenched her entire body. Three days did she thus pass, eating absolutely nothing. The many living creatures that populate the jungle heard and felt pity. The entire jungle began to fast in sympathy. For three days did the tiny fawn nestle under the protection of its mother, and each morning when it would awake the doe told it to suckle. But the fawn replied, "Listen, Mother, there is an important guest in the forest and she sits all alone, crying, clasping her lord to her breast. I will not drink any milk until this young woman stops her grieving and goes to bathe." These were the exact words exchanged between fawn and doe. Touched, the doe and her mighty buck wept together. Predators and prey alike gave up their food as they wept. The normal hunt of the forest was abandoned as every sentient being crouched down in sympathetic apprehension. For Lāl's sake alone did all the birds of the forest fold away their wings, like so much stubble, refusing to fly, roosting fast to branches like the roots dropped from the limbs of the banyan. At the foot of the *kadamba* tree the great steed neighed its grief loudly, for horses know these things. Three days passed and it would eat nothing at all. The flesh of the crown prince's body began to putrefy, giving off a wretched odor. The young lady sighed in exasperation, recognizing but grudgingly the condition of her lord and husband. Untold numbers of flies began to appear, multiplying into a frenzied swarm, while Lālmon tried in vain to cover the body with the ends of her own clothes. The young woman emitted a long, haunting wail of agony, which began to tug the heartstrings of Satya Pīr, who sat on his throne far away.

His seat, normally fixed and stable in this world, began to quiver and shake. Satya Pīr himself finally went to the rescue of his devoted Lāl. A wooden staff came to his hand when bidden, wooden sandals popped onto his feet. The Pīr picked up his worn and soiled shawl and wrapped it tightly around his withered body. By magic did Satya Pīr take himself to the place where Lāl wept, holding a severed head in her lap. As he watched her, the Pīr was finally able to get her attention and speak, "For what reason do you weep like this, stretched out on the ground?"

When she heard him, Lāl replied, "Listen, Wise One. In this jungle has my fate run foul. The lord of my life has abandoned me, leaving me unprotected, bereft of a husband. I have become the most unfortunate creature in this wide expanse of the world."

The Pīr listened and then advised Lāl directly. "It is only because of the irascible nature of Satya Pīr that this favorite son of the emperor met his death. Offer to Satya Pīr the *śirṇi*—a simple mixture of banana, rice flour, sugar, and milk—prepared with liberal doses of faith and trust, and your husband who is now suffering death will regain his life. With single-minded zeal attach the severed head to its body, and your intimate companion, Satya Pīr, will resuscitate the darling son of the emperor."

Hearing his words, Lāl concentrated on the proper preparation of the *śirṇi*, while the bestower of all pleasures quietly slipped away. She carefully placed the severed head, affixing it to the body just so, and by the grace of Satya Pīr, the head was firmly reattached. Life began gradually to stir and reanimate the body. When the vital breaths returned, the crown prince slowly came to consciousness. As soon as he was revived, the prince sat up. The young woman immediately threw herself at his feet. "Where did you go, my lord? When you left me behind, I became the most unfortunate creature this mundane world has ever seen." Overcome with emotion and blustery with tears, she held fast his feet. The emperor's son could make neither heads nor tails of her behavior. Then Lāl explained to the prince, "Listen, my lord, Madana the *phāsarā* decapitated you with your own sword. . . ." She then proceeded to describe all the ensuing events to the prince. "Listen, lord of my life, for three whole days you lay slain. . . ." The prince listened carefully to Lāl's vivid description, then the two of them went to bathe and to eat. The multitudes of living creatures there in the forest were relieved, finally able to take their food, and the prince said quietly, "Let us stay here and burden them no longer."

The poet Ārif sings the praise of Truth, Satya Pīr, whose feet I clasp in hard embrace, Gāzī, Warrior for the Faith, who is benevolent to our hero.

The couple saddled their horses and rode off, but they completely forgot to offer the promised *śirṇi*. So distracted were they in their romance they failed to honor the Pīr.

The Pīr declared, "I shall make Lāl suffer for this!" Filling with anger, Satya Pīr cursed her: "For six long months will you languish in prison!"

Just as Satya Pīr dispatched that curse from his place in Mecca, the city of Mogān could just be seen ahead. A lake lay hard by the city, and there the prince stopped and pulled loose his cummerbund. The son of the emperor made fast his horse to the trunk of a convenient tree. The prince then went off to shop in the local bazaar. The lady Lāl uneasily called out to him, "Go straight there and come straight back. Don't dawdle!"

The young prince took note and went off with high spirits. Along the roadside he spotted a woman who was selling flowers. Her name was Purṇimā—the Full Moon—and her beauty was that of a celestial nymph. When she in turn saw how handsome the prince was, she was smitten. When she started to stare at the prince, dangerous ideas cried for her attention, each asking, "How can I charm this attractive young prince?" The string of rose and magnolia flowers that bound her hair she pulled down around her neck as a garland. The hair that was wound tightly on top of her head she loosed, and deftly wove into it fresh jasmine and miniature magnolia blossoms. She pushed another flower blossom behind her ear, enhancing her already ample charm. Then, smiling coyly, she addressed the prince. This mischievous wench spoke suggestively, if not outright provocatively. She surreptitiously tugged the cloth from her body to reveal her breasts. The prince, understandably, quite forgot himself, and, his eyes riveted on this flower vendor, he muttered, "I'll take that garland of flowers hanging there around your . . . neck."

Purṇimā the garland weaver knew well the art of magical charms. Into the prince's outstretched hand she placed from her body those flowers so charged. With great delight the sporting young prince inhaled the fragrance of those flowers, and by the incredible power of that erotic magic, the man was transformed into a ram! Having made him into a ram, she took him home. She kept the charming prince in a specially constructed wooden deck and enclosure. By night she transformed him into a man to enjoy his fine company, but by morning back into a ram he was turned, to be kept for the day in his special pen.

Meanwhile, back at the lake, the minister's daughter decided to take a look around. When the prince was late, she began to fret. "The lord of my life has left me here without protection!" But there she remained rooted, both she and her horses involuntarily fasting. "My lord has brought me into a strange land and abandoned me—such is my luck! I do not know why fate makes me suffer yet again." Falling to the dust, disheveled, her breasts unbound in anguish, she lay weeping. Somehow the day passed and night stole in.

The ruler of the city of Mogān, one Sayyid Nehār—the All Seeing—had two horses stolen from him that night. When the king arose the next morning and sat in his court, he called for the constable to inform him of the event. "I want my horses returned now—and be quick about it! If you are slow, your head will roll!" Taking his cue, the brave young constable searched high and low. Meanwhile Lālmon was fast beneath her tree, weeping disconsolately.

It so happened that the exact coloring of the two horses that were stolen matched precisely the color of the two horses in Lāl's possession. While the noble Lāl was distracted in crying for her prince, the constable apprehended her as the horse thief. Finally waking up to what was happening, Lāl pleaded, "Where is your sense of justice? By what measure can you jail me, my brother, without hearing me out?" But he had no time for appeals and dragged her away. Screaming for her beloved lord, Lāl was swept away in tears. "Just when my lord abandons me, so too my fortunes. I have been made out a horse thief. My fate has turned fickle!" Lāl's cries fell on deaf ears as she headed for jail. Some of her captors struck her around the neck and shoulders, pushing her forward, while others roughly shoved her back.

When the king held his regular public audience, the report was handed over and the constable had her produced. Seething with anger, the king examined his horse thief, never dreaming she was a woman. "Beat him and behead him in the southern gateway!"

When the king issued this command, Lālmon became incensed and began to berate him. "Listen, you who are a king in name only! You have ordered me punished without granting me a trial. The true extent of your intelligence and wisdom have surely been exposed. Those who sit in your court are nothing but mindless ignoramuses. Your soldiers and servants are equally sycophantic fools. There is none among you worthy of being the king's spokesman!"

As her passions rose, her words fell over themselves until the king commanded, "Sieze this thief and take him to jail! It is the will of Allah that this contemptible creature be granted a reprieve! Tie him up in prison. I will try him later."

Receiving this order, the constable remanded Lāl into the jail for men. They bound her with ropes, hand and foot. An impossibly large stone was hoisted onto her chest. Lāl cried out in gut-wrenching pain, "As heart and hope wither, my chest rips apart." Her heart fluttered anxiously; she could hardly breathe. Endlessly she wept, at first counting each of her sorrows. But as her weeping could not be stymied, Lāl lost track of her miseries. Mentally she repeated the name of her prince—who can calculate just how many times? "Where have you gone, lord of my life? You have abandoned me! I am the most unfortunate creature in all of this worldly creation." But, exhausted, Lāl no longer registered the extent of her suffering. All this noble woman could do was to cry out for her lord and master. "If only I could meet my lord for a moment! There is no one who can fathom just how wretched I have become. This must be the suffering that fate etched so plentifully on my forehead at birth. Your beloved servant cries out, for she is dying—come to see me one more time! If you have not seen your Lāl by the time of her demise, then please, my lord, meet me in the next world! It was undoubtedly decreed that in this world we two would be estranged, and now here I lie in the dust on the floor of a prison."

In this way did two full months pass. The king had completely forgotten to bring her to trial. Endlessly did Lāl weep, lying in that awful jail cell. Finally, moved, the Pīr decided, "I shall save Lāl." And so the Pīr spoke to her from afar, "Be calm, cry no more, my child."

Shortly after that, a rhinoceros appeared in the city; it was a regular monster of the species. Everyone fled the city in great alarm and the news was duly reported to the king by his ministers. When he heard about it, the king immediately made it top priority: "Spread the word that the rhino must be slain!"

May everyone repeat the name of Allah, Refuge for the Anxious. Says the poet Ārif, "The Pīr will save you."

The king spoke with the full power of his office
  and personally went forth with great pomp and majesty.
He called this to the attention of everyone
  and ordered his cavalry to muster their ranks.
Bamboo mallets thumped smallish kettle drums;
  the ground reverberated with their message.
Horns, bells, and cymbals sounded
  to assemble nine hundred thousand titan warriors.
Then war trumpets blared and massive kettle drums boomed
  as mounted soldiers strutted forward their steeds.
Message drums and signal bugles ordered forth the assembly,
  while innumerable victory drums banged their support.
Again the horns sounded, this time with flutes,
  mustering the sepoy lines to the front.
Then waves of drummers lined up,
  reminiscent of a precision machine in action.
The cannons were then wheeled from the arsenal.
  Archers bristled with clusters of sharp-tipped arrows,
while other soldiers seemed to dance into their formations.
  Collectively they advanced, row upon row upon row.
They mounted one massive attack,
  firing on that place where the rhino rested.
Arrows and grapeshot rained down
  only to arouse that rhinoceros to defiance.
In a rage that rhino bull charged, head down,
  goring some to their grisly deaths.
It looked hideous, like a monstrous demon,
  forcing the rattled infantry and officers to flee.
No one could stand his ground
  as the beast gored horses and tossed riders to their ends.

Some fled on foot to escape being killed;
  others simply dived deep into the surrounding waters.
Like some frantic demon embodied,
  it scattered the nine hundred thousand soldiers.
Then the king anxiously announced,
  "Whoever can subdue this rhinoceros
I will make my son-in-law!
  To him I shall give my daughter's hand in marriage,
and in addition hand over one-half of my kingdom."
  Even Lāl, sitting in prison, heard this announcement. . . .

Lāl beckoned the guard to come over
  and engaged him in casual conversation.
"Take these twenty-five gold *moharā* coins
  and release me for two hours."
Greedy, he took the twenty-five gold pieces
  and cut her rope bindings free.
He brought Lāl her spirited charger and
  even supplied her with shield and razor-sharp sword.
Her body had grown thin, emaciated,
  but she saddled and mounted her horse herself.
Out she rode on her steed,
  passing the king, to whom she bowed.
She spurred her horse forward, out past
  the dispersed ranks of the nine hundred thousand soldiers.
Still no one had recognized that
  Lāl was a woman and not a man!
With great cunning she ensnared that nasty beast,
  slipping a noose around its neck, a girth of a dozen feet or so.
The rhinoceros charged, enraged at this act,
  but Lāl met him herself, head-on.
It forced her mount to rear up dangerously,
  but she wheeled and smashed the beast's head, cutting deep.
Its majestic head thudded hard to the ground
  and Lāl pulled up her horse, reining it to a halt.
The assembly of nine hundred thousand witnessed her feat
  and sang high her praises in gratitude and admiration.
Lāl then took herself straightaway to
that place where the king was waiting.
    Serving Allah and the feet of the Prophet,
    the poet Ārif composes his tale.

When he witnessed the event, the king was overjoyed. He began to inquire of Lāl, "What land do you call home? Who is your family? Please tell me now, do not make me wait!"

The daughter of the minister acknowledged the inquiry but hid her identity. She spoke, calling herself Lāl Shāh. "Remember that person you called a horse thief and had jailed—that is I, who am talking to you now!" When he heard this, the king was understandably engulfed in shame, but he bravely continued, "You are the horse thief?" Then the king recovered and said, "My son, what I said to you I still hold true—my daughter, whose name is Māhtāb, I will give to you in marriage."

Lāl countered, "Your Majesty, I beg you to reconsider. How can you possibly give your daughter to a horse thief? If I, who am a thief, were to become your son-in-law, everyone in your fair city will hold you at fault."

The king was not deterred, "You cannot be a horse thief! And I will give you my daughter, Māhtāb, in marriage! I have no male offspring; I am a king who failed to produce an heir. You will ascend the throne and become king!" The king was persuasive and managed to get Lāl to agree. Without wasting any time, he sent for the town's magistrate, the local *qazi*. Tents and canopies were erected and wedding music was played. And of course all the soldiers and their officers lined up for their share of the food.

The princess Māhtāb was waiting in her chambers, and the king then presented to Lāl that charming young woman. Somehow no one had discerned Lāl's real identity as a woman. So Māhtāb joined Lāl in the marriage hall. Lālmon's physical form was radiant as the full moon. To behold her dazzling countenance provided everyone with extreme pleasure. All those participating in the festivities had a truly delightful time. Drums, deep throated and double ended, kept time, while someone sang appropriate songs. When they had exhausted the spectacle, everyone went home.

Alone, Lāl began to shed tears for the lord of her life. She fell onto the bed in a fit of sobs and tears—which, needless to say, did not go unnoticed by the king's daughter. Being shy and somewhat embarrassed, the young bride could do nothing. For three days she endured, until finally on the fourth day she returned to their bridal chamber. Dejected and feeling the grief of her life mate, the young bride screwed up her courage and spoke, "What is the reason, my beloved, that you weep so disconsolately? Why do you not joke and play romantically with me?"

With tears flowing down, Lālmon could barely speak, "What can I say, my newly beloved, when my heart aches so? If you will be patient for one month, I swear I will tell you. My bride, I will explain everything, all there is to know. I will tell you this much now, however: When you hear my tale, it will surely break your heart!" And so somehow they got through the rest of that day.

Lāl then conjured the memory of the one they call Satya Pīr. "I promise to build a mosque, a permanent structure with exquisitely decorated walls. And when I get back the lord of my life, I will offer *śirṇi* to that Pīr." Within the hour she had fetched the building contractors and immediately started to lay the foundation of that mosque. And she commanded, "Let the singers sing and dancers dance throughout the holy month of Rāmadān! Let musicians and troubadours entertain without stop!" And to herself she thought, "If only my lord is alive somewhere here in this land. . . ." Thinking only of this, she kept the entertainment going day and night, for everyone in the country would eventually come to the celebration.

And, as these things happen, one day her prince heard about the great goings on, and of his captor, the flower vendor, he asked, "Who is putting on such long and lavish entertainment for the general public?" To which the flower vendor replied, "It is the king's son-in-law. He is a trained soldier, a foreigner of sorts, who lived in Karab City. The king has married his daughter to the one he accused of being a horse thief. Apparently the bridegroom suffered terribly in jail, branded a thief, but when he slew the rogue rhinoceros, he got to marry the king's daughter." As the prince listened, he slowly pieced together everything that had transpired. He reached for the flower vendor's hand and spoke. Holding her hands he pleaded with her earnestly. "Please take me to see this great event! I must see it for myself!" Seeing the obvious agitation of the prince, she was unable to deny him, so take him with her to the extravaganza she did.

When they attended the festivities, the two of them sat together—the emperor's son in front and the flower vendor right behind.

Ārif has composed his song, meditating on the greatness of God. With deep devotion repeat the name of Allah, my brothers, acknowledging no other.

The prince stayed for a long time and watched many interesting performances, but Lālmon had failed to recognize him with that magical garland draped around his neck. To himself the prince likewise lamented, "It has been written in my fate that I should be unable to meet with my Lāl. My luck has run out with the Fates conspiring against me. I shall write my name on the side of the mosque. . . ." Someone had conveniently spat out some chewed tobacco, so with that this heroic young man began to write. In addition to writing his name, this young man described his predicament, telling his tale of woe. "I have fallen into danger in the clutches of the flower vendor. If you are able to locate me, then please rescue me! O Lāl, my eyes long to behold you! . . ." And so he wrote his sad story, taking care to point the way for his beloved. As he returned with the flower vendor, he could not stop weeping. Purṇimā, that wicked garland weaver, led him back to her house and reinstalled her handsome prince on her special platform.

Sometime later Lāl went as usual to inspect personally the mosque's progress. Examining it from one end to the other, her eyes ran across that fateful wall. She noticed that the wall was discolored with dark blotches. And as Lāl began to decipher those marks, her grief overwhelmed her. The message she read rattled her brain; her mind raced, but overcome, she slumped to the ground, completely insensate. "O my beloved," she moaned, "You departed from me promising to return. What incredible miseries must you have suffered in the lair of that flower vendor! O my lord, it was written on our foreheads to suffer through all of this. May you once again physically return to join me!" Several soldiers and officers noticed that she had fallen and ran forward to assist her getting up.

Although deeply anguished, Lāl sat for her daily court audience. She called the sepoys and started to issue a series of commands. "Listen carefully, all you who are present. I have a mind to see staged an elephant fight. Also staged battles with tigers, water buffaloes, and wild horses. And better yet, search the land over for rams. Today, in fact, I want to see some rams butt heads and until then, everything else must stop—I'll neither eat nor bathe until I've seen them."

When it received its orders, that vast assembly quickly scattered to all the points of the compass. And collect rams it did, countrywide, all to present to His Majesty. Lālmon inspected all the rams, but found them lacking. She at last declared, "There is an extraordinary specimen of a ram to be found in the house of a local flower vendor. South of the city in Begam Bazaar you will find a ram, strong and spirited, in the house of one Purṇimā. As her name—the Full Moon—implies, she possesses the beauty of a celestial nymph. She has penned that special ram on a wooden platform made just for it. That platform lies in the northeast corner of the house, visible as you pass through the southern entrance. Go and fetch that ram from the flower vendor."

Taking their orders, the men assigned to the new prince hurried off, systematically searching out this flower vendor, whom they found and questioned. "Produce the ram you've got; we are here to collect it. And by the prince's decree, you too will have to come with us." When the flower vendor heard this she protested—it was as if the sky had fallen, crushing her head to pieces, such was her surprise. She had three or four other rams inside her compound, so all of these she handed over to the armed scouts. But these soldiers were not so easily fooled. "Pay close attention. We did not come after these rams. Bring out the special one!" The flower vendor swore, but recovered quickly and said, "If there is a ram inside, then you can bring him out." Receiving that go ahead, they all rushed inside. The ram that was standing on that magical platform they unleashed and brought out.

They took the flower vendor back, hurrying until they reached the royal and august presence of the prince. When Lālmon saw the ram, she was flooded with a sense of happiness and well-being. Then she turned her attention to the flower vendor. "Listen, flower vendor, turn this ram back into a man! If you do not do it right now, you will pay with your life!"

This flower seller listened incredulously to Lāl's demand and retorted, "What kind of nonsense am I hearing—that a man can become a ram? . . ."

When she heard this reply, Lāl flared with anger! In no mood to brook such impertinence, she wasted no time in giving the order to lash the flower vendor. She was flailed severely, the rapid arc of the blows resembling the up and down undulations of a yak-tail whisk. In the end the flower woman capitulated and reluctantly transformed her ram back into a young man.

All who witnessed this miracle were stunned. Lāl collapsed to the ground and began to weep. Her crying was uncontrolled and in the stress of the moment, she banged her head onto the ground. "Where had you gone, my lord, leaving me so utterly alone?" She cried like this for a long time, simply holding onto his hands. Then wrapping their arms around each other's necks, they slumped down into a heap on the ground.

Serving my spiritual preceptor, my murśid, the poet Ārif sings. Repeat the name of Allah, O brother, and take your place in the community of the faithful.

Lāl was overjoyed to see her young prince. She had proper royal clothes brought to her lord and, grabbing the prince's hands, she led him into the inner chambers of the palace. Everyone else who was present took appropriate leave. Inside, adjacent to the primary palace residence, stood a small annex. There she deposited the prince until all the servants in the vicinity could be alerted. Then Lāl escorted the prince into the palace's main residential hall. Māhtāb had been waiting there on her bed. Lāl explained and showed her who she really was. "I am not a man at all. In fact, I am menstruating right now. . . ." Listening with utter disbelief, that innocent young bride sobbed in shock, anger, and hurt. Lāl continued to explain, "That flower vendor, Mālinī, knows well the art of magical spells. She had placed in his hand a flower she had so charmed. With great pleasure and expectation did my handsome young prince sniff its fragrance, and by the incredible power of her magic, he, a man, was transformed into a ram.

"That flower vender then took him to her home. She kept the prince in a specially constructed platform, by transforming him into a ram—and so my lord lived in that flower seller's house. Now, using a number of strategies, I have recovered him from that ignominious fate. I have nothing but profound love for this prince. Listen carefully, my young lover, the jewel I had lost I have found again. Now I shall escort him back to our own country. You should remain here in the house of your mother and father." But when she heard all this, the young bride pleaded with Lāl, "How can you, my lord, go and leave me behind? You are the lord of my life; I am your female servant. If you abandon me I will hang myself in shame. Please stay right here for a moment, my love. First I want to explain everything personally to my mother and my father."

Having taken her stand, the young bride went deeper into the palace, where she found the king and his queen seated on the edge of their royal bed. Māhtāb addressed them. "Do you have any idea what you have done to me, Daddy? You gave me in marriage to someone you knew nothing about. And that young man is no man at all, but a young woman! She holds an abiding love for the son of another emperor.

He had been held captive in the form of a ram in the house of a flower vendor, and now that she has gotten him back, she wants to return to her own home! Still, she is the treasure of my heart! I cannot part with her. Summon her, please, and hand me over to her custody!"

"Where is this 'husband' of yours, show us!" boomed the king. Seizing that opening, Māhtāb called for Lāl.

Having anticipated the worst, the wazir's daughter was much relieved to hear the call, and she commanded that her own husband be fetched. Taking him by the hand, Lāl entered into the inner confines of the palace. Hosen Shāh and Lālmon moved as one. The king was deeply moved to see how handsome this young prince really was. He then seated the prince and held him by the hand. Taking his daughter's hand, he proffered her to Lāl, and Lāl in turn made her over to her husband, the crown prince.

The king announced, "I am a king without an heir. I have no one of my own. You must ascend the throne and reign as king." Having levied this royal edict, the king returned to his own chambers, while the three heroes took their seats together on the throne. Lālmon sat to the right, Māhtāb to his left, Hosen Shāh in the center. The two women plied the king with betel from their own hands. When the night had passed, what they all desired had been fulfilled. And, as promised, seven hundred thousand rupees' worth of *śirṇi* was given to honor Satya Pīr.

At his place in Mecca, Satya Pīr smiled benevolently, knowingly. And Hosen Shāh ascended the kingship of Mogān City. His desires continued to be fulfilled, death and misery held long at bay.

May Satya Pīr be merciful to all who join him.

That I may be worthy of your protection, O Gāzī, Warrior of the Faithful, I clasp your holy feet. May everyone repeat the name of Allah, as this fabulous tale reaches its end.

The Unwilting Garland of Faithfulness

Kiṇkara Dāsa's *Rambhāvatī Pālā*

May your mind be stilled meditating on the boundless grace of Satya Pīr. When you hear this song, your miseries will slip away.

Jayadatta the merchant owned a house in a city on the Ajaya River, and in this house he had many treasures and gems. This man was blessed, a man of great fortune, and that fortune included his wife, Rambhāvatī. Her name—She Who Possesses the Form of a Nymph—was appropriate, for this woman was the very embodiment of beauty itself. Quite understandably, the merchant was reluctant to leave her, even for a moment; he would not go outside his home, just as Śrī Kṛṣṇa kept watch over his wife Rukmiṇī. So dear to her husband was this woman that she could never get away to visit the house of her mother and father; and appropriately, she in response never failed to think of her husband alone as her lord. The merchant would not even leave to visit a friend—he was more than content to stay at home. So consumed was he by this conjugal love that he even managed to forget Satya Pīr.

Now the Pīr took note of this merchant's omission and, so offended, his anger grew. Just as Kamalā, one of Kṛṣṇa's many wives, stole from him, so the same befell this son of a merchant. Diamonds, sapphires, pearls, corals, strings of precious and semiprecious stones, silver, gold, and gold necklaces of fine filigree, exquisite yak-tail whisks, sandalwood and other unguents, carved conch shells, finely wrought musical instruments of many shapes and sizes—anything and everything did Satya Pīr pilfer.

One day Rambhāvatī felt compelled to speak, "Listen my precious husband and trader, how are we going to manage in the days to come? The wealth that had accrued to us when I joined my father-in-law's house has been completely consumed. I have begun to notice the sure signs of impending poverty and misery. Everyone in the house remains idle, but constantly consumes. Unless you undertake some new business venture, the storehouses will soon run dry. When water is constantly poured from a pitcher, there comes a time when no amount of coaxing will produce more. Why? Because the initial investment was never replenished. To each and every administrator and hired hand, and to the hundreds of servants—men and women—go two rupees for salary every day. Enormous quantities of money are distributed to professional genealogists, brahmins, and holy men, and quite a bit more goes to singers and dancers. Spend only what you earn, lest we come to ruin—that is my sound advice. Start stockpiling saleable goods and equip your fleet of seven ships, for you must act decisively and quickly. My advice has never proved false or misleading. You are certain to attain complete success."

Although he heard, the merchant's son could only smile. "Why do you say such things? In the end, one is always reduced to penury and suffering."

May Satya Nārāyaṇa be merciful. Bowing his head at his holy feet, the devotee calls for Satya Pīr to make his presence felt.

The trader was finally compelled to agree, for he really had no choice. "My good wife, you have spoken the truth. I will prepare my fleet of ships and venture out again to trade. Because I cannot escape the clutches of your natural beauty, let us prepare the boats and depart together."

Grasping her husband's feet, Rambhāvatī was terrified and earnestly entreated him, "Whenever a woman goes along on a the boat, misery is certain to follow, my lord! The wife of a merchant never accompanies him to sea on a trading voyage. I have never heard of it, nor have I seen it. It is a sure recipe for disaster!"

The merchant argued back, "Listen, my good wife, you belong by my side. Rāma went to the forest to uphold his father's promise, but did so together with Jānakī and Lakṣmaṇa. All three went. Why must you worry so about coming with me? Rāma chased into the forest after an illusionary deer and so Rāvaṇa, finding the palace unguarded and empty, stole Sītā away. Likewise, Śaṅkhāsura the titan demon went off to make war. So, disguising himself as Śaṅkhāsura, Kṛṣṇa entered his house. He made love to that man's chaste woman, plundering her virtue, and, having accomplished that, Lord Nārāyaṇa was able to slay Śaṅkhāsura. Lest you find yourself in such a predicament and forget me, I want to take you with me when I go."

Rambhāvatī quickly countered, "I may be lowest among mortal beings, but listen, O merchant, to the story of the incredible power of chaste women who are called *satīs*. The wife of the sage Gautama was the charming and youthful Ahalyā. When the lord of the gods spied her, he simply stole her for his own. But that chaste woman was made insensate and turned into stone by invoking her husband's name. She was liberated only by the touch of Rāma's feet. Draupadī, beautiful, chaste, and devoted, maintained chastity—as the result of her earnest prayer—while going with five different men. But there is no chastity in the triple world to match that of Sītā; yet why did she have to live with the demon Rāvaṇa? We hear in the *Rāmāyaṇa* story that Mandodarī is a chaste woman, a *satī*, so why then does she propitiate Vibhīṣaṇa to slay Rāvaṇa?[1] This is the way chaste and faithful wives have always been treated. I imagine myself to be the lowest of creatures on this earth, but if you still cannot fathom my intentions and trust me, then I shall provide you a crutch. I will weave a garland of *campakas*—those fragrant yellow moon-magnolias—and personally place it on your neck. As long as the flowers of that garland remain fresh and radiant, you will know that the woman you left is thinking only of you. But should that garland begin to wilt, then rest assured that your wife's interest has moved elsewhere." With this that jealous merchant's mind grew easy and he prepared to leave on his journey.

May everyone worship and meditate on Satya Pīr!

"I know what my husband desires. . . ." So the charming and seductive young wife of the merchant visited her garden. She picked a wide variety of flowers—magnolia and *vakula*, white and Arabian jasmine, star jasmine, red amaranth, and *kadamba* in great quantity; *kuruveli* and *kuñjalatā*, perfumed hundred-petaled- and moon-magnolias, *jai*- and *jui*-jasmine, and *aparājitā*. With hundreds of flower blossoms did this woman propitiate Śaṅkarī, Durgā, the model of chastity, and Pārvatī, wife of Śiva. Then she wove her special garland of magnolias, all of the favored *campā* variety.

When it was finished, she draped the garland around her husband's neck and made obeisance to him. Happy and content was this merchant's daughter. Then Rambhāvatī spoke, "Listen, master of my heart, this I vow to you. If this garland should ever become desiccated and wilt, then know that I have cheated on you. The value of these flowers is truly without equal, for if they remain fresh, day after day, then your Rambhāvatī—and you can know this for sure—remains faithful and is intimate with no other man. Keep it always around your neck and watch it ceaselessly; never cast it aside. For this *campā*-magnolia garland carries my vow. Now, my lord, you may make your journey."

This faithful daughter of a merchant slipped the garland from her own throat and gently secured it around Jayadatta's neck. Auguring an auspicious journey, the merchant took leave of his hometown and made his way to the river's bank. Dockhands were mustered, the ships' fitting out was completed, while the quartermaster loaded and secured stores. All the hands' womenfolk gathered around making the propitious *hulāhuli* sounds, which rendered the ships auspicious. All seven of the sea captains reassured those present, including the sons of the crew and the rest of their families.

Hoisting their green bamboo oars, these able Bengali boatmen took their places on the wide-beamed cargo boats. Rambhā returned home, while on the boat remained her husband. Raising their arms in salute, the boatmen cried out, "Sail on! Sail on!"

Glory be to Satya Pīr! Victory! I bow to Satya Pīr, destroyer of adversity. As the lord of the Kali Age, you alleviate the suffering of the wretched.

Massive offerings of flowers were made to the boats in the Ajaya River. They then floated past the Kamala Kulinī Ghat of Benāpura. By way of Navadvīpa, Pāhāḍapura, and Vaidyapāḍā, they came to Kāli Āḍā after a mere fifteen days. The boats floated past ghats on both banks of the Jahnavī, while the fort of Tribhāga Denā lay off to port. After twenty days they came to a fabled City of Jewels—Māṇik Pāṭana—and the ruler of that kingdom was the Rājā Mānsiṅgh.

They landed the boats at the ghat and climbed up to the bank. The merchant instructed the captain that they were to pay their respects to the king. The merchant culled some appropriate gifts as tribute, packed them up, and headed off with his captain to meet formally with the king. With the help of the gatekeepers, the collected items were assembled before that *rājā*. The merchant proffered selected goods as a generous tribute, while offering his profound and sincere obeisance. This greatest of rulers received him with grace and reassurance, and begged him to take a seat; and the seafaring trader did just that, right next to the king.

The *rājā* politely inquired, "Tell me, merchant, in what region is your house? For what purpose do you make the long journey to our fabled trading center, Māṇik Pāṭana?"

The merchant replied, "Lord of men, listen carefully. My city is Benāpura, which lies on the banks of the Ajaya. My given name is Jayadatta, and I am the son of a conch-shell merchant. It is only for purposes of commerce that I come to Māṇik Pāṭana."

The *mahārāja* was delighted to hear his response and could be heard quickly muttering, "good," "excellent" in approval. "I have no objection to your doing trade here, good merchant. The treasures of Māṇik Pāṭana will not disappoint you. Stay here at my palace for a month or so and I shall supply you with whatever marketable goods you might desire." The trader agreed to the king's proposal and was then shown to living quarters close by. An enormous quantity of food—fifty *kāhana*s worth[2]—was prepared for cooking, and that magnificent feast stretched well into the evening before it was finished. From that moment on, two times per day—morning and evening—did the merchant consult and converse with the king. And, quite conspiciously, that *campaka* garland always hung beautifully around his neck. During the merchant's many regular visits to the king's court, the garland never seemed to wither. The king, who remarked this day after day, was amazed and somewhat puzzled.

This campaka *garland had piqued his curiosity.*

Time and again the *rājā* wistfully cast his gaze on that *campā* garland that remained so brilliant around the merchant's neck. Finally he testily broached the topic with his own garland weaver. "Without fail you supply that merchant with stunning garlands, yet you routinely ignore me! Weave me an equally beautiful garland, one that is redolent of sandal!"

The flower vendor protested, "Why do you censure and implicate me? You should inquire directly of the merchant! Someone else is responsible for the daily stitching of that costly garland with its exquisite fragrance."

At this the *mahārāja* was momentarily mollified. Heeding his garland weaver's advice, he approached Jayadatta through lighthearted conversation. Then this lord of men broached the topic, "My brother, I want to ask you a serious question, and, merchant, I want you to answer truthfully. Your speech never distorts or hides the truth—on that everyone agrees. You are clearly an honest and righteous man."

The merchant cut him off, "Listen, my king, what good results from telling lies? Feel free to ask anything, honorable sir, and I will endeavor to answer."

So the *rājā* pressed on, "Merchant, my son, your neck is strung with *campaka* blossoms every single day. Where do you get them? Who is this special garland weaver? And where does she find such special flowers to adorn you day in and day out?"

The merchant promptly answered, "Your Majesty, this is not the work of a flower weaver, nor is the garland strung fresh each day. My wife offered me this *campā* garland along with her personal promise. Pay close attention, O jewel among men! Before my departure, she brought these fragrant flowers and placed them around my neck with the following solemn vow: 'Pay heed, my jewel of virtues. When I become adulterous and give myself to another man, only then will this magic garland fade and wilt.' As the lotus floats ever-fresh on the waters, so these precious flowers hang on my neck, always brilliant, day after day. I have spoken in truth, I swear. My wife is a virtuous woman, a *pativratā*, vowed to fidelity. Her heart yearns only for me."

Hearing him out, the king was moved in admiration and affection for the merchant, and—perhaps amused at his naïveté—honored him with rich gifts of clothing, perfume, and sandal. This best of men then granted leave and the merchant returned to his living quarters; but two aides were pointedly requested to stay with the king. They discussed for some time how they might positively determine whether the merchant was telling the truth or lying. The king just could not let it go; it had become an obsession. He worried himself to the point of being consumed by it: "What can I do to find out?" And so, in his anxiety, thinking of little else, the king's body began to waste away.

Being filled with mercy, may Satya Pīr fulfil the wish of our hero!

Pressing my palms together, I bow down to Satya Pīr. May you who are our father, perfect and pleasing to the eye, descend among us.

The king spoke, "Tell me, my trusted advisers, whom might we dispatch to determine the extent of this woman's chastity? We shall see for ourselves just how pure this beautiful specimen of the weaker sex really is. If she cuckolds her husband, she will wither that flower garland."

The minister smartly replied, "If this is what you have decided you really want to do, there are only two men capable of pulling off the job. . . ."

The minister's response pleased the king to no end, and he summoned those two reprobates—they really were dissolute and shameless. The king gave his instructions: "Both of you go quickly to the merchant's hometown. Seduce this trader's wife and undermine her severe practice of fidelity. If you can succeed in capturing this delectable young woman's heart through the pleasures of erotic love, then the merchant's *campakas* should dry up and die. Carry out this foul deed exactly as I have said; then the chief of security will confirm the real story of the magnolias."

One of those men was the chief of security, and it fell to him alone to execute the order. He made ready a swift boat with beautiful lines. The eye of silver was applied and the colorful bimini-canopy spread.[3] Striped canvas sails shone brightly, luffing gently in the breeze. On both sides, port and starboard, were stationed straight rows of oarsmen, precisely aligned like dots of reddish cinnabar and sulfurous yellow orpiment embedded in crystal. The agent of the king took his formal leave. Bowing deeply, he positioned himself proudly in the diamond-shaped pulpit of the boat. Rich carpets were unrolled and scattered about the cabin and gangway. The agent posed as if he himself were the son of a king.

When the boatmen pulled their oars in unison, the earth seemed to shudder, and the boat shot across the waves like an arrow. With one smooth, quick stroke of their blades, the boat leaped twenty cubits, some thirty-six feet, and with the steady rhythmic pull of those oars the boat seemed to fly. For the next twenty days the boat sailed on, until it reached the banks of the Ajaya River, where lay the merchant's town. Where he first sighted the city the agent chose to land. He moored his diamond-prowed boat and climbed the steps at the first ghat.

On that bank of the Ajaya perched the house of a flower vendor, named Mālinī, her name literally indicating her occupation, where paramours and other individuals of questionable character went to fetch garlands, and so on, as they headed for their nightly assignations. Mālinī presented a truly captivating garland to this security agent, after which he inquired where he might locate the house of Rambhā. Mālinī, eager to please, quickly responded, "Her house is close by, and a little later, I will provide you with all the particulars."

The chief took up her implicit invitation and said, "Since I was unable to follow the exact directions to the merchant's house, perhaps you could put us up in your house for three or four days instead?"

Sensing some money and possible adventure, Mālinī graciously responded, "You are most welcome to stay here until then." In return and as expected, the chief of security presented her with a fashionable silk sari. And so it was that Mānsiṅgh's security chief came to stay at the flower vendor's place.

May everyone make obeisance with sincere devotion to Lord Satya Pīr!

From the boat moored at the ghat, the agent collected jute goods, fine cloth, and his personal kit, and then moved in the house with Mālinī. This chief of security was impressed with the house of the merchant, and so he began to make inquiries, filling in his meager knowledge. He began rather innocently but effectively. "O radiant beauty, listen, my dear Mālinī! Whose house is it that lies just north of here? It is decorated with pointed bulbous finials, its banners and pennants sparkle in the breeze, and beside it lies a long and inviting lake. A covered pavilion juts up from the center of the compound, reminiscent of Indra's fine citadel. Tell me, what merchantman owns this fine house? There are so many people inside the buildings engaged in such a great many tasks, that it appears to me that the owner is quite a successful and fortunate individual."

Mālinī readily supplied the information, "Listen, my good man, he is a merchant by the name of Jayadatta. In wealth he is a millionaire and devoted to Lord Govinda. He is an endless repository of good qualities. But the merchant has left his home to go on a business trip. His wife, Rambhāvatī, stays alone in the house. She is totally devoted to her husband, a true *satī*, and she is maintaining a special vow in that regard. That woman wove together a garland of *campā* flowers, those special magnolia blossoms, and slipped it around her husband's neck. As a good wife, whose beauty and charm are legendary, she has vowed never to forget her lord under any circumstance. If this *satī* slips and forgets, the *campā* garland that hangs on the neck of that merchant will wither and die. As that severe promise attests, her mind is firmly committed and fixed on the feet of her husband and no one else."

The chief of security was mildly amused; after a moment he spoke, "Listen my beautiful Mālinī, this woman is a treasure, a priceless gem. And I crave treasure and want you to procure her for me! Listen closely to my plan, Mālinī. You must work on her day and night to convince her to stray. While she has been faithful until now, an endless barrage of suggestions is sure to weaken her, make her restless, and she just might forget herself and relent. . . ." Mālinī considered carefully what he said, calculated the potential reward, then started to collect flowers to stitch a garland. Soon she was off to see Rambhā.

The servant of Lord Hari sings his pāñcālī *tale in the three-footed meter.*

Mālinī confidently carried a garland that included white and star jasmine, but her nervous steps betrayed the unsettling of her mind. Mālinī entered Rambhāvatī's confines, keeping with her that jasmine-laced garland. She pulled the garland from her basket and presented it to this pure and chaste woman, who was sitting in all her beauty performing the worship of Lord Śiva. She took note of the lovely, indeed enchanting, garland Mālinī placed on the image of Śiva. Gauging her visitor's intention, this moon-faced woman spoke, "The chaste woman in me keeps her heart and mind firmly fixed on the feet of her husband, but when I see your garland, Mālinī, my mind is perturbed and grows uneasy. Listen, my friend, when it should be time for pleasure, my husband is never at home. So whom and on what occasion might I dress with a garland such as this? When will my charming lord show his mercy and return to me? I would gladly serve him as a slave, even as a courtesan. . . ."

Divining Rambhāvatī's condition, Mālinī began her seduction, coaxing her with sweet words, little by little, just as water dripping slowly on rock is reckoned to have such profound effect. "You are a devoted wife, yet you send your husband away on trip after trip. Why have you produced no son to stand at his side?"

Rambhāvatī bravely replied, "What you have suggested is all true. Life for a merchant has no meaning except through his trade. Nothing else matters."

Sensing progress, Mālinī pressed on: "You are still young and beautiful. In my house right now there is a man who is the very image of the god of love, Madana the Enchanter. This man is a gem, with an intoxicating physique. He is just the kind of youthful lover you should meet."

Rambhāvatī replied, "What you advise is sound and tempting; I will do my best not to turn your advice into useless words. Except for you, I have no one to whom I can turn for such help. My husband has gone to a distant land, so you must act as my helmsman. Besides, who remains truly faithful in the throes of this difficult existence? Tell your handsome young friend to come. But you must not come with him, otherwise you will find yourself in a terrible fix. Were my servant woman to see you, she would personally see you run out of town. Go and send him to my quarters tonight, and hurry, for in three or four days my husband-merchant could return. And listen carefully, my dear, I should be, but I am not the least embarrassed to tell you that if I am going to do this, it is my earnest desire that he come dressed to impress me, out to win my heart."

Mālinī took careful note of all of this, and hurried back to her house where she explained everything in great detail to the king's agent. Sensing greater reward, Mālinī somewhat embellished her work in the telling: "I clasped her feet and told her all about you. She said nothing at all nor would she look at me. Then I placed that jasmine-laced garland around her neck. Perhaps it was the combination of the magnolia and *vakula* flowers I had intertwined that made it so intoxicating and sweet. Suddenly she laughed and threw her arms around my neck. She then told me to send to her that man so skilled in the arts of love. She placed her hand on my hand and solemnly assured me: 'I have but a single female servant attending me.' She adorns herself with the most exquisite taste—necklaces of silver and gold, her hair held in place by golden clips. Gather up all your gifts and riches—jewelry, clothing, money—and carry them on your head to meet her. Have no fear; go directly up the path ahead."

The chief of security hesitated, "But, sweetheart, what are you telling me? You are familiar with the situation, the people, the place—you come along too!"

Mālinī replied, "That was certainly what I had intended, but that gorgeous creature anticipated my design and expressly forbade me come. She has a servant woman, an old bag of a widow. If she sees me, then I will be humiliated, lose my house, and be run out of town. Go alone and take no companion or porter with you. Carry your clothes, jewels, and expensive gifts on your head yourself."

Not overly sanguine with this change in his plan, the agent reluctantly agreed. He confidently told the old woman, "Somehow or another I will seduce the merchant's wife tonight. After I have met this chaste woman, I shall return to your safe haven, sometime tomorrow." So he began his toilet, dressed in expensive pajamas, and gathered all his gifts on his head. Once outside, he inched his way along with great stealth. With no one to accompany him, he soon found that he was trembling with fear, his entire body quaked. But fewer than two hours into the night he had successfully negotiated the path to Rambhāvatī's house. The ever-captivating Rambhāvatī, however, had anticipated all of this well in advance, and so it was that she dressed and made up her servant woman to meet her would-be paramour.

The agent arrived safe and sound, and soon he had gained entry to the merchant's house. He quietly deposited his treasures with the one female attendant and just as quickly found his object. The beautiful woman he had come to meet wasted no time, but said—in an uncharacteristically familiar and surprisingly forward manner—"Please come in. Do sit here on my bed. Please have a drink and eat some betel nut from my hand. With the merchant out of the house and my snooping neighbors always on the watch, I was reluctant to wait for you outside." And in her disguise, the servant—obviously enjoying her role—suggested all manner of things, but the chief of security was very ill at ease, so much so that he found himself unable to carry out the order of his king. He did, however, manage to sit beside the servant and hold her hand.

Rambhāvatī took in the whole scene from the door. Then the beautiful Rambhāvatī stepped forward and spoke harshly and contemptuously, "Tell me, Mr. Sneak, why have you slipped into my room in the dead of night?"

The chief of security, who was stretched out on the bed, nearly died from the shock. He jumped up and hid in the corner, cowering with fear. Then the servant began to berate him, "O noble gentleman, if you are so afraid, why did you come here in the first place?" But the chief of security had already bolted. He ran away and never looked back. To herself our heroine wondered, "Why was he so afraid? . . ." But to his flying backside she yelled, "You came to eat sweet curds and milk! Why do you run away in disgrace after tasting this bit of whey?"[4] But the chief of security, alas, heard not one word of this reproach, for he was hiding in the brambles, deep in the woods, his body convulsing in fear. His heart pounded uncontrollably and madly he could only think, 'I've nearly lost my life in this botched affair! How can I find the boat?'

Although he was wearing fancy clothes and a dress turban, he plunged directly down the forest path, oblivious to the thorns that tore at his feet. Certain prickly flowers and shrubs jumped out to tear at his fine pajamas. And in no time this dandy chief of security was shamefully disheveled. His misery knew no bounds. His pajamas were ripped to shreds and his heart pounded furiously as if to repent for his sins. He dragged his body through those thorny hooks without looking back or pausing for breath. Somehow he emerged from the forest right at the landing ghat.

It was well into the night's second watch—hours later—when the chief of security landed at the ghat. He awakened all the boatmen—pilot and oarsmen. "Brothers, I have accomplished my mission, now let us return home!" And having given that instruction, he boarded the boat to safety. "There are still some items sitting in Mālinī's house—someone must go to fetch them. But go carefully and call her quietly so that no one will hear you. But be aware—there is a large man on the road wearing a turban and carrying a staff who chased me and beat me! When you get to Mālinī's house, tread carefully and inquire of her the possibility of bringing back those precious items straightaway. Do not dally, brother. Go with great haste and remember my warnings." And so one lucky man set out on a dead run and, just like a thief, quietly entered Mālinī's house. He deftly awakened Mālinī without a sound, gathered up all the clothes and the stray pieces of jewelry, and, as commanded, returned quickly to reboard the boat.

Unfurling its golden canvas, the boat set sail. In the dead of night the boat pulled away swiftly, its smooth hull propelled by the running currents of the high tide. The oars dropped in rhythm and the boat lunged forward like an arrow. The chief of security gradually came back to life. Day and night the boat sailed, for twenty days nonstop, until it landed at Māṇik Pāṭana. The sails were furled and the boat anchored. It was with a light heart that the chief of security went straight to the king.

The *rājā* wasted no time in his inquiry. "How did you manage to meet this chaste woman in the middle of the night? Please narrate that exceptional event for me." And with great pride the chief of security began to tell his version of this encounter.

"Listen, my great lord and protector, I barely returned with my life! . . ." The chief of security continued, "My king, by your blessing I successfully reached the merchant's home region. Right near the landing ghat stood the house of a flower vendor named Mālinī. Mālinī was herself a delightful woman, an ocean of fine qualities. She spoke glowingly of Rambhāvatī's many fine traits. I used her house as my outpost. I bribed Mālinī by giving her a fine silk sari, whereupon she readily wove a garland and carried it without delay to our lovely lady in question. Employing an admirable array of tactics, Mālinī worked on that figure of beauty and quickly turned her head—so much for the faithful wife. Our rendezvous was fixed for the early evening hours of the first momentous night. One of her female servants, however, turned out to be a real mischievous brat. She came right out and announced that a royal security chief had come calling. When Rambhāvatī heard it so baldly and loudly proclaimed, she withdrew in apprehension. I managed to stay for something less than half an hour, before she agreed to slip away and meet me elsewhere. She slipped outside, onto the street. It was easy to spot this pure *satī* among all the lowlife, servant women, and prostitutes. In no time I easily won Rambhā over. Her superior beauty, which radiated with a hundred qualities, was exquisite. And so it was that we had our love tryst.

"When I returned to the boat, the seas and winds were favorable and transported us quickly. The boat landed here at the ghat, and I immediately presented myself to your royal Majesty. I found Rambhāvatī to be the most skilled of lovers; her words are sweet and well-chosen, her beauty truly astounding. . . ." And so his story grew.

The king listened keenly to this tale. He dismissed the chief of security and took himself directly to the merchant's personal quarters. There he found the merchant with the same *campaka* garland around his neck, bright and dazzling as ever. To himself the *rājā* observed, "I think I understand the chief of security's clever cover. He must have passed his time with one of her servants and then returned pretending success." The king promptly informed his chief minister, "I want to go and see her myself! You are deputized to discharge all royal duties in my absence."

The king then issued the order to make ready his boat. They brought around one of the special diamond-prowed boats and made it ready. The oarsmen and coxswain put on brightly colored dress uniforms—special hats and fine suits of finely woven broadcloth—all of which showed to great advantage. "Let her sail! Let her sail!" they boomed out in a traditional departure. The royal barge's twelve sets of oars bit into the water, seeming to chew it up. In a mere fifteen days they reached the city on the Ajaya and docked at the very same ghat next to Mālinī's house.

Mālinī, in best form, received them with her speciality: magnolia garlands. The king, always polite, queried her about local news and events. "Tell me, Mālinī, whose house is that just north of here? It appears that the owner is a wealthy man, a prince of some sort. . . ." And Mālinī, always ready to supply information, said, "My king, pay close attention. He is the son of a successful merchant and he is called Jayadatta. This trader has gone on a business voyage to Māṇik Pātaṇa, the Jeweled City, and his wife lives alone in that big mansion. Her name is Rambhāvatī and her looks are those of that class of celestial musicians so famous for beauty. So extraordinary is her form that she passes for a heavenly nymph, so her name—that of celestial nymph—is most appropriate."

The king offered, "If you can arrange for me to tryst with her, I will place on your arms the most elegant of conch bracelets." No sooner had she heard this proposition than Mālinī pledged her complete cooperation. The old woman began to devise many ways to charm this lovely neighbor who seemed to arouse so much interest in men.

Mālinī was delighted to receive the king's commission. She set about to weave a garland of many different flowers. Putting on that silk sari—which she had received from her last visitor—she went off to the trader's house and entered the premises while it was still morning. As soon as Rambhāvatī beheld those fragrant flowers, whose magnificance would shake even the minds of sages to the point of desire, she was moved to speak, and so preempted Mālinī.

"My husband has left me to travel to a land far away, and with each passing season, I waste away, neglected. Why, then, would you bring such enchanting flowers to me? Listen, my dear Mālinī, I no longer see my husband even in my dreams. The misery he heaps on me is unbearable and relentless. Before he left, I wove a garland of special *campā* flowers and placed it lovingly around my husband's neck. But when I think of it, I ache so! I could spend my days doing pleasant things in the company of my female companions, but instead, I only suffer through my nights alone, wide awake, worrying. In childhood we belong to our fathers, in our youth we belong to our husbands, and in our old age, we belong to our sons. In this way women can live their whole lives in pleasing comfort—but such is not my good fortune. Except for you, I have no real friends. I do not see anyone else as much. Help me, my friend, to find a way out! I only manage one day at a time. How can I maintain this precarious grip on life? My mind and will are slipping. . . ."

Somewhat unsettled, Mālinī composed herself, and with palms pressed together in respect finally said, "Listen, my widow-to-commerce! If such thoughts were bothering you, why did you not share them with me, for I am your best friend! It so happens that there is a *rājā* named Mānsiṅgh whose personal beauty and qualities are truly incomparable. And, as luck would have it, he has developed a strong attraction to you. If you will but consent, you can have this treasury of greatness all for yourself—I will deliver him to you in person."

Rambhāvatī listened intently and replied, "My husband stays abroad and I see no hope for having a family here. What else can be done to find solace for my misery and relief from my fears? Send me your king, my beloved friend! A king by the name of Mānsiṅgh, of incomparable wealth and virtues, comes to me for erotic pleasure—would anyone else do differently? I will serve this king personally. Bring him to me tonight!"

So this moon-faced beauty issued her decree, and that, needless to say, thrilled the mercenary Mālinī. She went straight to the *rājā*. Pressing her palms together in respect, she informed him. "Listen, O mighty and respected *Rājā*! Tonight you will have your vaunted tryst with the enchanting Rambhāvatī. . . ."

For her part, Rambhāvatī emphasized her womanly nature, which was already considerable. She selected an outfit sure to captivate and decorated her body with expensive jewelry. Her hair, beautifully thick and curly, she highlighted with the flowers supplied by Mālinī—so fresh they were that bees hovered to try and lap their nectar. The dot of vermilion on her forehead glowed like the rising sun of early dawn, while collyrium suggestively accented her eyes. The ornament that pierced the side of her nose reminded one of streaks of lightning when the light glanced off its pearl setting. Her sensuous, pouty lips shone redder than a fleshy, ripe *bimba* fruit.[5] Her teeth, in contrast, played over those lips like delicate beads of pomegranate. Strings of gemstones encircled her waist and breasts, golden bangles banded her wrists, a seven-strand necklace drooped gracefully from her neck. Above her feet jangled delicate anklets that put silver and pearl to shame. Her innocent glance shot from the side of her eye as true and deftly as an arrow. Finishing her adornment with more jewelry, she lay in wait on her bed.

When they finally met—and the king did come as promised that evening—this entrancing wife-turned-paramour completely befuddled the poor *rājā*'s mind. It was with effective strategy that this able woman, who still brandished the vermilion mark of marriage in her hair's part, sat down in apparent submission to cook. It was, however, a ruse to determine the real state of this *rājā*'s mind and heart.

As he sat on the bed, the king examined her closely. He soon found himself drowning in Rambhāvatī's beauty as he looked on her face. He lightly chided her with sweet but cajoling words, "You keep me waiting while you sit to cook. . . ." To which Rambhāvatī gently replied, "The lord of my life has gone to Māṇik Pāṭana. For that I reason I am grieving, dying little by little. By day I fast in honor of my husband; not until ten in the evening do I cook for myself and take my meal. She who serves her husband as if he were Kṛṣṇa is blessed with many good qualities and possessed of great merit. One's sins are effaced by recalling those five faithful women: Ahalyā, Draupadī, Satī, Rāṇī, and Mandodarī. The faithful and chaste Sītā was abducted by Rāvaṇa and carried to the isle of Laṅkā; and Tārāvatī was even stripped nude at his feet. The *Rāmāyaṇa* always speaks of Mandodarī as a faithful and chaste *satī*, but why did she propitiate Vibhīṣaṇa to slay Rāvaṇa? I envision only these five women in my meditation, and by that have come to understand something of their values. How can I fathom anything of the minds of men? Just as the aesthete can discern a true aesthetic, and the erudite can discern true beauty, pure women can discern true chastity—but what can an unfaithful, cuckolding wife discern? She who is born a woman but censures or casts aspersions on her husband, especially by being unfaithful, is the greatest sinner in the world, bar none."

Having made her point, Rambhāvatī finished her cooking. On golden dishes she served rice and fifty varieties of succulent curries—meat, fish, and vegetables. Watching the loving care and skill with which she prepared each dish, the king's desire to eat grew proportionately. Rambhāvatī meditated on Lord Nārāyaṇa with sincere devotion. Then she ate but five small morsels, at which point Lord Satya Pīr complied with her wish and afflicted the king with a ravenous hunger. As his stomach screamed for food, the *rājā* grew even more restless than before. Finally he called to her in exasperation.

"My good woman, explain to me how you can eat food and not offer any to me!" Rambhāvatī modestly replied, "Mahārāja, I quite simply forgot you. Please, please come and do me the honor of eating!"

Needing no additional prompting, the *rājā* bounded off the bed and quickly seated himself and began to eat. Unnoticed by the king, Rambhāvatī seated herself on his right side, while he sat firmly ensconced on the seat of honor.[6] This great king waded quickly into this feast, while Rambhāvatī sat quietly beside him, hands withdrawn. The *rājā* could not contain himself, such was his pleasure, "Such food as this I've never tasted! Anyone fortunate enough to eat this exquisitely cooked food is fortunate indeed! . . ." And so did the two of them eat, each in his own way. When the king had finished, he rinsed his mouth and hands. Chewing some betel, which had been freshened with a touch of camphor, the king retired to a cot, while Rambhāvatī stood obediently nearby.

Finally and inevitably the king beckoned, "Sit down, my loving nymph!"—but Rambhāvatī steadfastly refused. "I would like for you to first consider one small thing, your Majesty. You have eaten the food from my plate like my own son. How can you then ask me to come and sit romantically by your side?"

As soon as the words were uttered, the great king pressed his hands together with the utmost respect, called her "Mother," and fell fully prostrate at her feet. Rambhā graciously responded, "May you live a long life, lord of men. May your heart remain ever fixed on Kṛṣṇa's holy feet." With her permission this great king took his leave of Rambhāvatī.

Kiṅkara Dāsa has composed this story to serve Lord Nārāyaṇa.

Before parting, the *rājā* explained. "Rambhāvatī, the ruler of your life has gone to my city of Pāṭana. I could not help but notice that the special *campā* flowers that you wove together and placed so lovingly around your husband's neck went unspoiled and remained fresh every second of every day. I interrogated the merchant closely about the garland he wore so deliberately and, it turns out, he told me nothing but the truth. 'It was given me by my wife,' he said, 'who was fulfilling a solemn vow to demonstrate the extent of her fidelity.' In order to test your resolve, I sent an agent, the chief of security, whom you thoroughly and appropriately humiliated. Then I myself came, and you cooked food with your own hand, which I ate as if I were your own son. . . ." Rambhā stopped him.

"Please say no more! Go back to your own country and watch over your people like Rāma! Promise me that you will send my dearly beloved husband back to me, safe and sound, so that I may fulfill my intended object!"

The king assured her, "Rambhāvatī, your husband will certainly return. Do not worry yourself at all about that. Grant me your blessings, for I am off to my own country." With those parting words, he made obeisance to her. Offering a variety of gifts—expensive, finely crafted goods and clothes of delicate fabric—the king boarded his royal boat, whereupon he gave the order to push off. The boat rode the crest of the waves like a magnificent shooting star, which the king took as a sign. In but fifteen days, the boat docked at its home ghat and the king returned to his palace.

The mighty *rājā* recuperated that first night, but by midmorning of the following day he had the merchant summoned. He greeted the merchant very affectionately, and, taking him by the hand, seated him on his own throne. In a jocular tone, the king said, "You, my good friend, are a man truly blessed, for I have seen Rambhāvatī with my own eyes. There was a famous *satī* in the Satya Age; her name was Vṛndāvatī and her husband was the demon Jalandhara. By the power of Vṛndā's goodness and fidelity, her *satītva*, she won over the king's clan and, by that same power, claimed dominion over the three world spheres. Rambhāvatī is exactly in her image. You are her lucky husband and I have become her spiritual son, progeny of *dharma*. Grant me your blessing, merchant, and return to your family!" With these words the king bestowed on him wealth to a fabulous degree. They exchanged the traditional gestures of parting, but, being deeply moved, the king and the merchant spontaneously hugged each other, warmly and sincerely. The king turned and entered his palace.

The merchant made ready his boats and sailed off to his homeland, while those on shore sped them along with cries of, "Hari! Hari!" On his return trip home, the merchant and his crew reveled with much singing and dancing, which lasted day and night. From his heavenly vantage, Satya Pīr looked on, waiting to be acknowledged. After twelve days of this, Satya Pīr positioned himself on the far bank of the river and summoned Gaṅgā to bring the boats to him. The waves immediately rose up and hurled all seven boats in that direction. Weathering the apparent storm, the merchant, who had been dunked more than once, climbed sheepishly onto the bank. Looking up, he and his men quickly wrapped shawls around their necks, pressed their hands together in respect, and humbly clinched grass in their teeth. Each made his formal greeting of salaam as he stood directly in the presence of the Pīr. Lord Satya Pīr tried to calm them by saying, "Have no fear of my tiger-mount . . . ," but the merchant and his men had already beaten a hasty retreat. But when forced to stand in this august presence, the merchant in humility covered his shoulders with his shawl and stammered a few words. He was much distressed, as he anticipated the worst, but he was still in possession of his wits: "Please listen, you who are a treasure trove of compassion. If you slay this merchant, then who will there be to offer your service and promote your worship? Yet if you do take the life of this one who serves you, then—because you are the Lord and very fount of mercy—my life will have been made worthwhile and imbued with meaning."

Satya Pīr, who is Lord Nārāyaṇa, was favorably disposed toward this renewed devotee and granted the merchant not only a reprieve but also a glimpse of his true nature. "Proceed, my son, back to your family to institute the worship of Satya Pīr!" And with these simple words, he reassured him. As the merchant turned to leave, the Pīr flew off into the heavens, while his tiger disappeared back into the jungle whence he came. The merchant boarded his boat and pushed off, with the crew crying, "Hari! Hari!"

Finally to his own land Jayadatta the merchant sped.

When Jayadatta returned to his home, he placed the *campaka* garland around the neck of his wife, Rambhāvatī. As his boats were ritually purified, conchs and other instruments raucously announced the event. With great dispatch were the commercially tradeable goods transported and stored in his warehouse. He presented the local ruler with pleasing sandal and royal yak-tail whisks. And that great king in return presented him with jewelry and clothing. After conversing with the king about his adventures, the merchant returned to his family home, where he made formal gifts to brahmins and Vaiṣṇavas.

The merchant could not forget the majesty and greatness of Satya Pīr, and likewise that of the king, by whose favor the merchant could claim success. He desired to perform the worship of Satya Pīr, so he fixed a proper place and installed a golden seat. He purchased one hundred maunds of milk and one hundred maunds of sugar.[7] To this he added two thousand bananas, and, mixing them all together, concocted *śirṇi*. One hundred *maunds* of this *śirṇi* he offered to his divine Lord. Double-ended drums, large and small, along with a variety of other musical instruments punctuated the event. The merchant exulted upon completing the *pūjā* of Satya Pīr. He distributed flowers and sandal to all those present. When they took the Pīr's *śirṇi*, they prostrated themselves fully. After placing the *śirṇi* in their mouths, they brushed their hands up and over their heads, distributing the grace over their beings. They all cried out the name "Satya Pīr Sāheb" and then went to their respective homes.

Whoever listens to the song of Satya Pīr's benevolence will triumph on all fronts and have his adversities simply disappear. Lord Nārāyaṇa grants the protective shadow of his feet to all those who gather together for that purpose. Thus closes the long tale of Rambhāvatī. May everyone rejoice with the cry of "Hari! Hari!"

The Fabled *Beṅgamā* Bird and the Stupid Prince

Kavi Kaṇva's *Ākhoṭi Pālā*

Everyone listen carefully to the tale of the Pīr and the unparalleled adventure of the fowler without compare. In the western portion of the Bhilli lay the capital of a kingdom ruled by one Bhīmasena, a dispenser of law and authority. The court *paṇḍitas* were learned, well-behaved men of integrity, and among the brahmin priests, the king sat like the Lord of Law among the guardians of the eight directions. There in that kingdom one could find cowherds, gardeners, oil pressers, coppersmiths, low-caste *baurīs*, cultivators and husbandmen, sugar refiners, royal parasol bearers, and the usual itinerants and homeless riffraff. The various castes earned wealth sufficient to develop the metropolis. Everyone had proper housing, save the few constantly moving on the edges of society. In this land, too, there dwelled a young man who was a fowler, but a bit of a strange bird he was, for he only captured his birds, preferring not to slaughter them. Apart from trapping wild birds, he had no other means of subsistence—fate, Bidhātā, had decreed penury as his lot. Every morning he would head into the forest with a net fashioned with seven bent sticks slaked with lime and weighted for control, and he would entrap the birds and haul them home over his shoulder, his net serving as an impromptu bag. From a shallow-draft boat he would cast his nets across the marshes for spotbill and pintail ducks, for river terns skirting the banks, and even the occasional pallid harrier. He netted black-winged stilts and even a greylag goose. And from the hollows within trees he extracted owls of various types. Parakeets, flycatchers, and plovers he snared in quantity as he poled along, and drongos, kingfishers, curlews, cormorants, and the occasional hornbill likewise he netted. And in this simple way he would ply his trade as fowler, selling what he could when he could in the long market.

One morning he got up and dressed and picked up his nets and cage, as he always did. That same day, sitting in Mecca, the Lord Master asked his attendant to give him a progress report on his worship, his *pūjā*. The wandering fakir replied, "Listen carefully, O Hazrat. Listen to the details of the prospect of your worship as it stands today. There is a young man, a fowler, who enters the forest each day to catch birds. Why not be merciful and reveal yourself to him in your true form? Direct the fowler to go to that special tree where the *beṅgamā* bird dwells. From the mouth of that bird will your worship spread far and wide."

Kavikaṇva tells the essence of the Pīr's praiseworthy tale.

At the suggestion of the wandering mendicant, the Lord Master disguised himself as a brahmin priest. As the fakir went to reveal himself through this magical disguise, it was no different from Lord Vāmana going to see Bali.[1] He wore a sacred thread, a clean white *dhoti*, his forehead daubed with an auspicious mark. On his feet he wore simple sandals, his hand held a tattered umbrella above his head while he counted over and over the crystalline beads of his rosary. In his other hand he carried the digest of astrology and ritual, looking for all the world like a proper celibate or *brahmācārī*. And so he placed himself prominently along the forest path that the young fowler was sauntering.

Satya Pīr accosted him, "Listen, young fowler. Come close, my son, and listen carefully to the predictions of the almanac."

"I am sorry, I cannot listen to the almanac's predictions, for I am penniless, O Lord. There is no one in the triple world who is as luckless as I."

But the Eminent One, Hazrat, began anyway, "I make obeisance to Śrī, goddess of weal, and to Sūrya the sun . . . ," and the young fowler prostrated himself to listen to the digest's predictions. "It is Wednesday, the third day following an eclipse of the sun, and therefore auspicious for commercial undertakings. Today, my young fowler, you will meet success among the mangrove forests. Today you will find in the forest an abundance of wild birds. Now pay special attention to what I am about to tell you, my child. Deep in the forest in the cleft of an old *aśoka* tree[2] you will find living a *beṅgamā* and *beṅgamī* bird, a nesting couple. Listen, fowler, my son, should you capture that bird all of your troubles will soon be far away."[3]

"As you have commanded . . ." said the young fowler as he plunged headlong into the forest. This young prince of a fowler searched high and low through the dense creepers and undergrowth, traversing the depths of that dense forest until he reached that tree. He spread his net and broke off small branches and twigs to camouflage it and his body, but both the *beṅgamā* and *beṅgamī* saw through the ruse. The *beṅgamī* called to her mate, "Listen to what I'm telling you. The forest itself is moving, and that augurs something unfavorable. There are more leaves than is proper and the various flowers seem to move of some alien volition, there are no flower buds, and the branches are not right, not right at all. We have dwelled in the forest a long time, but I am not sure that we should not escape to some distant land where we can live unmolested." The *beṅgamī* continued, "O husband, I beg you, can't we shift to another forest today, right now? The trees themselves seem to be closing in—I have never seen that before. I do not understand what fortune has twisted today, my beloved, but let us leave this forest right now and flee to another. I sense that if we stay in these woods we will forfeit our lives." The *beṅgamā* drew near, but he had not even investigated the state of their territory, for the bird did not put much faith in his wife's warnings. The endless magical machinations of the Pīr are unfathomable. Ever so carefully did the fowler maneuver his net closer, when by the grace of the Pīr he flung it around the bird's neck. The bird fell to the earth enmeshed, and thrashed about on the ground. The huge bird was caught fast and was about to die, or so it seemed.

The twice-born Kavi Kaṇva sings the waves of this tale.

The *beṅgamā* pleaded, "Bird hunter, no matter what you are striving for in this existence, why do you persist in this sinful taking of life? This torture you inflict by catching animals in nets and binding them with leather will in the future return to enslave you in like fashion. I have no doubts whatsoever about your future affliction. The Lord Master seems to have set against me because I did not listen to the warnings of my wife, and so I was trapped in your net. Every time you kill or ensnare a beast or bird you incur an evil that bodes punishment in your future—and justice will in the end be done. You labor under a false impression if you think that your son, your wife, or anyone else you know will share in this retribution; it is reserved for you alone. Heed my words, faithfully worship Śrī Kṛṣṇa, and Govinda will drive your chariot into the future."

When he heard the bird speak with a human voice, this son of a fowler gently cut him free from the net. He held him in his hand and began to stroke his body, while the *beṅgamī* wept from her perch on a high branch. She said, "Fowler, you know nothing of *dharma* or *adharma*—those things that one ought and ought not to do. This time do the right thing by the lord of my life. When you trap wild game and birds, your actions go against what is proper and good and the effects accumulate. Please honor my earnest supplication and free my husband. In return I will give you a ring set with a ruby. You are the very incarnation of proper *dharma*, what else can I say to make you understand? Please set my husband free!"

The fowler said, "Listen, my fine-feathered friend, based on your word, it is hard for me to imagine that when I set him free he will not return."

Placing trust in the narrative of the Pīr, the twice-born poet Kavi Kaṇva cleverly composes this narrative in the pāñcālī *style.*

About this time that *pakṣirāja*, king of birds, the *beṅgamā* himself, spoke to the fowler.[4] "You should consider carefully, my child, the vocation of the fowler. You have caused the demise of many a bird in these forests. How can you escape the nets of Yama, lord of death, in the next life?" The bird continued his plea, "Listen to these words, fowler, humble yourself and listen to the tales of the acts of Kṛṣṇa. Early one morning Nārāyaṇa Kṛṣṇa was playing with his friends in the house of Nanda. While they were playing, Gopāla slipped away; he dug in the dirt with his nails and ate it. One of the other boys happened to see him eat the dirt and he went and told everything to Kṛṣṇa's foster mother, Yaśodā. As soon she heard, Yaśodā, matron of the house, ran quickly to him. 'Did you not eat curds and milk and clotted cream just this morning? Then why should you give up all that and go eat dirt?' Yaśodā spoke to him with anger and indignation, but Kṛṣṇa innocently replied, 'Please calm down. I have not eaten any dirt, my dear mother, so please don't rebuke me. Look, I am standing right in front of you with my mouth open and you can see for yourself.' Laughing loudly, Gopāla opened wide his mouth, but when his mother peered in she saw the whole of the universe! The sight stunned, perhaps frightened her, so she quickly scooped up Gopāla in her arms with a nervous laugh.[5] Now listen, fowler, to these and other similar stories. Worship Kṛṣṇa by taking his name and you will effect your salvation, O hunter."

When he had listened to the story of Kṛṣṇa from the bird, the fowler was moved to tears from his misery. He said, "Kṛṣṇa is the wishing tree for all one may want. From this day forward, O *beṅgamā* bird, you are my guru. You have purified me by telling me about Kṛṣṇa. And because of my chance meeting with you, I have reaped the rewards of tens of millions of previous good works. Now you listen, O king of birds, to what I have to say. I catch and peddle birds only because it is my calling."

The *pakṣirāja*, the king of birds, deftly replied, "Listen, son of a fowler, from today all your miseries will disappear."

He wishes to shower mercy by bestowing great wealth on the fowler. Kavi Kaṇva sings the emotional essence of this increasingly complex pāñcālī's *tale. With single-minded attention listen everyone to the glorious tale of the Pīr. This devoted servant makes a thousand salaams to the feet of the Sāheb.*

"Listen again, my child, the son of a fowler, I am going to give you a jewel, a ruby of incomparable value." Lodged in the massive throat of the *beṅgamā* bird were three rubies. He vomited them up and gave them to the fowler—and then he told a story. "Sudāma was a brahmin who lived in Dvāraka. He kept thinking that he should go and see Kṛṣṇa. He came carrying a small folded cloth bag filled with broken rice and offered it to Kṛṣṇa when he met him. When he gave the bag to Kṛṣṇa, that one eminent among men, who received it warmly, but then returned the broken pieces of rice to him. The glories of the Lord and Master Nārāyaṇa are truly endless, for by the grace of Kṛṣṇa those grains had transformed into priceless jewels.

"Something similar happened to King Parikṣit when he was cursed by a sage [to die by the bite of the serpent Takṣaka for throwing a dead cobra around the neck of his meditating father. Informed of the curse, the king invited powerful brahmins to protecct him, and one, Dhanvantari, the only one who had the power to reverse the death,][6] met Takṣaka on the road. As they exchanged pleasantries Takṣaka told him, 'If you go, then the curse of the sage will be proved false.' The *ojhā*, master of poisons, listened to Takṣaka's proposition and said, 'Give me the fabulous gem on your head.' And so Takṣaka parted with his gem, placing it in the hands of Dhanvatari." And having made a similar promise, the bird handed over the rubies to the fowler.

The inexperienced fowler could not recognize these stones as rubies and opined, "You have deceived me by giving me three pits from some forest fruit. All you want to do is escape, so you give me these worthless pits." So the fowler continued, "I will not release you."

The *pakṣirāja* replied, "Those are not pits. You do not even recognize something valuable when you see it. You must have gone mad. Since you, fowler, are incapable of recognizing them using your own devices, make yourself present in the king's court tomorrow morning with those in tow. O son of a fowler, I have promised you solemnly. If you encounter any difficulty, simply seek refuge with me. Once I, the *beṅgamā* bird, have made a promise, I never contravene it." And then, having received that promise, the son of a fowler released the bird and took his riches home. He abandoned his nets and sticks and taking the jewels headed home feeling released from his passions. He soon emerged from the forest and reached his own place.

With relish has Kaṇva composed this tale in song. Listen, each and every one, focus your attention exclusively, then all activities will be successful and your wishes fulfilled. May everyone repeat the name of Hari out of a sincere desire for gaining the Pīr. Without fail will the Pīr take upon himself your sorrows.

Here the fowler's wife was in a snit, worrying constantly, about the reasons why her husband had by this time not come home. "For seven days the two of us have had nothing to eat. My husband went into the forest today soon after he got up. Had he quickly snared some beast or bird in the forest, he would have come back to the house in a hurry." Rādhā Ṭhākurāṇī pined from the separation from her Lord Who Wields the Discus, Cakrapāṇī, when he lived in Madhupura, and in just this same way did the fowler's wife weep and worry. About that time, however, the fowler made his appearance.

When the fowler's wife saw that he had no game or birds, she wept bitterly, "Will I have to forfeit my life for want of a few husks of broken rice? And seeing that you have ditched your nets and sticks, you have returned like some wandering mendicant who has abandoned the homelife."

Seeing his wife's anger and frustration made the fowler weep, "Here, take these gemstones; I have brought three of them."

"How did you come by those, who gave them to you? I do not know how to tell if these things you call rubies are genuine at all."

"With considerable effort and skill I trapped a bird deep in the forest. He gave those to me with the promise that they were genuine rubies."

"Let me look for a second at those that you call rubies. May my two eyes be blessed with good fortune at their bounty."

Saying, "See for yourself, look!" he pulled the gemstones out of his shoulder bag and placed them in his sweetheart's hands.

With great care did she look at and finger the stones, turning them over and over. Finally the fowler's wife asked, "My good husband, are these really rubies?" The simple woman did not have the tools to discern what they were. Finally pronouncing them "FRUIT PITS!" she hurled them aside. Two of the jewels landed inside their little hut, but one of them fell outside. The fowler's wife turned and yelled at him, "Are you crazy? Are you seeing things? To bring home these fruit pits in exchange for releasing the bird! If you had bothered to bring the bird home instead, we could have sold it in the city today as we normally do. But instead you bring home fruit pits and call them rubies! . . ." And on the sweet woman went with her tirade, venting her exasperation with vile aspersions.

And in this manner the couple continued their altercations well into the night, when, exhausted, they fell into bed. While they were fast asleep inside their hut, the local constable was making his evening rounds through the neighborhoods of the city.

In the village of Papaḍyā near the metroplis of Kharggapura, the poet Kaṇva has composed this glorious tale of the Pīr.

The ruby lying outside seemed to glow in the moonlight. The constable saw it and gingerly picked it up with both hands, and contemplated, "Such an unusual item. I wonder where the fowler managed to get this? He must have thought it a fruit pit or something and tossed it aside." Then the venerable constable took the ruby and quickly left the vicinity. The constable soon found his way into his own neighborhood and house just as the night was coming to an end. All knowing, Satya Nārāyaṇa was wise to what had transpired and so he sat by the bed and spoke to the fowler as he lay asleep in the little hut. "Get your body up, my child, young boy of a fowler, get up! By what incredible stupidity did you get rubies and then in a tantrum hurl them away? That bird has bestowed on you jewels of inestimable value. How could you throw them out and then go to sleep in your hut? Take the two remaining rubies to the king straightaway and from this day forward your suffering will be over." This is what Satya Nārāyaṇa expressed in his dream.

The son of a fowler then woke up with a shiver and sat up. He took the name of Rāma twice before passing the rest of the night. In the morning the fowler sat up in his bed. The fowler queried his wife, "Listen, sweetheart, I gave you three gemstones, but where is the third?"

The fowler's wife replied, "I threw them down here, perhaps one of them rolled outside."

When he heard this, the fowler picked up the two remaining stones and made ready to leave, just the way Rāma and Kṛṣṇa headed off to the court of King Kaṃsa. When he came into the presence of the king, he stood before him with the rubies resting in his respectfully cupped hands. As soon as he saw the rubies, the king had questions for this hunter.

The poet Kaṇva constructs this glorious tale in waves.

The king spoke. "Listen, honored son of a fowler, to what end have you made these ruby gemstones over to me?"

The fowler replied, "Please give me some rice and a few cowries to take back to my humble hut."

The king listened incredulously and laughed at what the fowler had requested. "And just how many maunds of rice did you expect to sell them for?"

The fowler naïvely replied, "I have no idea how many to say. O great jewel among men, I'll take whatever you give me." The fowler boldly continued, "I lay this request at the king's feet: Be generous and give me enough so that I can eat for a good number of days."

The lord among men replied, "My young son, I say to you, if you do not give me the number of maunds, then I will not take the gemstones."

The fowler, somewhat nonplussed, replied, "Well if I must fix a price, my king, then perhaps you would be generous enough to give me four or five maunds?"

As soon as he heard this price the king was thrilled. He gave five hundred rupees to the fowler. Absolutely delighted, the fowler prepared to return home. "May you be successful in whatever you undertake," said the king. He continued, "Have no fear. Have no worries, you are a blessed man, for it is said, 'Who takes the life of a man on whom he has just bestowed wealth?' Take your rupees and go home happily." The fowler made grateful obeisance. The king blessed him and bade him farewell. The fowler headed home as happy as he could be. The king also ordered the chief of police to supply him with two large measures of rice, and no sooner had the order been given than it was handed over. The fowler then tied the rice up in a cloth and hauled it home. The fowler's wife was absolutely ecstatic over what he brought. She immediately fell to cooking and they ate sumptuously. The wife could only observe that indeed their troubles were finally over. The ailments and bad luck that had afflicted them seemed to have been shaken off.

Meanwhile, the king consulted with his courtiers. He was lauded for having upheld justice in the kingdom. He then retired into his own private quarters, where he was bathed and massaged. Afterward he ate and then partook of the customary postprandial palate cleansing. He sat on his bed and savored a betel quid with a touch of camphor. Then he made a gift of the two rubies to his queen. The queen accepted the rubies with great pleasure, and in this little exchange they passed the remainder of the day.

A thousand salaams to the feet of the Pīr. The poet Kaṇva composed this glorious tale of the Pīr.

The queen called for her servant girls to come before her. She gave the command that she be dressed. They combed her hair, and laced it up with a fresh garland. They put collyrium on her eyes, placed a bejeweled stud in her nose, and marked her part and forehead with vermilion. She was truly stunning. The two rubies—already carefully mounted—she had placed in her ears. Her brilliance outshone the moon itself. Around her neck they draped a double-braided necklace of some two hundred gold links. Onto her upper arms they slid conch bracelets, then on her forearm and again on her wrists. She was draped with an iridescent silk sari, and was transformed into the queen consort, so beautiful that she would pass for the heavenly consort of Indra himself. Her maidservant complimented her, of course: "You are beyond resplendent made up like this, but in the end there is one missing adornment that, were you to get it, would make you ravishing beyond compare, my queen. Hold up the mirror and look at yourself."

When she heard this the queen asked, "What other ornament is there? Tell me honestly."

Her maidservant replied, "I humbly place this before your feet as a suggestion, but listen carefully. Please request from your king one more ruby like the others. I have hung the two rubies in each of your ears, and for that your face is more brilliant than the moon itself. But should you hang one more ruby on your august forehead, your face would outshine more than a hundred moons."

When she heard this, the queen instantly wondered aloud, "Where can I find another one?"

The maidservant answered, "Ah, my queen, let me tell you. Beg one from the king. Just make yourself a little obnoxious and he will be happy to supply you with another one."

Hearing this plan, the queen consort was giddy with anticipation—and just then the king himelf entered her apartments. Placing herself before the king, she pressed her hands together in supplication and pleaded, just as Satyabhāmā had badgered Kṛṣṇa for the unwilting *pārijāta* flowers, or it could just as easily have been Haragaurī on the top of Mount Kailāsa begging Śiva for a new pair of conch bangles. "O do listen, lord of my life, I place this one humble request at your feet. Would you please give me one more ruby to match the others?"

The king quickly replied, "Ah, my dear queen, let me be perfectly honest. I do not have another ruby to give to you."

"But King, if you were really partial to me, if you really cared, then you would find another one to give me . . . ," and so she whined.

The king eventually began to soften, "O my queen, what are you going to do with another ruby?"

To which the queen replied, "Look, I will place it right here on my forehead. See how the two rubies work as earrings? Were I to have another ruby placed in the center of my forehead, then my fashionable look would be complete. If you do not give me another ruby, I cannot go on living. . . ."

When he divined the general direction the exchange was headed, the king quietly said, "A singular ruby like that is very expensive, about the wealth of seven kings. . . ."

The queen cut him off, "O King, I'm sure you can give me another one, because I am prepared to give up my life for the sake of that ruby. Find a ruby somewhere, my king, if that's not too much trouble to show you care for me."[7]

After trying to console his queen, the king of justice spoke to all of his many ministers and courtiers. The dispenser of justice called for his constable.

The poet Kaṇva has composed the glorious tale in the sweetest of tones.

All of you—friends, beloveds, brothers, companions—listen to more of the glorious story of Satya Pīr.

When the king called the constable, he came quickly, made his obeisances, and stood respectfully in front with his hands pressed together in submission. The king explained, "Listen, all who are gathered, ministers and courtiers alike, the queen consort cannot live without getting another ruby. The queen has been ranting and raving, making quite the fuss that she would die for the sake of that gemstone. Listen, my good men, the queen is as good as dead. What a mess, all because of ruby. Tell me, my advisors, what is the way out of this mess?"

One attendant suggested, "Why not summon the fowler? Haul the fowler back into the assembly and he, O King, will explain how to procure another ruby."

The lord among men then gave the order, "Listen, my constable, fetch the fowler and do it now."

In much the same manner that King Kaṃsa summoned Akrūra to go and fetch Govinda from Gopapura, or the way Hanumān set off at the command of Lakṣmaṇa, the constable and his henchmen headed off to seize the fowler. Roaring and breast-beating, they went down the road, a commotion like that of Aṅgada when he entered Rāvaṇa's assembly. With much venom in his voice, the constable yelled for the fowler, but it was about as effective as Aṅgada looking at Rāvaṇa when the latter had magically assumed a hundred forms that sat there in his court. The fowler managed to hide himself as effectively, even though he was close by. The fowler's wife informed her husband, "My lord, you have a summons from that good and just king who gave you the wealth." The fowler replied, "My dear wife, you go on out and speak to the rabble and see what they want; I will follow along behind."

Anxious with distress that good woman addressed the constable and his crew, "Just who are you?"

The chief constable replied, "I beg you to hand over the fowler, your husband."

"He is not home today," the wife covered, "he went out, but I do not know where."

When he heard the faithful wife's dodge, the constable grew quite animated and bellowed, "Where has he gone, you little slut of a whore!" . . . at which point the fowler came out of the little hole in which he had been hiding. With his hands pressed together in supplication he greeted the constable.

When the constable confirmed it was the fowler, he informed him, "The king has issued a summons; you must come at once." And so off the fowler went in the custody of the constable, and not too long after they entered the king's court. In abject submission the fowler prostrated himself.

The poet Kaṇva has composed this glorious tale of the Pīr.

The fowler made his obeisance, and then stood with hands pressed together, while the king offered him some consolation, "Listen, what I have to say to you is simple, my son, bring me another ruby just like the two you brought before."

When these words tumbled out of the mouth of the king, the sky crashed down on the head of the poor fowler. The fowler stammered, "I will go to that place where I got the gemstones and will bring to you the one who supplied them to me."

The *mahārāja* replied, "If I can locate that individual, then you are exonerated and free of the responsibility to supply the ruby."

And hearing those parting words, the fowler headed back to his own home. He gathered together a new net and sticks, and when he entered the familiar forest he let out a long sigh of relief. "The bird that lives in the *aśoka* tree had given his word," and with this thought he headed for that same tree. As soon as he saw the hunter, the *beṅgamā* bird took off and flew high into the sky; the fowler in turn plopped down at the foot of the tree and began to weep. "O *beṅgamā*, you gave your word! And realizing that you are bound by that promise, you are about to be cast into the depths of hell. The *gopīs* extracted a promise from Kṛṣṇa Gopāla and he kept it, but at your risk you seem to have reneged on your own promise to me. For the sake of a ruby the king is willing to kill me and should that come to pass, O King of birds, the responsibility falls squarely on you."

"Because of her insatiable sexual desire, Uṣā kidnapped Aniruddha, but her father King Bāṇa found out Aniruddha was in her quarters and had him bound with ropes of cobras. Aniruddha meditated on the feet of Kṛṣṇa, and shortly Govinda arrived there riding his mount Garuḍa. The cobras, *nāgas*, fled as soon as the snake-eating Garuḍa came."[8] The *pakṣirāja* thought about this story of a promise kept, and promptly returned.

The bird landed on the fowler's outstretched hand. Taking the name of God, Hari, the fowler realized his life had been spared.

Said the *beṅgamā*, king of birds, "My son, the good son of a fowler, why do you worry so needlessly?"

"It is my wonderful good fortune that you have shown yourself to me. I need to take you to the king."

"Why would you need to take me there?"

"This lord of justice desires another ruby." The fowler continued, "Tell me truthfully, can you produce another ruby?"

And so, at a particularly auspicious point in time, the hunter took that *pakṣirāja* and entered into the presence of the king in his court.

The twice-born poet Kaṇva sings the glorious tale of the Pīr under the generous patronage of the Yaśovanta Siṃha.

The fowler bowed to the king, and, after making his obeisance, stood stiff as a stick with hands pressed together. "I submit to your careful consideration that this is the individual who provided me with the rubies."

The king, turning to the bird, commanded, "Please produce another gemstone from your hidden trove, and do it without delay."

The bird replied, "If it please your Majesty, O Mahārāja, I have no other riches about me save the name and tales of Kṛṣṇa."

"Well then, let us hear the tales of Kṛṣṇa pour from your mouth. . . ." And so the bird began to speak much, to the delight and amazement of all.

"Listen carefully to the scriptures, O great King, with undivided attention. The son of Devakī, Kṛṣṇa, came down in the house of Nanda. Upon his birth the most revered Kṛṣṇa was propitiated [to slay demons . . .].[9] The Disc-Wielder Cakrapāṇi slew the demon Jāmalā Arjuna and took the life of the antigod Baka by ripping its flesh.[10] When they witnessed these events, the cowherd boys were thrilled and drove their herds of cows to the banks of the Yamunā River. Finding there soft grass, they let the cows graze freely, but the lord of the gods, Brahmā, stole the cattle, whisked them away, and stored them in his waterpot. At this miraculous disappearance, all the young cowherd boys were agitated. 'Tell us, Kṛṣṇa, who stole our cows?' to which Kṛṣṇa smartly replied, 'It was Brahmā who took them.' Understanding exactly what Brahmā was thinking, he created a new herd of cows fashioned from his own body. And in this way Nārāyaṇa ground Brahmā's pride to dust.[11]

"And listen carefully to more of the scriptures, O King, focusing your mind. In order to ensure the general weal of the cowherds and the boys who looked after them, Nanda, Kṛṣṇa's foster father, proposed to worship the feet of Indra, king of the gods. Kṛṣṇa alternatively suggested, 'Let us do *pūjā* to Mount Govardhana, where our cows graze so contentedly.' When the worship of Indra had been aborted, the king of the gods was furious, and unleashed from the heavens a torrential storm. Kṛṣṇa simply picked up Mount Govardhana on the tip of his finger. Hari, the son of Nanda, hailed from the clan of Govardhana and so protected everyone by picking up that mountain with his left hand to serve as umbrella.

"You must listen, Mahārāja, to these tales of the holy books. You who are inclined to violance should devote yourself to Kṛṣṇa."

The king responded favorably, "This bird has lived in Vṛndāvana, but how did he manage to get here from there?[12] If he has not passed time in Vṛndāvana, how can he possibly know the stories of Kṛṣṇa? O great *Pakṣirāja*, you have had me listen to the stories of Kṛṣṇa and I have gained from meeting you the fruit of an incalculable merit, riches of a different sort."

The king of birds followed, "Now I beg you, O King, please release this good son of a fowler and send him on his way."

And so the king granted the fowler the revenue from five villages as reward, and the fowler gratefully bade farewell and returned to his home.

Such is the wondrous mercy worked by Satya Nārāyaṇa and the horrible tribulations brought by the poverty of the fowler were permanently relieved. Listen, everyone, to the song of the glorious tale of our Lord.

After listening to more stories of Kṛṣṇa, the king was so overcome he felt woozy.[13] When he came to, he announced, "O *beṅgamā*, I am not going to free you. I shall take care of you as if you were my own son."

The nonplussed *pakṣirāja* objected, "But why would you imprison me, O King?"

"So that you can tell me stories of Kṛṣṇa." Then that giant among men summoned a goldsmith and commissioned him to fabricate a golden cage at once. So in this golden cage did the king imprison the *beṅgamā*, king of birds. Every day he repeated the name of Kṛṣṇa and his work was satisfying and succesful. Eventually the queen requested her ruby once again, but the king offered the queen the bird instead.

The poet Kaṇva has composed the glorious tale in its sweetness, whose abode was constructed by patron Sadar Caudhurī.

The king said, "Alas, my queen, you should take this *pakṣirāja* and relieve me of the burden of having to give you another ruby."

The queen retorted, "O great King, what does this bird do?"

"The bird will tell you stories of Lord Kṛṣṇa."

The king continued, "We might die today, we might die tomorrow, but die we certainly will. This body is like a bubble on the water that could disappear at any time. What can you do with riches, with sons, with family, because any day you might die. If you want to avoid the miserable machinations of Yama, the god of death, then abandon everything and worship Kṛṣṇa, who is the essence of everything."

Humoring the king, the queen then spoke to the bird, "I beg of you, please share with me some of the stories of Kṛṣṇa."

The *pakṣirāja* began, "Listen attentively, my queen, to the stories from the holy texts. This is the one where Nārāyaṇa playfully steals the girls' clothes. There lived then some sixteen hundred cowherd girls in Gokula, and, while they were playing in the waters, they dropped their clothes on the banks. While these young women were playing in the waters of the Yamunā, Kṛṣṇa Nārāyaṇa surreptitiously stole the garments of each and every one. Kṛṣṇa then took the clothes and climbed into the branches of a *kadamba* tree. And each of the *gopīs* had to climb out of the water onto the banks and beg him for her clothes. But those *gopīs* managed to extract a promise from Kṛṣṇa in return, and later they experienced the joy of the round dance, the *rāsa* dance, deep in the forests of Vṛndāvana. Kṛṣṇa Nārāyaṇa embraced each and every one of those women and fulfilled their utmost erotic longings. And so it was that Nārāyaṇa provided the pleasure of the round dance. Pay careful attention, O Queen, to this tale from the sacred scriptures."

The queen was overwhelmed, and swooned from the mellifluous song of the bird. When she came to, she declared, "This bird has surely lived in Vṛndāvana. . . ."

The king and queen then sent for their son, Prince Kāmodara, and handed over the bird to him for safekeeping. "Display the bird to the two of us twice each day, every morning and every evening." And so, taking note, Kāmodara made arrangements to care for the bird. Kāmodara took the bird away and cared for it—and every morning and evening the bird had them listen to stories of Kṛṣṇa. And the routine went for twelve years, until one day. . . .

Listen all present to the marvelous story of Pīr who is God.

As luck would have it, suddenly one day the kingdom was beset by a dangerous and disruptive invasion of tigers. The king made ready nine lakhs of soldiers—an inordinately large number—and then he marched them into the affected area of his city.

Listen everyone and have complete faith in the Lord, for Satya Pīr worked his magic on Kāmodara. Extending his magical web of illusion, the venerable Pīr sang to Kāmodara, for He Who Fills the Void himself sat in the bird's throat.

When the *pakṣirāja* was telling the tales of Kṛṣṇa, his voice sang with a music like that of the *kokil*, the cuckoo. Kāmodara was completely smitten with the beauty of that singing and he observed, "O King of birds, you must have lived long in Vṛndāvana."

The bird suggested, "You should listen to me, Kāmodara, fill yours eyes, for I am going to dance!" And the magnificent bird danced, spreading his plumage to fill the cage just like a peacock. Kāmodara fell under the sway of that enchantment; he was infatuated. Then the *pakṣirāja* complained to Kāmodara, "It is impossible to dance properly in the confined space of this cage. Release me."

But even Kāmodara was leery, "But you will just fly away."

The bird cleverly replied, "Why should I fly away? If you set me free then I will be able to show you a proper dance."

Not able to fathom just how ingenious the bird was, the naïve Kāmodara made a terrible miscalculation and freed the bird. Now out of the cage, the bird spread his feathers and danced, laughing to himself at the success of his subterfuge. The sonorous voice of the bird again worked its magic, and, when Kāmodara was sufficiently mesmerized, the bird took wing and flew, alighting some distance away on the top of the compound wall.

That the bird flew away spelled certain doom, no less than if the sky itself had fallen on the crown prince's head. The prince earnestly, but respectfully, pleaded with the bird, "The king will execute me all on account of you."

The bird reassured him, "Whenever the king threatens to kill you, you need only think of me and I will come to you."

The prince countered, "You must take me with you. Nowhere can I manage to live without you. But now that you have slipped out of my hands, what will I do?"

"It is written that the individual who fails to honor a promise once made, even if in the form of Śakru, king of the gods, will be reckoned no better than an animal." Then the *beṅgamā* bird swore to him three times.

And the prince muttered, "I am finished."

But the bird pressed on, "I have been imprisoned for twelve long years, and today finally that sentence is complete and I am flying home." And with that farewell, the bird up and flew away.

The twice-born poet Kaṇva sings the glorious tale of the Pīr.

The bird soared across the expanse of the sky, but as soon as he had gone, a great tumult arose in the palace, for all the retainers and ministers of the court cried out in exasperation and fear. For them too it was as if the sky had broken on their poor heads. Naturally it was just at that moment the *mahārāja* returned from his hunting and entered his own private quarters. He immediately gave the order to have the bird fetched, "I want to see with my own eyes, and I want to listen to the beautiful retellings of the stories of Kṛṣṇa."

A brave retainer stuttered, "Listen, your Highness, there is a problem. Your son Kāmodara has set the bird free."

The king was furious when he heard those words of his courtier, and he summoned the constable to drag in his son—and so he was fetched.

"Explain to me, Kāmodara, just exactly how did the bird get free? And who now is around to relate the beautiful stories of Kṛṣṇa for our edification?"

Kāmodara sheepishly reported, "Father, the bird has flown away."

The king responded, "Why, oh why, my son, did you release the bird?" The *mahārāja* flared with anger and called out to the constable. "Hack off the head of my son Kāmodara in exchange for the bird." No sooner had he heard the order than the constable grabbed the prince by the arms. It was no different than when Hiraṇya levied the curse on Prahlāda.[14]

The crown prince pleaded, "Father, I beg you reconsider. What a contemptible act to take a human life for the sake of bird. If you do the unthinkable and slay me, you will be famous in this world as a killer of your own son. I wish you only happiness after you have taken my life. And now I am going to be sacrificed in exchange for a bird." He continued, "I take my leave, Father."

The king sat unmoving, with his head down, unable to raise it to look at him.

Then the prince added in exasperation, "You have looked after me for many long years, so how can you have me killed? Do you have no mercy whatsover?"

The constable was about to take him away to be executed when the crown prince told him, "First, I must go to see my mother. If I can see her I know I will be able to breathe a sigh of true relief because she will talk to my father and effect my acquittal." And so the constable took him to his mother.

The crown prince fell down on the floor in complete prostration. "My father is a raging inferno of anger because I released the bird. Now the constable is taking me away for execution. If you could just talk to the king it could be rescinded. What awful fortune have the Fates written on my forehead."

The queen replied, "Why did you let that bird escape? It will be ill advised and to no avail for me to attempt to persuade him." These were the harsh words the queen consort spoke.

The prince began to weep as he hung on her. "I had thought that you would be merciful. How can you bear such a hard heart? As my mother, how can you bear your son's affliction? Why then did you even bother to give me birth from your womb? For ten lunar months and ten days I gestated in your womb. You call me your son, so do you not harbor at least a shred of compassion for me?" His mother the queen sat motionless, her head down, unable to look him in the eye. Then the prince resignedly bade his mother farewell.

When Prince Kāmodara had taken leave of his mother, the constable escorted him deep into the forest. The prince stalled a little longer, "Brother, I have a favor to ask. I need to bathe properly in the lake and then perform *tarpaṇa*, the ritual of offering water to the manes and deities. I shall worship the feet of Kṛṣṇa to effect my liberation, and *tarpaṇa* offerings for my family and community."

When he heard this reasonable request, the constable led him to the lake. The prince bathed properly, dunking himself in the waters. He ritually rinsed his mouth and then, placing a few drop of Gaṅgā water in his hands, he declared, "I am going to be executed," then lifted the water up in *tarpaṇa* offering to his revered guru, to Vaiṣṇavas, and to Kṛṣṇa individually and collectively. Then he called to mind his mother, his father, and his friends and fellow students. Again he offered the *tarpaṇa* water with his hands. "Accept my water offering, O Mother who bore me, so that I might be born again into your womb in some more salutary future situation." And to his closest friends with whom he played he made water offerings to each by name. He then recalled the many subjects in his kingdom and proffered similar water offerings to them. Finally he called to mind the *pakṣirāja*, the *beṅgamā* bird. . . .

The poet Kaṇva writes with relish the glorious tale of the Pīr.

"O King of birds, you have abandoned me! You seem now to be completely carefree in spite of that conversation we had earlier. Uthānapāda's son Dhruva gained Kṛṣṇa in the Madhuvana forest after his mother spoke with him. At the suggestion of his mother he entered the Madhuvana forest armed only with the one-hundred-syllable *mantra* given him by Nārada. He recited the *mantra* to Nārāyaṇa with unwavering ardor until Madhusūdana himself granted his grace to Dhruva."[15] And thinking these kinds of thoughts, he directed his mind toward the feet of the bird. "How could you simply forget such an important promise you had made? That you just up and flew away was like a blow to the head that led to this mess. You are living without anxiety, while I am going to my execution. Come, O bird, and save me this one time. . . ."

Through his meditation, Satya Nārāyaṇa came to realize the situation. He ascertained that the king's son was going to die for the sake of that bird, who pretended to practice religion. That *pakṣirāja* had in fact promised and had now forgotten, so the Pīr began to cross the vast reaches of the firmament. "You slipped away, you little scoundrel, and in so doing have created an intractable predicament. Simply on account of you, Kāmodara is going to his execution." The Pīr roared and spat with anger, casting his eye about the world, and commanded, "I dispatch you to find the crown prince, place him on your back and carry him here."

When the Lord Master spoke, the bird understood then and there, "It is truly because of me that young man is going to lose his life." Khaga, Viṣṇu's mount Garuḍa, in order to free his mother from slavery, promised that he would bring the nectar of immortality to the serpent *nāgas*.[16] The *beṅgamā* had himself made such a promise, and so he flew with the wind, and the higher he rose the more he thought about the nature of that promise. Riding the wind, the bird came to the young man and, while creating a diversion, he picked him up and placed him on his back. Everyone at the lake cried out in surprised protest, "What has happened to the crown prince, where has he been taken?"

Eventually the king heard that the bird had flown away with his son, and those in court were moved to tears, very much aggrieved in their sorrow. In mourning for the king's son, his parents did not dress or have their hair coiffed, while the people of the metropolis wept till their cries filled the skies. Meanwhile, the *pakṣirāja* carried the couple's son Kāmodara on his back, riding the winds higher and higher into the heavens. The bird headed in a westerly direction, and, when deep into the forest, spotted a dwelling. It was a derelict structure, an open-sided pavilion right in the middle of the forest. There the bird deposited the king's son.

The bird advised him, "Listen to what I say, my child, you stay here and I will go fetch food."

The young man replied, "What else can I say? You may fly off again and never return."

The bird took a moment to reassure Kāmodara, and then flew off in search of food. Close by was another kingdom, this one ruled by King Bīrabara. The *pakṣirāja* entered that capital city and headed straight to a confectioner, where he procured some sweets. With this food in tow, he flew back. When the *pakṣirāja* flew over the fort, he happened to look down and see the young daughter of the king. The king's daughter was named Sūryamaṇi—"Jewel of the Sun"—and, true to form, her body was as effulgent as the glowing sunrise. She was drying her thick mass of long hair and that struck the bird dumb, completely enchanted. The bird instantly began to plot, "I wonder how I can manage to get this beautiful maiden married to Kāmodara?" And having taken special note of the girl, the *pakṣirāja* flew on.

As the bird flies to the prince, the poet Kaṇva sings.

The bird, who had carried food back to the hungry young man, landed and entered the deserted shelter. When the *pakṣirāja* gave the boy the food and sweets, their hearts and stomachs grew content. The king of birds began to think about the young woman, and so he began to describe her to the prince. "Sūryamaṇi is the name of the king's daughter, and her qualities, her body, rival Rāmā, the lover of Indra, king of the gods. This young woman is in the first blush of youth, superlative in every way, and that thick hair on her head hangs all the way to the ground."

When the young prince heard this description his heart grew restless, his thought turned to love, until he found himself saying, "Please show me favor and introduce me to the young woman."

"The palace is surrounded by a magical spell—Indrajāla, the net of Indra. Tell me just how do you propose we enter?"

The young prince insisted, "Concentrate, figure out a way. My heart soars at the prospect of seeing this young maiden."

The *pakṣirāja* listened and relented, bent down and slipped the crown prince onto his back. With the prince firmly on his back, he soared, finally landing on the perimeter wall of the palace. Then the bird cut through the Indrajāla, counteracting its magic with a spell of his own. He took a passage that led directly to the princess. She lay there asleep. The prince put his hands out to touch her body, but withdrew so that her sleep was not disturbed; he only looked. This was his first visit, and a growing uneasiness began to tug at his heart, so he retreated, climbing onto the back of the bird.

The morning broke with the resounding sounds of the name of God, "Rāma, Rāma," and the servant girls came to tend Sūryamaṇi.

Listen, one and all, to the mischief caused by the Pīr.

This good king had established a peculiar routine. The servants would enter and set up a pair of scales and day after day weigh his daughter against the measure of seven weights. Recently she had pushed beyond the seven weights, which she noted was simply because she was growing into her puberty and filling out. And so the next two days passed as usual until the bird carried Kāmodara back to the capital city.

By the magical power of the Pīr, the entire city fell insensate in sleep. The prince went straight to the young woman. A bejeweled lamp burned inside her rooms. Kāmodara deftly sat beside the young woman and embraced her—but the sleep did not flee from the eyes of this beautiful young thing. The prince then let the princess down and lay down on the bed beside her. "It would be a great sin for me to wake her, how can I? But how can I make this girl aware of me, how can I let her know I was here?" Taking the cloth that wrapped his upper body, he placed it on hers, and returned to his own abode. The bird carried the young man back to the open shelter and entered.

Now listen to the tale of the glorious Pīr as he complicates things.

In the early dawn the young lady got up from bed only to discover that she was covered with a strange blue cloth. She stared at the cloth and whispered, "Rāma, Rāma," the name of God, and thought, "Someone must have entered my quarters last night." And so the beautiful young woman worried this thought over and over again until the the maidservants entered to weigh her.

"Today your weight has doubled the standard daily measure, my princess," the maidservants informed her with their hands pressed together in respect. One maidservant opined, "How can you have gained double the normal weight?" To which Sūryamaṇi simply replied, "A girl blossoming into her youth grows bigger every day." And so she put them off and somehow the day finally drew to a close.

The poet Kaṇva sings the glorious tale of the Pīr with relish.

Then the young man placed before the *pakṣirāja* the following request: "Today, Father, I beg you to take me to the house of that young woman. I have left her signs that she is sure to have reckoned, and she will ask, "Why did you come furtively?" Then I will tell her the sad story of my youth, which is no different now from King Raghunātha wandering through the forests."

The bird considered what Kāmodara said, and, finding it reasonable, agreed. He picked him up, placed him on his back, and flew off to the young woman's home. Then the prince entered the private quarters of the princess, and that young woman, when she saw him, was visibly agitated. "Who are you? Whose son are you? And in what country lies your home?"

Hearing this jumble of questions, the son of a king replied, "Bhīmasena is the name of the king who rules the land of Avantī and I am his son, called Kāmodara. The good son of a fowler gave this *pakṣirāja* to him, and my father in turn entrusted his care to me. I let the bird escape and my father directed his wrath at me. He ordered the constable to take me out and cut off my head. Guarding me heavily on all sides, soldiers took me to be executed. The bird swooped down and lifted me to his back and rescued me. He deposited me deep in the forest, where he takes special care of me. Please believe me, you who are such a beautiful young woman; that is the full and honest explanation."

She listened to his tale, and was gradually overwhelmed and unsteady. The prince took her by the hand and guided her to a seat on her bed. The prince then sat himself down close beside the young lady, who presented herself just as Rādha had in the groves of Vṛndāvana. Kāmodara was as beautiful as Kāmadeva, the god of love himself, so Sūryamaṇi instantly infatuated, her heart flutttering. She was overwhelmed with the desire to touch him, to embrace him, and the thought of the touch of a man on her body transported her into the madness they call love. She was aroused, her mind and body burning from the arrows of love.

The glorious tale of the Pīr the poet Kaṇva composes with relish.

The touch of his hand on her body maddened her with desire to the point that Sūryamaṇi decided to embrace him. As her voice choked with the heat of love, the young woman whispered to the prince, "Take me into your arms, but be kind, gentle."

The young man rightly inferred the intoxicating rush of passion—a young deer had fallen into the claws of a hungry tiger. Such was the delight of lovemaking that the princess, daughter of a king, rode waves of rapture until she felt her arms could reach out and touch the sky. The young prince made love to her steadily and unceasingly. When they stopped, the prince gently suggested to her, "Now that the night has passed and it is daylight, listen carefully to what I say. You must stay here for I will soon return. . . ."

"Please show your mercy to me and to me alone. Do not abandon me," replied the young woman submissively. "Keep me at your feet."

And with that exchange, the bird placed Kāmodara on his back and off he flew. Soon they got sight of the abandoned open shed that was their home. In this way did the comings and goings of the prince become routine. It was by the mercy of the Pīr that no one ever discovered him.

Listen, everyone, to what the Pīr effected the next day.

Sūramaṇi's belly began to swell, a little more each day. When she discovered the pregnancy, the first maidservant was downcast to the point of grief; it was as if the sky had fallen and smashed her head. One by one the other maidservants confirmed it, their cries signaling their distress. Then one of the servants ran out to inform the queen. She made deep obeisance with palms pressed together in a show of respect to the queen. "Please listen, my queen, Sūryamaṇi is unexpectedly expecting. . . ."

The queen was mortified and ran, her mouth agape. She went and stood next to her daughter. Putting her hand on the girl's nose, the king's consort observed, "Sūryamaṇi, I see that you show all the signs of pregnancy."

The young woman innocently protested, "But how can that be true? I never even see the face of a man."

"You sigh and yawn, I see your breasts are swollen. Why have you allowed this awful stain on our world?"

"My body shows large and I'm yawning and sighing a lot because for the last two or three days I have suffered gas pains and flatulence."

The queen retorted, "I am not going to argue!" And off she rushed to find the king, the wielder of justice.

The queen chided her husband, "What are you doing just sitting there? Your daughter, Sūryamaṇi, the Jewel of the Sun, has become a little slut, a blight. The little ingrate stays in her quarters with her servant girls, so how can we find out how she has gotten pregnant?"

The news he heard made the king drop his head in anguish. It was as if the sky had suddenly come tumbling down. But he soon gathered his wits and screamed for his constable.

The poet Kaṇva has composed a beautiful tale of glory.

Summoned by the king, the constable asked, "What is your command, sire, tell me what you want me to do."

"Apparently you have taken to drugs or drink! How else could you allow a prowler to enter the women's apartments of this palace? By the end of the day you had better produce the intruder, or else you will find your life over, my son, when I have you thrown into a lime pit."

Terrified at heart, but with a cool smile on his face, the constable replied, "Give me three days, Sire, and you will get satisfaction."

With a simple, "Good," that great king, protector of the earth, agreed, and the constable beat a hasty retreat. He put on the disguise of a Vaiṣṇava fakir[17] and searched out every block of the city while pretending to beg. One watchman diligently gave up eating and drinking while he looked, but the intruder was nowhere to be apprehended. For two days they searched and turned up nothing substantive. The constable began to grow apprehensive; in fact he was worried sick. Then he hatched a plan. That night he sprinkled vermilion powder on the floor all around the princess' private quarters, leaving no spot untouched.

The long hours of day finally passed and late that night Kāmodara mounted and rode the bird to his assignation. Sūryamaṇi forbade him to enter through her door until she had shown him what was planned, then advised, "You must go back now!"

Kāmodara brashly responded, "Whatever has happened can only be because of the Lord, Gosāi. I've come this far and I'm not turning back now." And with these brave words, he sat down on the seat of honor, and his clothing was soon and thoroughly stained with vermilion. The young couple spent the entire night pursuing the pleasures of the flesh, reveling in the youthful exuberance of their lovemaking. When the night came to a close, he mounted the bird's back and flew away. Eventually the bird made it back to the abandoned shelter that was their home.

Kāmodara sheepishly approached the bird, his hands pressed together in respect. "My clothes are all stained with vermilion. . . ." And so the bird carried them to a local washerman, where prince innocently instructed the him, "Here, please scrub clean this filthy clothing."

The washerman replied and pointed, "Yes sir, just dump them there." The prince did as instructed, left his clothes, and returned to his abode.

Meanwhile, the constable had entered the quarters of the king's daughter. He inspected Sūryamaṇi's bedroom, moving back and forth, and then headed without delay into the city to the house of the local washerman. He spotted the stained clothing piled in a heap in the doorway, and immediately took the washerman into custody. The washerman complained, "What crime have I committed that you should apprehend me like this?"

The constable then inquired, "How did you come into possession of those clothes?" To which the washerman eagerly indicated that the man who had handed them over for washing would return that evening.

And so the constable hid himself on the premises of the washerman-now-collaborator, and, as promised, Kāmodara arrived to collect the offending articles. The washerman whispered, "O lord of night, Mr. Constable, that thief of love has come to collect his clothing." The constable identified Kāmodara and took him into custody.

The poet Kaṇva recites the pithy essence of the glorious tale of the Pīr.

Binding the crown prince in chains, the constable was ecstatic and relieved, and hauled him to His Majesty the king. Looking at him, the king lashed out in anger, "You are a despicable daughter-fucker! Take away this son of a bitch, this common thief, and cut off his head!"

With this invective-laden command, the constable hauled him away. Naturally the news found its way to the young daughter of the king. Striking her head with her fists, she cried out, "O lord of my life, you have abandoned me! Why did you not listen to my warning?" The king's daughter wept bitterly and her hair and dress soon were disheveled, but the constable continued to march the crown prince to his death.

When they reached the banks of the lake, Kāmodara fell down and grasped the feet of the constable and courteously requested him, "Brother, I beg your indulgence.

Could we please pause here a moment? I would like to bathe and purify myself in order to offer a small worship to Lord Govinda, for these last few days it would seem that fate has turned against me."

The constable gruffly allowed, "Go, then I'll cut off your head," and he stood on the bank and waited for him.

The prince submerged himself in the waters and spoke the rites earnestly, contemplating all the time the *pakṣirāja*, the king of birds. He raised the water in his hands, offering it as oblation, and wept for his misery. Standing facing the east, he touched a small dot of Gaṅgā water to his forehead, and thought to himself, "O Bird King, my father, perhaps you have not heard the news that right now I am on my way to be decapitated." The prince meditated, "Please come and save me." That unsettled the mind of the *pakṣirāja*, who divined that the young man was again in trouble. He quickly took flight, and not long after arrived. The bird swooped down to where the prince was standing, and, flapping his wings roughly as he hoisted him onto his back, flew away.

"You have saved me again, O Father, for the constable was preparing to sever my head. You plucked me from a terrible situation. Now I would like to see with my own eyes the woman who has caused me so much pain and grief. Please fly me there."

When his grief-stricken lover saw Kāmodara on the back of the bird, she cried, "Why, my lord, did you abandon me? If you go after promising not to abandon me, then I will kill myself and you will be responsible for the murder of a woman!"

Kāmodara turned to the bird and said, "O Father, pick up this king's daughter and place her on your back and fly us both away!" And just as Kāmodara had requested, the bird dropped down its wing and raised Sūryamaṇi onto his back, and off they went.

The good citizens of the king's citadel cried out in distress and grief. The queen cried copiously and writhed on the ground. They all wondered where the couple had escaped to. The bird rose up and flew until he reached the abandoned shelter. The bride and groom together made a home of that place, and lived under the care and provision of the bird.

Wherever the Pīr may be he listens. The twice-born poet Kaṇva says everyone should wish for the couple's prosperity. "May you be merciful to the hero. Grant the shadow of your feet, and in the future save me." Now listen, everyone, to the whim of the Pīr.

Sūryamaṇi's womb grew larger day by day. This moon-faced beauty strived to get comfortable lying down, and was of course beset with certain cravings. Pressing her hands together in supplication, the beauty said to the lord of her life, "Look, I am weak and withering, my health is disintegrating, and I have this insatiable craving for an unusual fruit, a special nectarine mango."

Kāmodara was nonplussed, "I am just a mere human, where could I possibly find such a fruit?" When she heard his unhelpful response, the young lady began to cry uncontrollably, her affliction great and her pain of pregnancy pressing.

But the king of birds also heard the young lady's desperation and said, "I promise you with all certainty, I shall bring you that mango. The trip will take me at least twelve days, but then I shall place before you that rare fruit you so crave. Stay right here, you have nothing to fear. I must cross seven oceans to the isle of Laṅkā to bring back the fruit." And as soon as he instructed them he rose up and was off.

It was not long before the bird made landfall at the citadel of Laṅkā. He found the fruits, ate one for himself and picked up two more to carry back. He passed over Candana Dvīpa, the Island of Sandalwood.

That extraordinary majesty that is the Pīr's, no one can possibly fathom. Working his magic, Satya Pīr inflicted a terrible disease on the beṅgamā *bird. The disease progressed rapidly and the* pakṣirāja *was spent, giving up his life.*

For many long days they waited without news of the bird until finally the couple struck out along his trail, tears in their eyes. They searched everywhere throughout the Sandalwood Forest. Then they spotted the *pakṣirāja* where he had fallen dead. Lying beside him were the two special mangos. Kāmodara observed, "He gave up his life to procure these two fruits. Take these two rare mangos, you who are the daughter of a king. It is for your sake that everything I ever had or was has been lost." The couple set up a soulful lament. The prince washed the body of that great bird in the Gaṅgā, and then performed the requisite ritual of the *piṇḍa* to ensure the safe passage of his soul and for those of his ancestors for seven generations in the past and the future.

The beautiful princess finally sated her desire and ate the nectarine mangos just as she reached term, ten lunar months and ten days. A handsome son was born at an auspicious moment on an auspicious day. They raised him with the name of Bīrabara—He Who Is Most Valiant—Sūryamaṇi's father's name. As the young couple entered the river with their son, a raft of plaintain was floated down the river by the Pīr. Holding the baby tight, they headed back to their own country, paddling and steering the boat with their hands, oblivious to everything else. Free from strife, the three floated along on the raft.

By the command of the Pīr, a Nepāl mouse[18] floated by. Kāmodara saw it and said, "I am going to pull it out and keep it."

His beautiful wife objected, "No, do not do that."

The prince replied, "I will keep it and raise it as a pet."

His wife continued her objection, "It could be a wild mouse from the forest and not given to domestication."

But the prince had already scooped the mouse out of the water and onto the raft.

He did not detect or understand the severe magic of the Pīr. The mouse hid itself, and gradually burrowed and gnawed its way through to the inside of the raft. Suddenly the plaintain raft separated into three different pieces which quickly drifted apart. Sūryamaṇi cried out in terror. Clearly it was the magic of Satya Pīr that sent the three rafts, each with its own passenger, floating in three decidedly different directions.

The good son of the king found himself floating to the northern country, where he found work on the plantation of a jaggery and treacle manufacturer. Sūryamaṇi floated a different way and finally landed in the garden of a professional flower grower. The gardener's wife saw her and took her into their own home. These two, husband and wife, going in two very different directions, managed to float to dry land, but Kāmodara's son continued his journey downstream until he was rescued by a merchant who was returning from a trading venture.

The poet Kaṇva has composed this beautiful and glorious tale.

The merchant Gaṅgādhara was returning to his home when he happened across the raft of plaintains carrying the infant boy. The merchant hoisted the baby onto his cargo boat and announced, "From this day forward I will be known as the one who celebrated the birth of his son just by throwing the eight cowries on the eighth day, a father at last."[19] The merchant guided his ships into the landing ghats, and then transported his riches and his new son home. The merchant looked after the boy with affection, just as Nārāyaṇa grew up in the home of his foster father, Nanda. Day by day the boy grew more beautiful in form, the very image of Kāma himself, and this handsome form he would retain for the next eighty years. One, two, three, four—the years seemed to roll by—and in the fifth year he had his ears pierced according to custom. The boy was fond of playing games with his friends—but back in the flower gardener's house his mother, Sūryamaṇi, toiled endlessly. As luck would have it, the gardener's compound sat in the eastern portion of the merchant's estates, and whenever she encountered that group of boys, Sūryamaṇi's heart ached in despair. One day she saw her son in the company of a moon-faced woman and she was mortified by the sight. She started to speak to her son but held back. When she saw her son with the other boys this beautiful woman could only weep and recount the names of Lord Rāma.

About this time Mahandara, the attendant, told Satya Nārāyaṇa, "Kāmodara was floating on the plaintain raft, but by your trickery a mouse nibbled apart the raft and the three people on board suddenly found themselves on three different rafts floating in three separate directions. The mother and the father both landed up safely and live separately under the care of others. The baby was rescued by a merchant who is raising him. The beautiful daughter of the king weeps inconsolably for her husband and for her child. You must restore her son to her. Should you wish to receive the honor of *pūjā* in the Kali Age, O majestic Lord and Messenger, Qādir, then you must act quickly.[20] Go there as Satya Pīr."

At the advice of Mahandara, he become a fakir, and, wasting no time, presented himself to Sūryamaṇi as the Pīr. The Qādir said, "Be calm, my dear, and accept my cordial greetings. Tell me, my little mother, what causes you such sorrow, for I oversee the distribution of the general weal, I am a powerful fixer."

Sūryamaṇi meekly replied, "Listen, Sāheb, to the reasons I cry. I weep for my son and husband. How much longer must I suffer so?"

The fakir promised, "For your son there is an immediate solution. I can help you to see your son."

When she heard this, Sūryamaṇi fell down and clasped his feet. "Please properly introduce yourself to me. Who are you really?" And so he did then explain himself to her.

"I am Satya Pīr. And look, here is your young boy. Call him quickly. . . . And I have another piece of intelligence: it regards your husband. He lives in the city in the house of a dealer of sugars and sweets." After revealing these tantalizing tidbits, Satya Pīr, in the wink of an eye, simply disappeared.

Sūryamaṇi headed off to present herself to her son. Crying, "My son, my son!" she threw her arms around his neck.

"How can you say such a thing?" objected the gathered children.

The child himself said, "The merchant is my father and I am his son. Why are you muttering such lies, pretending to be my mother? Are you crazy? Do you suffer from brain fever?"

Sūryamaṇi, undeterred, patiently replied, "It is true, I really am your mother. So tell me, how did you became the son of a merchant?"

The little boy sagely countered, "How can I know to call you Mother, what proof do I have?"

So this moon-faced beauty began to narrate her story to the young boy. "Some time ago we climbed onto a raft and were floating down the river when a malicious mouse gnawed the bindings of the raft, splitting it apart. By the magic of the Pīr, the raft broke into three pieces and the three of us were separated, floating on separate pieces in separate directions. I floated along until I landed up at the house of a flower vendor. You were picked up by the merchant."

At this the boy dashed into the house, full of questions.

The poet Kaṇva tells the mainstream of the glorious tale of the Pīr.

He burst into the house, "Father, I have some questions about my mother." The boy continued breathlessly, "Tell me the truth, who are my mother and father?"

The merchant queried him, "My child, what is the cause of all this? Why does your face look so dark today?" But sensing something, the good merchant continued, "I will tell you the truth about everything."

The child interrupted and pressed him, "Tell me, Father, the story of my birth."

As he listened, the merchant realized with a sickening certainty that the child was not going to remain in his house much longer, but he continued. "One day I was returning from one of my trading ventures and there you were, floating down the river on a plaintain raft. And so it was that I rescued you and raised you."

The child responded, "Yes, that is true, my dear father, but I have a request to make of you. My mother now lives in the house of the flower gardener. You are a paragon of virtue, Father, so I beg you to grant me leave to go to her."

The good merchant replied, "When you polish brass, does it ever become gold? If someone outside my family has given you birth, you will never be mine completely."

But the boy consoled him, "You must give your mind over to the sacred texts. Why did Yaśodā raise Śrī Kṛṣṇa as a foster son?"

The merchant conceded and bade him farewell, but with much anguish and grief. It was just like Kṛṣṇa, who lived in Gokula for so long and who then left for Mathurā. The young boy consoled both of his foster parents and then took himself to meet his birth-mother.

The child said, "O Mother, I have a proposition for you. Let us go together in search of my father. . . ."

Satya Nārāyaṇa understood through his meditation what had just transpired, and right before the break of dawn, he spoke to Kāmodara in a dream. "Listen, listen, Kāmodara, pay close attention. In the morning you will recover both your wife and your son. Take everything and set up shop at the foot of a particular tree, and during the time of the Car Festival you will be reunited.[21] Then, with your wife and son in your care, return to your original abode. When you reach there, establish in your home the ritual worship of Satya Nārāyaṇa." As soon as he had finished speaking, Satya Pīr disappeared into the heavens. In the morning Kāmodara jumped out of bed, took his wares, and set up his stall at the foot of the promised tree.

Meanwhile, the mother and son spoke affectionately to the wife of the flower gardener. "You have been very gracious in looking after our well-being for so many days. Now as mother and son we must go to search out news of his father." The wife of the gardener naturally was pleased, and bade them a proper farewell. The mother and son fell down in grateful obeisance at the woman's feet.

The mother and son headed off, discussing the recent events. It so happened that at just that time the great Car Festival of the king was about to take place. Soon the mother and son ambled right past the place where Kāmodara had set up his sweetshop as instructed. As he looked at the beautiful woman and the young child, he thought back to the conversation in the dream and wondered whether it was possible for it really to be true.

Sūryamaṇi, however, said confidently to her son, "My child, listen to what I say. See that man sitting at the sweetshop? He is your father."

At the cue of his mother's words, the child ran forward to question him. "What is your name? Whose son are you? Tell me truthfully."

Hearing the child out, he replied, "My name is Kāmodara."

Sūryamaṇi then came closer and tried to speak. This winsome daughter of a king wept as she looked carefully at his face. "How have you managed to survive and remain incognito? When on those dangerous waters of the sea the three of us drifted apart, I never imagined the good fortune of us ever reuniting."

Kāmodara listened, and then flung his arms around their necks and cried, "The three of us are united again. Let us all take the name of Lord Hari!"

And so it was that Kāmodara got back his wife and his son, all due of course to the good graces of Satya Nārāyaṇa. That night they passed in the hospitality of the confectioner's home.

The poet Kaṇva is borne along the waves of pleasure of the glorious tale of the Pīr.

Sūryamaṇi said, "My lord, I propose to you that the story of my trials and tribulations is one that cannot be described. Whatever was written on my forehead by the Fates is simply my fortune. But why are we staying here? Let us return straightaway to our own ancestral home."

The prince listened to her proposal, and, after thinking it through, agreed. He bade a proper formal farewell and left the house of the confectioner. The three of them together cooked and ate happily, then Kāmodara headed them back to their own country. They traversed the vast realm of King Bīrabāhu, fierce antagonist of enemies, and through that of King Kṛṣṇaketu, King Viśvajaya, and the ferocious King Bīr Mahātejā. After moving carefully through all these different lands, Kāmodara finally reentered his own country.

The prefect of police had been searching every village and town in the kingdom in search of the crown prince. He finally espied him, and immediately sent word back to the king. "Listen, O great King of men, to what I submit. After so many long days, your son, the crown prince Kāmodara, has returned."

Hearing these sweet words, the *mahārāja* was borne onto waves of rapture, as if by merely extending his arms he could reach the heavens themselves. Together with his courtiers and a company of soldiers, he headed out joyfully to meet Kāmodara.

Kāmodara made obeisance at the feet of his father the king and then said to him, "First we must perform the *pūjā* of Satya Pīr in gratitude, then we can go back to the palace."

The king promised with a simple, "We will do the *pūjā*." Then he began to dance with his arms up swaying in the air.[22] Everyone from the surrounding towns and villages came. The word spread that Kāmodara had returned. He took his wife and son back to the palace, where the king formally handed over the rule and responsibilities of the kindom to him.

Then they began preparations for the ritual worship of Satya Nārāyaṇa. The king summoned *kulin purohits*, brahmins of documented status trained in the ancient rites. In one of the halls of the great palace, the king fixed the *āstānā*, the ritual space dedicated to the deity. In the four cardinal directions they fixed an arrow demarcating the boundaries of the sacred area. A high platform seat made of gold was covered with a canopy of gold silk. Betel quids, betel leaves, and condiments were placed on a perimeter marked on each corner by one of the arrows. They brought one and a quarter seers of sugar, 125 flower garlands, one and a quarter seers each of milk, molasses, and sugary bananas. Everyone in the neighborhood was called to attendance, and there they mixed together the cooked and uncooked ingredients concocting *śirṇi*, the ritual offering. Conch shells blasted, bells clanged, drums resounded in a cacophony of celebration. The brahmin priests recited from the Veda and performed the ritual *pūjā*.

This was how the ritual pūjā *of the Pīr came to be performed in the palace of the king.*

Let everyone shout the name of Lord Hari with faces beaming. Let us contemplate the future well-being of all those assembled here. The poet Kaṇva sings, "May you be merciful to our hero."

The Disconsolate Yogī Who Turned the Merchant's Wife into a Dog

Dvīja Kavibara's *Bāghāmbara Pālā*

Listen, beloved, friends to the divine message of the Pīr. May you circumambulate him with dexterity and offer a thousand salaams.

The king in the city of Śrīhaṭṭa was one Mādhava. He had under his command countless regiments of battle-hardened soldiers.[1] The king would listen to the narration of the exploits of Lord Kṛṣṇa, just as King Parikṣit used to listen to Śuka-deva. As this jewel among men was sitting on his throne one day, like Lord Cakrapāni residing over the court of the gods, the quartermaster appeared before him with his palms pressed firmly together in supplication. He reported that there was no sandal, nor were there yak-tail whisks in the royal store. The king promptly issued a written summons to his adviser and began to issue commands. "Bring the merchant Sadāgara to me, and be quick about it!"

Now the king's personal purveyor was named Hīrānanda, whose name means "The Bliss of Diamonds,"and whose wealth was so great that it could be reckoned the same as his name. His brothers numbered five. When the adviser received the royal order he summoned the chief of police, who slipped the royal decree in the breast of his tunic and departed, just as Akrūra had gone at the command of Kaṃsa to Gopapura to fetch Govinda. This emissary made himself known in the house of the merchant and promptly handed over the king's written missive. And just as Nandarāya received the letter from Kaṃsa, the good trader read it and touched it to his forehead. The chief of police spoke, "My good merchant, please waste no time! Go quickly to meet with the king. Hurry! . . ." Hīrānanda, the oldest brother, was followed in order by Purāndara, Gopāla, Mukunda, Vidyānidhi, and finally the youngest of all, Jayānanda. The chief of police had addressed Hīrānanda and Purāndara, so they mounted their carts and rode off to meet the king. And so the merchant brothers journeyed to meet with the king, just the way Balarāma and Kṛṣṇa made their way to Mathurā City. They prostrated themselves fully before the king and then waited off to the left. The king greeted them cordially and had them come up and sit beside him in an intimate gesture. "There is no sandal to be found in my royal store, nor are there even yak-tail whisks. You six brothers must go for trade to the city of Nairāṭa. . . ." And so with these simple words did he command them, a royal commission. The merchants then returned to their home extremely pleased at the prospect.

Their mother had been waiting expectantly for their return. "Tell me, did everything go well? Was there good news to be had? . . ." and so forth. In response to his mother's queries, the merchant replied, "The king has ordered us to go to trade." His mother exclaimed, "My son, how can you even breathe such words? They strike my heart like a poison-tipped spear!"

Jayānanda, the youngest of all, responded, "I am much afraid to go, for somehow this smells of danger, much as a body under stress cannot shake the redolence of turmeric. Sumitrā had but one son, yet that Laksmaṇa never parted from Rāma. There was nothing Śyāma could not do, and yet his brother stuck to him like a *tilaka*, the ever-present mark on a woman's forehead." At his brother's announcement and admonition, Jayānanda publicly had this to say: "What you command, my dear brother, I will do."

So there and then the ship's captains began to outfit their ships. Meanwhile, Jayānanda consoled and comforted his mother. "Listen, dear Mother, at your feet do I earnestly beseech you to take good care of your youngest daughter-in-law, my wife, who must stay behind." Then the merchant and his five brothers fetched their wives and placed each and every one in the custody of their dear mother. "Protect them with your very life, for all of us must go, leaving the house totally devoid of male protectors." Campāvatī wept at being separated from her new lord and husband, just as the girls did when Hari abandoned Gokula to go to Mathurā. In fact, Campāvatī wept to the point of total distraction, much as Viṣṇupriyā could not control herself after being cut off from Caitanya.[2] Looking hard into the face of his wife, Jayānanda tried to console her, but it did no more good than when Govinda reassured the *gopī* cowherd women of his return, which never occurred.

Six ships were quickly made ready to sail, each loaded with assorted cargos of gifts, tradeable goods, local rarities, and clothing. Each son made obeisance to his mother's feet, and the mother in turn entrusted her children, all six of them, to the skill of the captains of the fleet. The boats were rendered auspicious with collyrium and vermilion, while offerings of gold were proffered and a goat slaughtered in sacrifice. The auspicious blast of the conchs joined the shrill of the women's *hulāhuli* trilling. Instruments were played while people danced and clapped their hands. The boats were launched with the benediction to sail well, a separation that clove the hearts of the women, not different from the *gopīs'* ache at Govinda's departure. Many of the weeping women clung to the boats to impede their progress, mirroring the cowherd girls clinging to Kṛṣṇa's chariot to inquire of Hari's intended journey. "Go back to the house and shed no more tears for the duration of our journey, for it would be inauspicious," commanded the merchant. And with these final instructions, which were intended to console, they quickly pushed off.

That merchant, a veritable treasure trove of virtues, headed for the landing ghat at Tripura. Let everyone sing the praise of Lord Nārāyaṇa's name.

The merchant called out according to prescription, "May we sail safely." The face shone magnificently on the boat's prow, its iridescent eyes shimmering like golden orbs. The ship saw its way quickly to the Kākada ghat and soon landed at Tripura ghat. There the king who had dispatched them sallied forth for final instruction. They followed the course of the Padmāvatī River, sailing past Raṅgapura, while in the heavens Dāśarathi Pīr charted carefully their steady progress. When the six had rowed their dinghies ashore to go into town, he thought, "Now I shall go there and test the hearts of each and every one of them. Should they honor me by offering me *śirṇi*—that favorite mixture of rice flour, banana, milk, and sugar—I will grant them my full blessings and return here right away. Should they be of two minds about me and waver, then rest assured that I will vex them in terrible ways." The Pīr then smeared ashes over his body in the manner of ascetics and transformed himself into a brilliant and charismatic form. He pulled his hair into a topknot like that of a peacock, strung a rosary through his hands, and wore a necklace of glittering gemstones. He cinched a cummerbund of knotted flowers round his waist and carried a waterskin. The fakir then appeared at the Padmāvatī ghat, and, to solicit alms, displayed a popinjay parrot in an ornate cage. A leather wallet was slung over his shoulder, a broad-blade machete in his left hand, like Vāmana the Dwarf come to deceive King Bali.[3] A ragged patchwork quilt wrapped around his body made the fakir menacing. He approached the merchants, doling out expansive benedictions of grace. The volume and clamor were like Brahmā chattering the Vedas with all four faces simultaneously, but the actions were those of the baby Kṛṣṇa begging butter from Yaśodā. The fakir spoke, "My child, may my blessings be upon you. I beg your charity to ferry me across the river."

The young and inexperienced Jayānanda cut him off, "Listen, you stupid fakir. As soon as we shove off from where we drop you, you will turn and call us back again without consideration . . ." The fakir retorted heatedly, "Listen, you disrespectful ingrate. Your words and tone are insulting to anyone forced to hear them. It is clear that neither Bali nor Māndhātā have anything on your arrogance, for you no doubt consider yourself equal to Jarāsandha, Mahāvīra, and Duryodhana.[4] I can find untold numbers of other better traders among the traditional ranks of Bāṇiks. . . ."

"You, ignorant fakir, are the most ungrateful, disrepectful son of a bitch. . . ." And so the war of words escalated as the young merchant heaped abuse after abuse. The fakir's anger welled up until he picked up some dust and flung it on the merchant with this curse: "If I am indeed the Pīr of Truth, called Satya Pīr, then may my words come true. I will give your dear wife to some magic-working yogī."

And having levied this awful curse, the Pīr disappeared. May everyone chant loudly the name of Hari with a joyful heart.

After the youngest merchant clashed with the fakir in a battle of insults, they all decamped from the Padmāvatī, shouting, "Hari, Hari!" Traveling past Ajaya's landing ghats, Ujani passed by starboard. After navigating past Rudrāpūra, the merchants then entered the realm of Icchāni. Sometimes they resorted to eating yogurt curds and banana, while at other times they feasted on sweetmeats. Eventually they entered the commercial precincts of Nairāṭa. When they docked at the landing ghats, the merchants sent their formal greetings to the local king, and the king made his usual inquiries when they met: "From where do you hail? What is your name? Why have you come here?" To which the eldest merchant replied, "O great King, I submit to your royal feet that my home is located in the fair city of Śrīhaṭṭa, where Mādhava rules as the lord of men. For many long years have I resided in that kingdom. My own name is Hīrānanda. But please listen, O greatest of men, the king's royal stores are depleted of all sandal and fly whisks, among other royal accoutrements. The king dispatched me, saying, 'Your mission is this: Go and procure the necessary sandal, fly whisks, etc., and bring them back to our country.' " The local king was well disposed, and laughed and joked with them in good-natured banter. The six brothers found lodging and settled in.

Now the Lord arrived and manipulated the magical veil of worldly illusion. Right in the middle of the road, he happened upon a yogī who was headed into the famous Fig Market when the Pīr accosted him with lighthearted cheer. "Tell me, O Nātha Yogī, why are you so miserable? My heart is unsettled to see the extent of your suffering."

At the kind solicitation of the fakir, this lord of yogīs replied, "Six months have passed since my mate and yogic companion departed for the heavens. The suffering I endure no one is capable of describing. The resulting condition from this grief is known only to the Master of Dance, Lord Śiva. . . ." The fakir listened attentively to the extreme distress of this yogī. Before doing anything, he got the yogī to agree to offer *śirṇi*, the special mixture of banana, rice flour, sugar, and milk. Then he said, "I will see to it that you meet a stunningly beautiful young woman who will become your lover." The Nātha Yogī replied, "Where is the home of this young thing?" To which the fakir replied, "Listen carefully and heed the details. I will give you complete and accurate intelligence about the place where this young lady resides. There is a famous seafaring merchant named Hirānanda Sadāgara. His youngest brother goes by the name of Jayānanda, and that young one's wife is called Campāvatī. I will provide you with a magic formula, a *mantra*, that will make her come with you. If anyone else tries to offer you alms—and they will—refuse to be satisfied with them at that time. Campāvatī, however, will try to give you an offering of garbage, detritus fit for no one. As soon as she passes off that garbage as alms, Campāvatī will turn her back on you. Right then you must throw on her body some magical dust, energized by the *mantra*. She will be transmogrified into a black dog, a cur that will follow you anywhere. You should take that young lady deep into a forest grove where no one else is around. You should then slap the body of the dog with the dew from wildflowers, and before you know it, your beautiful young lover will be standing before you. If you want to achieve your desires, mind the offering of *sirṇi*." The yogī then went his way, and the Pīr disappeared.

At the home of the merchant, the yogī sang and danced. The women of the household all crowded around to see him dance. The wife of the eldest merchant sent for alms for the yogī. The old withered yogī laughed and then spoke to all who were gathered. "Listen, all you lovely ladies, to what I have to say. Only after Campāvatī offers me alms will I leave." The daughters-in-law scurried off to convey the message to their mother-in-law, and the old woman rushed out to meet the yogī. That hardened yogī soon captivated the old woman with his mesmerizing stare. The old woman said, "Let Campā give alms to this greatest of yogīs." The hearts of the other five women skipped a beat, their right eyes twitching in omen. The youngest wife wondered aloud what the Fates had written on her forehead. All of the sisters-in-law recovered and encouraged her not to worry. Campāvatī gathered up the offering and went to the yogī. She had the innocent face of a deer, but her body broadcast the forked electricity of sexual lightning. Just to gaze at her wondrous form agitated the old yogī with pure delight. The women of the household flanked her on all sides, and as soon as she proffered the meager offering Campāvatī quickly turned away. The yogī hurled the magic dust, sprinkled liberally with the special *mantra*, and the fresh young girl suddenly transformed into an ugly black dog. The elegant women of that distinguished house simultaneously let out a loud cry of lament, but the yogī had already headed off to the town of Ijvillī.

The yogī reached the village of Ijvillī and scouted the all sectors looking for a place to stay. He gravitated toward the western portion of the village, and there he entered the Daṇḍaka Forest. The yogī sprinkled and then rubbed the entire body of the dog with the dew of wildflowers and there, in the dark depths of the forest, stood before him the most seductive of sexual creatures. The yogī was instantly aroused at her sight, while Campāvatī pleaded with him, "O Yogī, listen carefully to what I have to say. Rāvaṇa lost his life for the sake of another's wife and Gautama cursed the moon because of a tiny little stain. I am in the midst of a twelve-year vow to the goddess of the morning, Uṣā. After I have completed my observance of that vow, then will I become your personal servant. Do not try to force yourself on me or touch me with your hands in any way, for during this time I am your offspring, your daughter, and you are my venerable father. . . ."

When he heard this, the yogī secured her for sakekeeping in the Daṇḍaka Forest, much as Rāvaṇa had installed Sītā in the grove of *aśoka* trees. Each and every day did this beautiful young woman perform Śiva worship. And in this fashion she managed to pass the first four months without incident. But one day the king of Ijvillī, one Raṇajit, ventured into that forest on a hunting expedition. When the young damsel espied this ruler of men deep in the forest, she lost no time in escorting him to her quarters. The yogī intercepted them along the way and tried to waylay the king, but the king ordered his constable to apprehend the yogī. The constable instantly understood and carried out his king's command, and right away caught the yogī and tied him to a tree. The king then took the young woman where the yogī was bound. In absolute terror the yogī called out loudly for Lord Satya Nārāyaṇa. Suddenly the Pīr materialized before him and severed the restraints. Then he gave him a magical rope. Speaking through gestures, the ascetic indicated for the yogī to run after them, and the yogī did, catching up with the king and demanding the return of the woman. The king cast aspersions on the yogī, who instantly struck back with his rope, which turned the king into a palmyra or fan palm and his mighty steed into a lump of earth resembling the broken-down ruins of a mud dwelling. It was no different from the great demon Rāvaṇa smearing ashes on Rāma. And in this fashion did the yogī slay one and all in the entourage and eventually the kingdom. The only one he spared was a flower vendor, a weaver of garlands, and her for the sake of supplying flowers. Soon the old yogī became the ruler of that fair land. And each day the beautiful young woman performed her worship of Śiva and managed in that way to pass another four months.

Meanwhile, the six merchants concluded their business in Nairāṭa, and, after making ready their seven boats, returned to the fair city of Śrīhaṭṭa. When they approached the ghats a great tumult broke out, with drums and instruments announcing their arrival. With the arrival of the boats, the womenfolk rushed to greet them with their auspicious benedictions. The five wives dutifully welcomed their husband's five boats with celebrations of success, after which they together performed the same ritual for the boat of the youngest merchant brother. Jayānanda protested, "Listen to me. What are you doing? My wife will perform the welcoming rituals for my boat. . . ." His mother evasively replied, "Your wife has gone to visit her father. . . ." Jayānanda instantly announced, "Then I will go and fetch her." Then his mother tried to explain, "My dear child, she was devoured by a tiger as if she were a tasty confection made of butter and shaped like a doll. I do not lie to you."

Jayānanda proclaimed, "Mother, I will go out of my mind and die if you, the woman who carried me in her womb, were to lie to me. . . ." His mother relented when she heard the extreme distress of her youngest son, "It is even worse: a yogī magically transformed her into a dog and took her away. . . ."

That terrible fellow, insane and consumed by lust and sin, escaped in this direction . . . so Dvīja Kavibara sings the verses of the Pīr's great book.

When he finally heard the tale from his mother's mouth, the young merchant was stunned, as if a poison-tipped spear had rent his chest. Tears gushed from his eyes like the monsoon rains of July and August. He could have been confused with Rāma, that gem of the Raghu clan, weeping in grief for his Sītā. His brothers approached and promised in consolation that they would bring him another woman, young and equally beautiful. But Jayānanda would have nothing of it. "I will not marry again, but will abandon this way of life to search for her and bring her home."

Hīrānanda protested, "Now she has become the wife of a yogī, a magic-working witch. How can you even consider bringing back a woman who will be a permanent stain on our family lineage?"

Jayānanda replied, "Listen, all five of you brothers. Do not try to prevent me from going in search of my beloved. When Rāvaṇa abducted the daughter of King Janaka, Rāma went so far as to construct an earth-bridge across the sea to Laṅkā in order to rescue his Sītā. . . ." And so he outfitted a fiery steed, put on pajamas and tunic, and adorned himself with ornaments truly divine. Tears of love streaked his face as he thought about beholding his beloved's face, much as Rāma grew agitated at the loss of Sītā. Hīrānanda said, "If you are overmuch delayed in your return, we five brothers will strike out in search of you. . . ." And so, meditating on Lord Mādhava, the youngest merchant headed for the forested regions, just as Rāma went in search of Sītā.

For seven days and seven nights the merchant traversed those regions, never once tortured by the pangs of hunger or thirst. The merchant searched far and wide for his beloved wife, visiting Gayā, up the Gaṅgā to Kāśī, then Kāñcī, back to Prayāg, and to Mathurā. He went through Aṅga, Vaṅga, Kaliṅga, Tailaṅga, and Gujarāṭ, then through Bhorāṭ and Korāṭ he searched, even to Pāṇḍava Ghat. He queried every tree and creeper of his wife's whereabouts, just the way Rāma had been agitated on account of Sītā. He scoured any number of regions, until he came to Kākathoṭa. The young merchant had come a great distance in his search for the yogī's dwelling place. Finally he reached the city of Ijvillī. All he could see around the place were fan palms and lumpy earthworks scattered about. About this time the garland weaver—the one person still around the place—was returning home after delivering some flowers. When she spotted the handsome sepoy, she began to question him. "What is your name, my child, and what is your city and country? . . ." To which he replied, "I am an inhabitant of Śrīhaṭṭa town and I'm abroad on business."

When she heard those words the old woman's hand moved instinctively to her throat as she pondered the incredible power of the yogī's magic rope.

The garland weaver spoke, "Listen, my child, to what a singular and extraordinary tale I tell. Since that hardened yogī arrived in our region he has created havoc. There was a famous merchant named Hīrānanda, who with his brothers and their wives lived in the fair city of Śrīhaṭṭa. The yogī captured and hauled back here the beautiful woman Campāvatī, whose husband was Jayānanda. With a magic yogic rope in his hand, he subdued the local king and confined Campāvatī there in the forest. All those groves of palmyra palms are those inhabitants. That is the yogī's claim to fame. All these earthenworks are all the horses and elephants. And that is how the yogī became king. I have been spared only for the sake of supplying fresh flowers, for each day the young woman performs the ritual worship of Lord Śiva and needs them."

When he heard what she had to say, the merchant began to weep uncontrollably. "That yogī is hard-hearted, and by stealing away Campāvatī has caused me much personal misery. He can worry all he wants, but I have finally found my wife after a taxing search. . . ."

The garland weaver advised, "You may as well return home, for you will never get back your wife. As soon as the yogī sees you he will subdue you like all the rest, and you, my son, will lose your life, too."

"When Lord Rāma, jewel of the Raghu clan, lost his wife, he went and slew Rāvaṇa. So listen carefully to my plan, O gracious garland weaver, you must inform her of every detail. If you do not communicate everything to her, I shall simply die, and in vain. You tell her what you think best. . . ." And so Jayānanda laid out his scheme and then entered the yogī's lair.

The faithful wife Campāvatī was overjoyed finally to lay eyes on the lord of her life.

Worrying about the love of her life, Campāvatī asked him, "Why on earth have you come here to the very seat of death? All the palmyra trees you see around us are humans. As soon as the yogī spots you he will subdue you. I have become an indelible stain on my lineage during this birth, yet you, the lord of my life, would lose your own life on my account. This cruel yogī has effected my ruin. The lord of fate, Bidhātā, has granted me the same sorry circumstance as Jānakī. O merciful one, please grant me, this wretched and unfortunate woman, the dust of your feet, then wash your hands of me and go."[5]

Jayānanda replied, "Better that I should die, for I will not return home so shamefaced. . . ." Jayānanda was no different from Rāma, the scion of the Raghus, grieving over Jānakī—such were the extremes of agitation that shook his heart over his wife.

As this husband and wife declared their love in the midst of their bereavement, that Nātha Yogī overheard them talking. Grabbing his magic rope, he ambushed them with a bloodcurdling cry. "Who the hell are you? And where the hell are you from?" Jayānanda stammered, "My name is Jayānanda and I hail from the city of Śrīhaṭṭa." Having heard enough, the yogī lassoed him with his magic rope and—poof!—Jayānanda had become a fan palm and his mighty horse nothing more than a mound of earth. The misery from losing her husband a second time was too much for the merchant's young wife, and she wept inconsolably in her grief day and night.

Jayānanda's five older brothers began to wonder about the situation when he failed to return home, and soon they set out in search, just as they said they would. The wife of the oldest, Hīrānanda, pleaded with him, her hands pressed together in respect, "I am six months pregnant. Fortune will turn her back on me and everything will go to ruin if you leave town. I shall have no choice but to go live in the forest, abandoned. . . ." And so she lamented.

"Don't cry, please don't cry, my dear, for you are my companion for life. Before I go in search of my brother Jaya I will write special instructions for you. If we have a daughter, name her Candrā, 'With the Beauty of the Moon'; but if we have a son, call him Amara, 'Immortal.' As the boy grows, see to his formal education, and if I am delayed too long, send my son in search of me." And with these instructions he handed the letter to his wife. Looking at his face one last time, the distraught woman broke down in a flood of tears. "In a few days we shall all become widows, separated from our lords. . . ." And so the wives of the merchants wept together, as just as the cowherd women wept when they were separated from Kṛṣṇa. "We go in search of our brother, so please do not weep"; but the consolation was no better than Kṛṣṇa's when he left for Mathurā.

At the time of departure, they equipped five good horses. All together let us sing the name of Hari.

Extraordinary steeds were brought in pairs and put into traces. These horses flew like the wind. First they searched to the north, then to the west. Eventually they wound up in the settlement of Ijvillī. Hīrānanda reined in his horse in the middle of the road, for all around them they saw fan palms and mounds of earth. About this time, the flower vendor was returning home from her daily delivery and she saw this particularly handsome sepoy there in the city. As she gazed at his face her eyes welled with tears, and she said, "When I look at you I see a close resemblance to Jayānanda. . . ."

At this first piece of information connected to his brother, the merchant began to inquire of the garland weaver, his speech controlled and gentle. "My name is Hīrānanda and Jayānanda is my brother." The garland weaver needed to hear no more before she began to unburden herself of Jayānanda's sad tale. "He appeared here at the yogī's abode to search out his wife. But the yogī spotted him and quickly turned him into a palmyra, a common fan palm. I warned him repeatedly but he ignored everything I said. It seemed his wish was, like the moth, to fly directly into the flames. Before he left, the young man gave me a message: 'Should my brothers come for me, tell them that Jayānanda has died.' "

When they heard this sad tale directly from the mouth of the flower vendor, all five brothers were utterly distraught and began to cry, venting their great misery. They shouted out, "Brother Jayānanda!" and wept profusely, their bodies soon covered with dust and their hair flying, let loose in their grief. Individually and together they cried out, "Brother, brother! On account of this one woman we have lost our brother."

Hīrānanda said, "Take care to hear out my plan. For the sake of our brother, we still should go and risk being turned into palm trees ourselves." And so in the frenzy of their grief, they mounted their horses and rode like men possessed until they reached the perimeter of the yogī's dwelling.

After she had performed her daily worship of Lord Śiva, the beautiful woman Campāvatī had seated herself in the entryway and wept uncontrollably, unable any longer to bear her burden. When she looked up and saw the brothers of her husband, the good woman admonished them, "Why have all of you, too, come here to this place where death resides? Go now, flee, quickly, and save your lives! For as soon as that nasty yogī finds you, he will kill you. . . ." Then they understood the fan palms and began to weep, but the yogī spotted them and came forth to question: "From what country to you come? What is your name? Where exactly is your home? . . ." and so forth.

"Hīrānanda is my name and Jayānanda is my brother. . . ."

When he heard this much, the old yogī went for his magic rope, but Hīrānanda and his brothers jumped on their flying horses and took off into the skies. Flying through the air, they showered countless kicks on the body of the yogī, a veritable rainstorm of stinging blows that made him stagger and fall. For eight days they battled, but in the third watch the yogī began to realize that his strength was waning and he was nearing death. With this realization he feigned defeat by falling down. Hīrānanda immediately announced that the yogī had lost the battle. The five brothers rode up and dismounted around the body of the yogī, who suddenly jumped up and lassoed them with this magic rope. He stood triumphant, amused at the unexpected change of their fortunes. All five brothers were soon made into fan palms, while their horses were reduced to mounds of earth. The yogī declared his own greatness: "I have exterminated the entire clan of my greatest enemy. There is no one left in the triple worlds who can challenge me now. I no longer have to worship the Pīr, so I will not make the offering of *śirṇi*. Should he object, I will turn that fakir into a fan palm as well. . . ." And so he ranted.

A thousand salaams to the feet of Satya Nārāyaṇa. May everyone sing of his wonderful qualities gladdening the heart.

The fair woman's eyes were awash with tears from incessant weeping. She worried aloud, "There is no one left in my entire extended family to perform the sacred obsequies with flower offerings in the waters of the Gaṅgā. Why has the Wielder of the Discus, Lord Viṣṇu, dispensed such awful misery? I, a woman abandoned by fortune, am drifting along in fathomless waters. What other tribulations does fate have in store for me? I shall drift aimlessly now that the entirety of my extended family has died. You once showed your mercy to Draupadī by exercising your magic over the phenomenal world, Narahari, yet you have denied it to this unfortunate wretch. With the strength of your own arms you once took Prahlāda onto your lap and extended your protection, and you saved the elephant by wielding your famous discus. My immediate family and my extended family, O Lord, you have consigned to become ill-fated lineages. I am now cast adrift in a sea of sorrow. . . ."

This beautiful young woman wept in her misery, for her fate had taken a nasty turn. Lord Nārāyaṇa then predicted that her heart's desires would be fulfilled.

Nārāyaṇa spoke from the endless void of heaven, "Listen, my dear Campāvatī. There is in your lineage one who is about to take birth and he will save your husband. His name will be Bāghāmbara, meaning 'He Who Wears the Tiger Skin.' I will see to it that he liberates your family. . . ." It was as if that illustrious Pīr had himself spoken those words from out of the sky. And so she passed four more months in this anxious-but-reassured state.

Hīrānanda's wife went to her family home for her pregnancy. And finally she reached the full term of ten lunar months and ten days. When the labor pains became acute, she squatted down like a wrestler, and in her fear and anxiety she meditated on Lord Vasudeva. She delivered a child that glowed like the morning sun, its limbs and body more effulgent than pure gold. It was no different from when Lord Kṛṣṇa was born in Gokula, or when Śaci gave birth to that golden-limbed Gaura, the jewel of virtues named Caitanya. In great joy, double-headed *dundubī* drums were resounded, conchs were blasted, and women made the auspicious *hulāhuli* sound. Heavenly nymphs danced and sang and clapped their hands. The umbilical cord was ceremonially severed with a special oyster-shell-shaped golden knife and then the navel was tied off with a canvas cotton thread and fresh medicinal *durbbā* grass. Lightly fragrant sandalwood paste was smeared around the frame of the lying-in room, and with great merriment the mother was seated and fed assorted hot and savory curries, the likes of which she had not eaten for months. Some women brought vermilion and collyrium, while others gave to the merchant's son gifts of sacred grass and special rice. After five days the special "rituals of the fifth" were completed, then on the sixth day, the women worshiped the goddess of children, Mā Ṣaṣṭhī, in the local temple.

It was about then that the Pīr, dressed in tattered rags and his complexion the color of a thick dark rain cloud, arrived. He entered the primary dwelling of the merchant himself. "I heard the great tumult of *dundubī* drums coming from your house, so I have come here in order to collect alms."

The mother-in-law asked him, "Do you know anything about calculating astrological signs?"

And the prescient seer of all things replied, "Why do you ask?" Then the fakir continued, "I do indeed know how to forecast horoscopes by reading the stars and planets and auspicious marks. Precisely what kind of reading do you wish me to do in your house?"

The mother-in-law replied, "A son has just been born to this household. It is to foretell his prospects that I ask you to exercise your astrological skills." And having negotiated this, the woman blossomed with good cheer and placed before him a spread of rice and betel nut.

Drawing out the horoscope on the ground, the Pīr calculated the various vicissitudes, risks, and confusions that loomed in each of the houses of the planets, after which he placed in the hands of the good woman a written horoscope. "The chalk revealed that among the events foreseen he is destined for truly heroic deeds. Everything attempted will turn out well; there were no inaupicious indicators. He will be held in high esteem and his name will be resonant with fame throughout the world. This son will be the salvation of your family and lineage." Then the dark-complexioned Pīr blessed the baby boy and bestowed on him the name Bāghāmbara. "I am acting just as the ancient sage Garga did when he entered the house of Nanda and bestowed the names of Rāma and Dāmodara on the two boys. This boy will surely save your family." And with this prediction, the Pīr abruptly departed for his own abode.

Day by day the young boy grew a little bigger there in the house of that trading family. After three months he was able to roll over by himself. After five months his voice had grown sweet like the cuckoo's call. And at six months he was stuffing dirt into his mouth on his own. Then, as dictated by tradition, he was given his first solid food, a ceremonial eating of rice, after which gifts were made to brahmins as directed in the sacred texts. Crawling about on all fours this way and that, he brought joy to the heart. And so the boy grew during his first year in the home of the merchant. They sent for the barber, who ceremonially pierced his ears, and again great wealth was distributed to brahmins and holy men. The child continued to grow for the next seven years, and was soon playing all over town with his friends.

Amara was very strong, restless, and perhaps a little mischeivous; he yielded to no one. Kavibara recites the message of the Pīr's great book.

Being obstinate and minding no one, the young boy grew up street tough and earned his way in countless fights, beating his young friends mercilessly. All the boys complained bitterly to Amara's mother, saying, "See for yourself the bruises he has left on our bodies." Yet the young merchant boy grew up in princely comfort, wanting nothing. And in pure physical might there was no one his equal. Endowed with nearly superhuman strength, his physical presence was extremely imposing, equaled only by his courage. No one could match such raw power as he possessed. When the other boys complained, they were pacified with expressions such as, "Don't cry, my children, don't cry," liberally sprinkled with various sweets and other elegant foods before being sent on their way.

The child would crawl up on a stool and slip into someone's room, prompting the women of the household to complain to his mother, just as the wives of the cowherds complained to Yaśodā about the child Kṛṣṇa: "Your little jewel of the Yadu clan has messed up our rooms."

Amara's mother would reply something like this: "Please go easy on him, for my son has grown much too contrary, too naughty, to remain confined at home."

But the reply finally came, "O my dear friend, may I suggest to you something about this one who is so dear to your heart: Why not send your son to study with a brahmin so that he may be disciplined to stay at home?"

The advice hit home and the official family priest was summoned right away. Amara's mother handed him over to the custody of the best of twice-born. "Please work diligently and give him an education incomparable. I formally remand to your custody my darling boy, my very life." After paying homage to the five deities, he was ceremoniously inducted into formal study. The new student fell at the feet of his teacher and prostrated himself in full obeisance. It was no different from Rāma and Dāmodara going for their education to the city of Avanti and entering the house of the sage Sandipanī.

The alphabet was chalked out on the ground and the guru said, "Now, young man, recite. . . ."

Amara, the son of the merchant, studied eighteen forms of conjunct consonants, after which he began the mastery of the ritual texts called Brāhmaṇas. The boy studied the *Bhāgavata Purāṇa*, where one finds the stories of Lord Kṛṣṇa's many exploits, then he worked through other Purāṇas, then the *Tantrasāra*.[6] He learned hundreds of auspicious *mantras* designed to hold Kṛtanta or Yama, the god of death, at bay. Then this epitome of virtue was initiated into the *Tritantra*. Single-mindedly did he learn those works that were quoted as authoritative and then mastered both the *ṭīkā* and *ṭippaṇī* commentaries for each. The young scholar soon learned all eighteen of the classical Purāṇas, the *Bhagavad Gītā*, and a host of other great scriptures for preserving life. He studied the *Bhāṣya* commentary of Vedānta and related texts, but also mastered the corpus of the Tantras, focusing especially on the mysteries that govern the auspicious and inauspicious times of the day and the means of destroying demons and other powerful beings. Like Brahmā's ever-vigilant guard against the wicked, or the righteous innocents who oppose the goddess Caṇḍī, he completely assimilated the details of the astrological scriptures. And so Amara shone like the sun among those assembled and was recognized as a master poet, no longer regarded as the pretender all students naturally must be.

When one dedicates oneself wholly to the feet of Nārāyaṇa, his mind is cleansed of all misery and suffering.

One day Bāghāmbara said, "Teacher, now please explain to me how precisely a drop of semen falls from heaven to impregnate the earth. . . ." All the students present were aghast at this singular behavior, and even worse in the presence of the guru. When he heard Amara's impertinence—not only because of the inappropriateness of the subject matter but worse, that he should think he knew enough to declare the time for such instruction—the brahmin was incensed, and, seething with anger, replied curtly and with malice. "You inexperienced and uneducated fool, how dare you smart off to me in this manner! So you want to know the details of how you came about? Well I'm your family's priest and I know everything about your origins. I know how you were born and who your father is. Go ask your mother by whose medicine and ministrations your birth took place, who your father is. Fie on you, I know you to be a bastard child. . . ."

When he received this tongue-lashing from his guru, the boy began to fret and so he went and queried his mother about it. "Tell me truthfully to my face, dear Mother, how was I born and who was my father?"

When she heard this from her son's mouth she was caught off guard and became quite agitated. Then, from safekeeping, she handed over her husband's letter about Jaya. As Bāghāmbara read the letter over and over, his eyes gushed with tears of sorrow and anguish, and he announced simply, "Listen, Mother, I must go to rescue my father. . . ."

His mother replied, "My child, what I hear from your mouth strikes me like a bolt of lightning crashing from the sky. You can't do this."

"Listen, Mother, with your own ears to what my father has written. For what reason would you, my own mother, try to dissuade me? It says that the Sagara royal lineage was destroyed by the curse of a brahmin. One particular son, Bhagīratha, single-handedly saved the lineage. Even Govinda saved his own mother. Even though I am just a mere mortal, just so much worthless dust and ash, I am duty-bound to try to find him. And if in that process I should die, then my life will have been made fruitful. I simply must try to save my father's line."

When the news spread, untold numbers of people quickly gathered there. Amara then said before all assembled, "Treat my mother as if she is the mother of you all." To his longtime playmates and friends he said, "Please honor my words. All of you must call my mother by the name 'Mother.' When he left, the disc-wielding Viṣṇu sent the whole of Gokula into paroxysms of agitation, and the young women, the cowherd girls, all wept bitterly." Then the young boy took formal leave by touching his mother's feet, just as Bhagīratha had done when he went to bring back Gaṅgā.

The crowds followed him, just as they had followed Nimāi when he renounced the world to become an ascetic.[7] His mother wept and cried out, "Why have you inflicted this misery on me? . . ."

A thousand salaams at the feet of Satya Nārāyaṇa. Shout 'Hari, Hari!' with all your heart.

Bāghāmbara's mother wept without respite, becoming disheveled, her now unkempt body covered with dust, just as Kauśalyā wept at Rāma's departure for the forest, or as Yaśodā and Rohiṇī were bathed in tears of grief when Kṛṣṇa left Gokula for Mathurā. As the local women rolled in the dust in their agony over Nimāi's renunciation when he became an ascetic, the whole of Śrīhaṭṭa city rushed to express its heartfelt grief. The citizens of Ayodhyā would not let Rāma depart, and so did the good women run out, crying, clothes only half covering their breasts in their rush. It was no different from Murāri consoling the cowherd women when he departed. Amara's mother wept, "I do not have five or six sons, I have but one. When I don't see my son I have no cause to live, everything goes completely dark. Don't go, my child, please don't go! Wait just a little longer, please! I would rather die drinking poison than to see you go. . . ." And so she lamented. Amara reassured her saying, "O Mother dear, I humbly submit this to you: I promise to return for your joy and prosperity." Then the young man begged leave, bowing at her feet, just as Bhagīratha had done when he went to retrieve Gaṅgā.

Amara moved off quickly, crossing over the mountains, just the way Rāma went in search of Sītā. After a while this young man of the merchant clan began to suffer from a severe thirst, but no water was to be found until the Lord Khodā, in the form of a fakir, sped forth bearing water from the Gaṅgā River. The young man whispered, "Without water I can stand up no longer."

The fakir said in return, "My dear child, drink this water from the Gaṅgā."

Amara replied, "Please hand over the Gaṅgā water, for should I drink it straight from your hand I will lose my caste standing."

The fakir rebutted his observation by saying, "Do not observe such niceties, for there is no difference, no difference at all between among the Vedas, the Purāṇas, and the Qur'ān."

"Even though I can confirm fully that your words correspond to what is written," the young man said, "still with my eyes I can only envision the manifest and true form of Govinda."

The fakir quietly rejoined, "Then shut those two eyes of yours, my child, and you will behold Lord Śyāma, blue-green as rain-laden monsoon clouds." And when Bāghāmbara Rāya closed his eyes, he embraced the true and essential form of Govinda, the Lord replete with all mercy. That dark-skinned fakir, wearing a tattered patchwork garment, suddenly sported a peacock-feather crown, which wafted gently in the breeze. The conch, discus, club, and lotus—all emblems of Lord Viṣṇu—shone majestically in the hands of his four arms, and a golden crown graced his head. Then he was the Lord Banamālī, who indulged in many hundreds of unpredictable exploits, Kṛṣṇa, who had assumed his trademark stance of three bends—at the knees, the waist, and the neck—playing his flute named Muralī.

With his own eyes, Bāghāmbara looked upon his Lord Govinda, and then the young man declared, "In this one day have all the austerities of my previous lives come to fruition. That which I have seen, my eyes filled with the image of the all-compassionate Lord, was no different from what Akrūra, Kṛṣṇa's paternal uncle, saw reflected in the waters. When Dhruva was but five years old and practiced terrible austerities, Kṛṣṇa recognized the desire of his devotee and granted him a vision." Speaking like this, the young boy fell down and grasped the feet of Govinda, who shed that form and again stood before him as the fakir.

In proper order the boy ate clotted cream and bread, and then drank the Gaṅgā water. Kavibara sings the inspired words of the Pīr's book.

Off Bāghāmbara went to the city of Ijvillī to meet with the supplier of flowers and garlands, but not before making sublime offerings to the Pīr for the welfare of family and lineage. "Whenever there is danger, just think of me, my child." And with these few words the disc-wielding Pīr vanished from sight.

With each of the hundreds of regions he traversed, the young man grew increasingly unsettled, indeed worried. But finally this young merchant entered the municipality of Ijvillī. Under a flowering *kadamba* tree on the banks of the flower gardener's own lake, the young merchant's son, Bāghāmbhara Rāya, came to rest. The garland weaver came down the path with a large clay pot wedged between the crook of her arm and her waist. When she came upon the young merchant boy she inquired of him, "From what far away place have you arrived here, my child? What is your name? Please tell me everything, spare no detail."

Amara replied, "Since you have asked, listen, Mother, to my sad tale of misery and strife. Some time ago my home in the city of Śrīhaṭṭa was swept up and away by a deluge. I abandoned that place in search of my kin and have now arrived here. For the sake of family and lineage I have searched through untold numbers of wild tracts and forests, searching for that one household that might provide news of my father." When the flower vendor heard his story in his own words, she took him in as her own foster child or godson. She showered his face with kisses. Just as Yaśodā had enveloped Devakī's child [Kṛṣṇa] in her bosom, the garland weaver pulled him onto her lap. The old woman confided in Bāghāmbara, "Terror reigns in this land, terror of a notoriously powerful yogī. Don't venture outside this compound, my child, for no sooner does the yogī see you than your life is destroyed."

"How does this yogī appear? What exactly does he do, how does he act?"

The crone replied, "Pay attention, my dear one, to these details as I relate everything I know. Once there was a merchant who hailed from Śrīhaṭṭa, one Jayānanda.

This yogī abducted his wife and spirited her here. The yogī has become a necrophagous ghoul, for he has destroyed the entire lineage. He magically transformed the king and all the inhabitants of his kingdom into palmyra palm trees. But he has spared me alone because he has a desire for flowers and garlands. For that I am a most unfortunate woman, my Child, so please, I beg you to pay heed to my warning."

When he heard this dire speech of the garland weaver, he quite naturally became unsettled and even wept a little, for he was just a young boy. "All the suffering I have endured, the misery I've borne in search of my family, has come to naught. Better I should enter the searing flames of the pyre here and now."

When the old garland weaver heard this boy's lament, she said, "Not one watch of my day is exempt from fear of the yogī. Even after the eighth *daṇḍa*—but a few hours after day's start—when he journeys to the isle of Laṅkā. . . ." The child queried, "Why can't Campāvatī make good her escape then?" To which the crone answered, "How can she get away? The yogī transforms her into an inert lump of flesh and keeps her secure in his compound."

"Tell me, my dear mother, how is it possible that this young woman is made to die and then miraculously is brought back to life again as the same Campāvatī?"

"Ah, he has two rods, one made of gold, one of silver. By the touch of the golden rod, Campāvatī's body is animated and brought back to life. But when the silver rod is touched to her body, she dies, and she remains lying on a special pallet, an unformed lump of dead flesh. Every day the yogī takes the life of the young woman and heads off to Laṅkā. In the evening, the yogī returns and once again awakens her. He keeps these two magic wands in the same place every day," the garland weaver confided, "right under the girl's pillow." When he heard this, Bāghāmbara was overcome with dread of the yogī, and because of that fear hid himself inside the flower vendor's house. Just as Lord Hari had hidden in the village of Gopapūra out of fear of King Kaṃsa, this special young man sought refuge in the garland weaver's house for several days.

And so it continued. Every day at precisely the same time the yogī left for Laṅkā. From his secret hideaway the young merchant boy registered the yogī's comings and goings. Then one day the merchant entered the yogī's compound to familiarize himself with it. When he found the main door locked tight, he began to meditate, concentrating his mind. The youth struck his hand hard on that impenetrable and indestructable door and the Lord of the Expanse of the Universe released and opened it. When Amara entered, the room was dark, but upon the pallet lay Campāvatī, a lump as good as dead. The young merchant then recalled the exact words of the garland weaver, and retrieved the two magic wands from under her pillow. The golden wand he struck lightly against her forehead, and Campāvatī sprang up reanimated, chanting the name of her Lord Kṛṣṇa. Amara stood rooted at the side of the pallet and Campāvatī instantly asked, "Who are you? Whose son are you? Where is your home? And what is your name? Tell me everything, my child, I am all ears."

Amara spoke, "Listen to my tale, Mother. My father is Hīrānanda, and Jayānanda is his younger brother. My name is Amara, my father's youngest brother's wife is Campāvatī. They are all traders by birth and station, operating out of the city of Śrīhaṭṭa." No sooner had she heard the words flowing from Amara's mouth than her eyes gushed tears like the rains of the month of Śrāvaṇa, the monsoon season. With the exclamation "Oh my dear child!" Campā fell to the ground and writhed, then, saying, "Come here, my boy!" she smothered him with kisses. "I had finally concluded that there was no one left alive in my extended family. It is my lineage's good fortune that the Lord has kept you safe and sound. This foul flesh-devouring yogī, a *piśāca*, brought me to this desolate forest and every member of my family who came in search has been transformed into a palm tree. I do not know by whose curse such fate has come to pass. . . ." And so Campāvatī spoke of her sorrows between bouts of tears. "By the curse of a brahmin was the line of Sagara destroyed, yet it took but one son, Bhagīratha, to save that entire lineage. Perform the ritual offering of water for the deceased and abandon any attempt to save me. Go home, I beg you."

Amara calmly replied, "Auntie, please listen to what I have to offer. If the yogī can kill and then revive, he must be enlightened to the most secret knowledge. Do not hold anything back, my dear aunt, speak nothing but the truth. If you tell me the unwavering truth, then I can search out the this great lord's work and return. If you tell me, my dear aunt, the secret of the yogī's death, then I shall return you to our ancestral home and rescue our lineage."

Campāvatī replied, "My child, the answer to the question you have asked I do not know. I have no idea how the yogī can be killed. . . ."

Amara countered, "Listen very carefully to what I propose. Being an attractive woman, you command an array of weapons to excel in the wiles of sensual and erotic manipulation. You must beguile that yogī's heart with the deadly arrows of your coquettish sidelong glance and he will eventually tell you himself the means of his own death." Looking hard at her face, Amara concluded, "Use any means necessary to get him to give you the information. . . . Lie back down on the pallet, my dear aunt, and remain here in the compound. I must return quickly to the garland weaver's house." And with those words he touched her with the silver wand, and the enchanting woman fell in a lifeless heap back onto the bed.

All the way back to the flower vendor's enclave, Amara pounded his forehead. Fate had turned sour, for the phrase, "Use any means necessary to give you the information . . ." reverberated in his head like the dull ringing of bell metal.

The woman would melt the hard resolve and body of the very one she had come to fear as her mortal enemy.

Later that evening, the Nātha Yogī reentered his house and touched the golden wand to Campāvatī's head. Her life breath regained, she stretched herself out on the couch. Her face was a radiant moon, glistening like a female Śiva with the moon adorning her hair, the passions strung in her bow. With a subtle wink from her lotus eyes, she smiled suggestively and greeted him. "Welcome, Nātha Yogī, you appear youthful and rejuvenated." To which he replied, "So many days have I returned here to my home, but never have I seen you smile to the extent you do today." And so it went. . . .

Campāvatī baited him with a coquettish laugh, "Would you keep your promise to hold to the truth were I to ask you something personal? It has been twelve years since I came. Recognizing that the time is nearly up, you continue to honor my vow. But I am growing a little apprehensive and must ask you something. Because I am a woman dependent, and struck with misfortune, will you not show compassion?"

The Yogīnātha replied, "You are the queen of my existence. I will provide whatever you beg of me."

When she heard this, she smiled suggestively and looked demurely from the corner of her eye and said, "Explain to me how you manage to avoid death, tell me."

"Now that you have asked, listen and I will tell you the only possible cause of my demise. For four ages have I eluded death. From Kumbhakarṇa Rājā, Yudhisṭhira of old, Kaṃsa, Śiśupāla, to the valiant Jarāsandha, and all the rest—how did all these great heroes forsake death?"

Campāvatī responded, "Tell me all the details. My suspicions will be allayed once I hear your explanation. . . ."

Witness the wiles of this charming woman pitted against this worldly Nātha. The power and control of a woman is evidenced by the way Satyabhāmā finagled Kṛṣṇa into getting her the magical pārijāta *flower that never wilted, and the way that Śaṅkarī subdued Śaṅkara—you too should never underestimate the beggar along life's road.*

And so, continuing to charm with her flattering speech, the seductress placed her hand quizzically upon her cheek and smiled meekly, lips slightly pursed—and soon the hapless Yogīnātha's tongue was loosed and he spoke of his mortality. "Rāvaṇa's citadel in Laṅkā is surrounded by a high enclosing wall and along its perimeter grow banyan trees of the Ajaya variety. Listen carefully, my beauty, only when the owl that resides there is slain do I die, otherwise, queen of my life, I am impervious to death." After revealing his secret, the yogī prepared for bed. As soon as dawn came, he headed off to Laṅkā as was his wont.

Amara then returned and entered the yogī's house. "Wake up!" he urged as he looked at his aunt. ". . . In the same way that to reveal his brother Rāvaṇa's secrets Vibhīṣaṇa came to Rāma, so did he tell me the manner of his death." And so Campā told Amara everything she knew about the yogī's mortality. From the mouth of his aunt he lapped up every detail of the yogī's mortal vulnerability, just as Dilīp Kumāra had listened to the words of Jānakī. To enter the yogī's enclave, Bāghāmbara girded himself with armor and slung his shield. Picking up additional special weapons, Amara set his heart on the citadel of Laṅkā, just as Hanumān had once brought relief. Amara said, "May Hari join forces quickly, just as Akrūra came to fetch Govinda to oust Kaṃsa."

He traversed the forests and scaled the mountains, so Dvija Kavi has composed this sacred tale of the Pīr.

Along the tops of the mountains were numerous banyan trees. In the highest branches of one of those dwelled a pair of birds, known as Beṅgamā and Beṅgamī. They were raising two babies in their nest, and they hunted throughout the southern reaches of the isle of Laṅkā. While they were away a giant poisonous serpent spotted the two *beṅgamā* hatchlings and began to slither up the tree to eat them. Just as the king of cobras is called upon to protect children, calves, and the young of all animals, the *beṅgamā* hatchlings cried out, "Protect us, O Lord!" In the same manner that mother earth calls down torrential rains to quell raging fires in order to save young from the flames, so did the Lord Who Wields the Club, Gadādhara, espy the two nested birds amidst the sulfurous poison of the serpent. To Amara, who was close by, he commanded, "Slay that serpent!" Protected by his shield and armor, the young man rescued the two hatchlings, just as Hari would have any young cow or child in Vraja. He hacked the serpent to pieces, trampling its head, just as Govinda had once slain the antigod Agha.[8]

In the evening Beṇgamā and Beṅgamī returned to their nest carrying in their mouths game they had killed for their young. The young *beṅgamā* hatchlings instantly announced, "We cannot eat anything now. A young man from a foreign country just snatched us from the jaws of a serpent. Only when we can properly acknowledge our debt to him will we will eat the food and water you have brought." When they heard their children's story, the two birds sought out Amara. They fell at his feet in prostration to offer thanks. Beṅgamā and Beṅgamī concentrated their attention on him and spoke, "Because of you we have received the gift of life for our children. Anything you desire we will provide."

The young man thoughtfully replied, "Please show me around the isle of Laṅkā. Hidden deep within this forest of countless banyan trees lives a great owl. Fly me safely around the isle of Laṅkā so that I might find him. And as we tour please show me all of the dwellings and abodes of its people. That is the nature of my humble request. It is my desire to see the great citadel of Laṅkā."

The great bird sitting in the tree replied, "Listen, Amara, I will show you everything within the dark old-growth forests. Come sit on my back and I will fly you around Laṅkā. I will fly high into the heavens, but you need have no fear." And so, with a running commentary that lasted until nightfall, they toured the isle of Laṅkā with Amara perched on Beṅgamā's back.

Finally, and much to the delight of Amara, they espied the great owl sitting comfortably on the branch of a banyan tree deep within the forest. They had traversed deep into the southern part of Laṅkā, where they found him, sitting in the top of the tree with freshly slain game in his beak. Uttering the name of Govinda, the young merchant struck him. The owl was knocked out, and at that same instant Yogīnātha cried out. The young man quickly grabbed the owl and bound him around his waist, just as Hanumān had bound Rāvaṇa in Laṅkā long before. When Amara firmly cinched his rope around the owl's middle, a fever suddenly broke out in the body of Yogīnātha, who was at home. Beṅgamā then took wing, heading quickly to that very place, but he questioned Amara about his actions. When he heard what was going on, he said to Amara, "Come here and sit on my back." He then flew from the tree and fetched some food in his beak, while Amara sat serenely on his back. That evening Beṅgamā brought Amara across the mountains to the house of the garland weaver, and then returned to his own home.

The Mālinī called out to Amara, "Where have you been to, you lovely child?"

Amara replied, "I have been visiting the isle of Laṅkā. I have brought back the owl that controls the life of the yogī."

The old hag then said, "You must have gone crazy in the head to risk my position, because my family has been bound personally to the yogī to supply flowers. I have just come because the yogī has fallen ill with fever."

Later that day the young man departed, just the way the valiant Śyāma headed off to slay Kaṃsa. Amara entered into the compound of the yogī; the yogī was inside, but his magic rope had mysteriously disappeared. The yogī called out, "Who comes calling? I am not feeling well. . . ."

And now the poet enters the yogī's house with the hero.

Amara said bravely, "Listen carefully, Yogīnātha. Come out here and meet me face to face."

The yogī slapped his head in disbelief—he still could not find his magic rope. Yogīnātha worried that perhaps his past karma had created this diversion and delay. When he could not locate the magic rope anywhere in the house, he was at a loss what to do. Finally he emerged, an old and decrepit man, limping, holding his knees. When he beheld Amara he questioned him, "Where do you come from? Whose son are you? . . ."

The young man replied, "My home is in the municipality of Śrīhaṭṭa. My father is named Hirānanda, and I go by the name of Amara. Jayānanda is my uncle, my father's brother, and his wife is my Aunt Campāvatī. I have come to search out news of my family, which has undergone such a strange twist of fate. A yogī once visited our estates to beg alms. But this yogi was cruel and obnoxious and stole away my aunt instead. One by one the members of my extended family struck out in search of her, but not one returned to our ancestral home. As I in turn searched out clues along the way I found this bird. No one recognizes it, but you certainly must. Look here and see. . . ." And as he said that he pulled it out. The first glance struck the yogī like a thunderbolt.

"The wiles of women are nefarious. She tricked me with her questions. That sweet young girl Campāvatī has brought me my doom. I am dumbstruck, I don't know what to say. I feel like Kīcaka, who was slain because of Draupadī's trickery."[9] The yogī continued, "I shall revive the members of your family for you—but in exchange give me back the owl, for it holds my life force." And with these words, the decrepit old yogī sprinkled a magical flower-scented water and suddenly the six brothers and their six horses appeared.

This son of a merchant was overjoyed to find his family restored and alive; he fell down in prostration at the feet of his father. Hīrānanda spoke, "Tell me all of your particulars. Whose son are you? Where is your home? What is your name, my child?"

The young man replied, "My residence is the municipality of Śrīhaṭṭa. My father is Hīrānanda, and my name is Bāghāmbara."

As soon as he heard this, Hīrānanda embraced his son and showered him with kisses as the tears gushed from his eyes. "It is just the same as when Nārāyaṇa saved his mother and father and Bhagīratha rescued his lineage in days gone by. But how were you able, my child, to overcome such incredibly complicated and dangerous difficulties?"

The boy said, "The bird lived on the isle of Laṅkā and the life force of the yogī lives within the bird. I was able to save you by capturing the owl." He continued, "Father, I am now going to turn all of the fan palms around us back into humans."

As he promised, he turned to the yogī and commanded, "When you have brought the king and his subjects back to life, let them go home!"

No sooner had he heard than the yogī once again sprinkled the magical flower-scented water, and the king, along with all of his subjects, was resuscitated. It was no different from the time the cows had been hidden in Brahmā's waterpot and Kānu returned them after a year, or the time when that famous son of Vraja brought back to life the children of Vraja who had been poisoned. And as everyone began to return to their homes, the young man wondered, "Shall I give the life-bird back to the yogī?" But no sooner had he said this than it struggled free and headed to the ocean, and there on the banks Bāghāmbara struggled with it. He thrashed the bird along the shoreline, but it escaped repeatedly as they moved down the beach and into the sea. Finally he plunged directly into the ocean to catch the wayward owl and did, but a monstrous bottom-feeding sheatfish, a *rāghava boyāla*, thought he was food and swallowed him whole.

Inside the belly of that sheatfish, Amara called for Kṛṣṇa, and Hari, who is affectionate to his devotees like a parent, appeared to extract him from this bind. Just as he had when Bhīma raised his head to call for Kṛṣṇa's help, Hari plunged into the waters to save his devotee. He grabbed hold of the fish and slit his belly end to end. He extracted Amara and held him tight. Amara sang the praises of his Lord, who once held the Blue Mountain on the tip of his finger, "You are the one who once saved an elephant from the jaws of a crocodile." He continued, "Listen, O Lord and

Master of the Triple World, I shall now hand over to the merchant the owl I have caught." It really was no different from the time Kṛṣṇa returned the stolen gem, Syamantaka, to Satrājit,[10] or when Bhīma took the life of Jarāsandha.[11]

But the Lord replied, "Why have you saved and protected this owl? I command you to crush this evil owl under your left foot as insult."

The young man then began to stomp the owl underfoot, but did so with a troubled heart. The yogī cried out in agony, "O Father of my father, I am dying!" Yogīnātha then turned to the boy and said, "Please, my child, don't kill me. I beg of you, just leave me here alone. . . ."

"Why do you plead with me now? You were the one who murdered the king and his court and then arrogated to yourself their powers as ruler." The merchant then killed the owl, at ease now with the decision. And there, in his own house, the yogī fell slain. By slaying the owl, the boy had alleviated much suffering and agony, just as Govinda relieved the cowherds by killing the demoness Pūtanā.

The gardener Mālinī's two sons—these three having been spared in order to supply the yogī with flowers—then entered the house and together they explained to the king with great relief and joy all that had transpired. "This young prince of a boy from a land far away came and restored everyone to life." To which the king promptly and appropriately replied, "Then I shall give him the hand of my daughter, Sumati, in marriage." He brought the young man before his royal advisers, ministers, and priests, who then called the astrologers, who, with arcane calculations, fixed the auspicious time. The drums were sounded throughout the halls of the king's palace and hundreds upon hundreds of subjects gathered to witness the wedding.

The bride and groom passed their first night in a house set aside for their use and the well-wishers were thrilled at the auspicious start for the couple.

The auspicious postwedding functions
the brahmin priests performed
  for the purification of Sumati.
The conch sounded, the kettle drums pounded
as the heavenly courtesans danced;
  Lord Śrīnivāsa himself was conspicuously present.
Worshiped were Lord Gaṇeśa like the sun,
Hari-Hara, half Śiva and half Viṣṇu,
  and obeisances made to the feet of Pārvatī.
Indra and all the others
were worshiped with grandeur,
  according to the sixteen scriptural injunctions—
Offerings of natural fragrances from the earth,
and bunches of paddy and sacred *durbbā* grass,
  each according to the auspicious custom.

With the undying matrimonial thread
the best of the twice-born bound the knot,
  as the conch screamed and *hulāhuli* trill rang out.
Plates were set to propitiate ancestors,
the walls marked with special symbols,
  as the small *dundubī* drums sang in the back.
Mixed were the seven special substances,
jeweled lamps were lit,
  and the praises and hymns begun.
At the most aupicious part of the ritual
the faces of the bride and groom
  were decorated and perfumed.
Brought out on a sanctified platform,
and seated facing west,
  the bride was formally given over.
Wedding crowns and special vestments,
jewels and other riches were bestowed,
  as Sumati was garlanded.
Other blessed women
bound their hands together
  with a special cloth.
After the radiant young bride
was given away by her father,
  Amara spoke in the traditional manner.
When they sat facing south,
a thin cloth draped over their heads,
  the bangles were slipped on her wrist.
Done according to scriptural injunction,
flowers rained down upon them,
  the wedding rituals were executed.
After the wedding was complete,
to the flowered bedchamber they went,
  to the praise of Lord Hari's qualities.

The couple was seated in the palanquin amidst a feeling of general weal and charm, a pleasant madness such as the bee feels when immersed in the flowering lotus. In this manner two more days of wedding festivities passed. On the third day the young merchant begged leave to depart. The words of his son-in-law struck the king like a thunderbolt, as if Indra himself had hurled one of his mighty bolts from atop the highest mountain. But the king heeded the measured request of the young merchant and so, with much love and affection, bestowed on him even more jewels and riches of various sorts. The king also furnished his son-in-law with several personal servants, both male and female, and happily sent along a contingent of foot soldiers and cavalry on horseback and elephants. Hirānanda and the other six lords rode atop majestic elephants, while Campāvatī rode in a comfortable silk-and-jute litter. The king offered good words of parting, and the son of the merchant paid his respects, "With your most generous blessings we take our leave to our own home."

They formed a train of about a hundred thousand people, many singing, while the king and queen wept, rolling in the dust to express their inconsolable grief. Sumati gently consoled her mother, "O Mother, why do you weep so? A son belongs to the household, but doesn't the daughter always go to the other family's home? Why do you grieve for me? You tell me yourself, in whose house do you reside?" With these final words they took their leave of all assembled. And Amara took special leave of Mālinī, the garland weaver who had helped him.

Passing through hundreds of small kingdoms and principalities, the young prince of a merchant finally entered the municipality of Śrīhaṭṭa with his entire clan in tow. When King Mādhava heard and fathomed all that was told, he sanctioned appropriate gifts to mark the occasion. The citizens of Śrīhaṭṭa all strained to get a look at Amara, just like the time Rāma returned to Ayodhyā and dispelled everyone's misery. Jananī was thrilled to look on the face of her son, just as Kauśālya had received Rāma back into her fold.

Amara spoke, "Listen carefully, Father and all his brothers, my uncles, this suffering befell our house because we failed to worship Satya Pīr." Hīrānanda unhesitatingly replied, "Then let us do what I am about to propose: Let us together prepare a ceremonial worship of the Pīr without delay. . . ." And so invitations were issued to the king and his court, all the family friends, and with great joy and celebration did they perform the ritual honoring of the Pīr. A small shrine was constructed, marked on the four corners with arrows. With an offering of 125 betel leavels, Satya Pīr was formally installed. Flower garlands, a canopy of cloth, and a golden oversized chopping knife, along with another 125 betel quids were placed upon the shrine. One and one-quarter maunds of wheat flower were mixed with another one and one-quarter maunds of sugar to form the raw base of the *śirṇi* offering, which they cooked and offered to the Pīr. The brahmin priest offered the ritual worship of the five deities, then the conch rang out and the *hulāhuli* trill resounded. After the *kalimā* was recited, the *śirṇi* was made beneficent. All assembled consumed a portion of the Pīr's *śirṇi*. Big and small, young and old rose up and exchanged their salaams: "May the Pīr Bhagavān bless your home." Then the son took his new bride to the mansions of the merchant's family.

May everyone cry out, "Hari, Hari!" showing the joy on their faces. And so this tale comes to a close. Place your mind at the feet of Hari—feet that remove the miseries from all those who remember.

The Mother's Son Who Spat up Pearls

Kiṅkara Dāsa's *Matilāla Pālā*

In an act of contrition,
cross both arms over your chest and
bow to pay your respects to Satya Nārāyaṇa,
the one imagined in the calculus of the Veda,
the avatāra *of the Kali Age here on earth as*
the Lord God Khodā, Nirañjana the Stainless One.

Rāma and Rahim—these two are but one;
they are distinct neither in the heavens,
nor in their qualities enumerated in the Qur'ān and the Purāṇa.
To navigate this vast ocean of sin
may Satya Pīr be your helmsman—
allow no other thought to enter your heart.

View the strife and conflict of this world as devoid of substance,
ultimately arising from an attachment to the ephemeral world—
this is the unprecedented teaching of Lord Sāheb.
He suspends stone arches in the sky,
He holds up the walls of the fort so they do not fall—
the very heaven and earth exist at his command.

To the Pīr goes the essence of the śirṇi *food offering;*
the land and the sky belong to him,
so too the play of fire and movement of water.

Along the bay he makes the sands of the shore stable,
glinting a fiery red from pearls and diamonds,
the nearby jungle replete with tigers and bears.

The Sāheb's appearance glows elegant and fine,
in his hand a golden staff; mellifluously
this preceptor to the gods mutters the kalimā *creed,*
a white cap on his head,
lustrous as the deer-carrying moon,[1] *as if*
Cakrapāṇi the Disk-Wielder himself appears before your eyes.

When the Lord shows favor to someone,
what he bestows produces
an experience that has no compare.
Friend to those who are his devotees,
this ocean of mercy looks favorably on the downtrodden.
May you, my dear father, come to my worshipful gathering!

Always pleasant in speech and demeanor,
the name of the Lord Sāheb should issue forth
seven times from the mouths of those gathered.
The satisfaction and pleasure of the Pīr bears fruit—
and so the twice-born poet Kaṇva speaks
in total submission, offering a thousand salaams.

Listen, everyone, open your ears to the joyful play of the Lord Sāheb. All desires will be fulfilled, sweeping the body in waves of pleasure. Nārāyaṇa had been seated in Mecca absorbed in meditation when he inquired of his courtier about the ritual prescriptions of his worship, his *pūjā*, out in the world. "In this Kali Age the power of reason and custom are severely tested in the public domain. In the east I have continued to receive worship, but people there in the west are befuddled and forgetful. In the southern lands people have proffered the *śirṇi*, but show me anyone in the north doing this."[2]

Hearing this, the wazir replied with his hands pressed together in respect, "While there are many there, only a few in the north worship. In the city of Āraṅga in Rāṅgpur region lived a prosperous merchant with three others—his wife, his son, and his son's wife. About a year ago the father was killed by a bolt of lightning.

Although he worshiped Lord Śiva, the young son of the merchant never went out to ply his trade. By the good grace of the Lord they had accumulated great wealth, and hosts of male and female servants tended to the young merchant's wife, Śīlāvatī. Should he be the one to celebrate your worship in ostentatious public display, then your fame would spread throughout the world. Go and make yourself known through the dreams of this young trader. You must assume the guise of his father and go to that city to speak to him. Afterward you will undoubtedly receive great and affectionate worship. If he will but leave his home and head out to foreign lands to trade, your popularity will definitely increase. . . ." When he heard this, Satya Nārāyaṇa was truly pleased at the prospect.

During the last dark of night, Satya Pīr went to the city of Āraṅga, and appeared above the young man's head dressed in the garb of his father. In this guise he said, "Listen to me, you black mark on my lineage. You have squandered my riches bestowed by Kubera, the god of wealth, by never observing the custom of boarding a ship to trade, wasting your life idly, and eating as if that wealth were as endless as the grains of sand in the ocean. My name was renowned as an able trader and through my travels I increased my personal wealth twentyfold. Were you to carry on this trade, your fame would likewise reign supreme, but the wealth accumulated in my household you have let slip away like offerings of water and flowers. In the city of Āraṅga my name meant something and I guided my seven boats hither and yon. All seven of my boats are still in working condition. First thing in the morning when you arise, you must call your pilot and helmsman." And with these words Nārāyaṇa disappeared, and the young merchant was jolted from his sleep and became instantly alert.

The young merchant sat up and bewailed his lot with mournful cries of "Hāya, hāya." This servant Kiṅkara sings as he bows to Lord Nārāyaṇa.

As soon as she heard the anguished cry of the merchant,
that blessed and beautiful Śīlāvatī jumped up and,
  weeping, clasped the feet of her husband.
"O lord of my life, what started you awake,
why do you cry out so suddenly? I can't tell,
  have you seen something in a dream?
Always have we been favored by Lord Śiva,
for the wealth of Kubera sits in our house,
  our stores are filled with rubies and other gemstones.
What misery could possibly invade our home?
Serving men and women meet our every need.
  Who could say anything hurtful or critical?"
Hearing her response, the merchant was filled
with the desire to console his lovely wife, so

he hugged her neck and smothered her with kisses.
"Listen, my beloved Satyāvatī.
What I am about to order
you must never try to countermand."
The good wife replied, "Listen well, my lord,
whatever you say I will not only listen, but
will hold it dear like your feet as my truth.
Whatever you say is what I will do,
otherwise I would give up my life.
How could I oppose my husband and master?"
The merchant then replied, "So pay attention, dear one.
In my dreams last night I beheld clearly
my father, who severely rebuked me.
I hold my father's words on my head as sacred,
so tomorrow shall I outfit his seven trading boats
and make ready to trade!"
His wife was dumbstruck to hear this so out of the blue.
The skies had fallen on her head, such was
the bitter gall borne of her husband's words.
"If what you say is true, how can you even contemplate it?
You, my lord and master, plan to abandon me,
making me one without a protector!"
She uttered these words in smoldering agony
and with much weeping fled
to tell her mother-in-law as she clasped her feet.
Before the morning was done, the merchant's mother
had heard the whole story
that Kiṅkara Dāsa now relates.

Upon hearing the news of the impending trading venture, the old woman took her daughter-in-law straightaway to see her merchant son. The elder woman blurted out, "My child, what are these crazy things issuing from your mouth? Are you going to make me suffer the same grief as Caitanya's mother, Śacī Ṭhākurāṇī?[3] Stay right here at home, my child. What's the point of this trading enterprise? . . ." It was no different from the time Kauṣālyā wept and pleaded with Rāma.

Grasping the feet of his mother, the young merchant explained, "If I continue my ways of remaining idle and not trading, in no time everything will go to ruin. The Veda, the sacred scripture, is also called the mother of the Dharma Śāstras and the Puraṇas. Those two sets of *śāstras* are in turn the eyes of the knowing and the wise. Were you to follow just one, you might manage, but listen to what the *Bhāgavata Purāṇa* predicts should both sources of authority be abandoned: Anyone who abandons family and traditions of righteous action, even though born in the Gaṅgā itself, becomes the living epitome of pride inflated with envy and malice. Should one dwell only on the superiority of one's birth, the *Bhāgavata* gives no credence to that, good or bad. Why else after the cow sacrifice did the aspiring sage Viśramila take birth as a *yavana*—a non-Hindu foreigner—from the womb of the seer's wife? Diti, the daughter of Dakṣa, was the wife of the sage Kaśyapa; so how could an antigod, an *asura*, spring forth from her womb? Look in which caste Mucirāma Dāsa took birth—who gets the morsel of benefit when the bell rings in sacrifice? However brilliant he might be, one who casts aspersions on others is considered of the lowest social rank. How can I possibly call him an enlightened or high-souled one? Between the highest and the lowest there is virtually no difference, for wisdom and honor are reckoned precisely the same in the body of each. When a person born of a low caste applies himself and purifies his mind by practicing devotion to Kṛṣṇa, no longer is that individual considered lowly. Now try to understand, my dear mother, what I am about to say." The merchant then informed his mother, "I am going out on trade. Mother, you absolutely must not try to block me in any way. If a practicing farmer sloughs off in his indolence, he grows only misery and perpetual shame. And so it is that my own path of proper conduct falls to trade. That, Mother, is unmistakably the traditional activity to which my clan is bound—and that I must observe."

With this justification the merchant consoled his mother, then quickly sent for his East Bengali helmsman and crew. Recalling the ways of his father, he made ready his seven cargo ships, and in no time the boats were set to ply the swirling waters of adventure.

He had summoned the astrologer, who made the necessary calculations—the boats set sail with all auspiciousness, as narrated by Kiṅkara.

The merchant's young wife assembled there all the prescribed items for ritual, and went off issuing auspicious trills to imbue the boats with a proper weal. The seven wave-runners rested magnificently, making her heart beat with excitement. It was just at this time the merchant was pleading with his mother. "Mother, please take my young bride and return home. Look after her and be sure to keep her close. When you prepare to sleep, lock the house up tight, for the merchant's wife is a devoted, true, and virtuous gem of a woman, making her highly desirable. But if you ever find evidence that her door is open, her chambers violated, then right then and there strip her of her the eight ornaments and finery that define her high status and banish her to the jungle. . . ."[4] Carrying on like this and issuing other instructions for some time, the merchant knelt at the feet of his mother to take formal leave.

When the most auspicious moment struck, the merchant launched his ships. The helmsman, grasping the boat by the ear, its prominent rudder, set sail. Gradually they watched the familiar banks of their own country slip by. Quickly they entered the confluence of the great rivers, and within a day and a night had reached the waters of the Gaṅgā. With a thrill pounding his heart, the merchant sailed toward Śāntipura, but soon both Śāntipura and Navadvīpa were left far behind. Eventually to port lay Hāliśahara, the point of the southern Triveṇī,[5] and all the seasoned adventurers remained hushed in their places, for there multitudes of powerful sages and holy men performed rituals for ancestors and austerities for their own release. To witness this in person brought joy to the young merchant. Anchoring his fleet of ships, the trader took a ritual bath and dispensed alms according to custom. Then, there on the banks of the Jāhnavī, he prepared a great feast for those holies. The rest of that day was passed on the Jāhnavī's shore, and only in the evening did the sages finish the rituals on the crew's behalf. Untold numbers of holy men gathered in that one spot, and they sat along the bank enigmatically consulting among themselves and each said in his turn: *Makra śūkla trayadośī nakṣatra* . . . which interpreted meant "When the fourth great star, Rohiṇī, the Moon's wife, sits in the constellation of the *makara* beast,[6] it will be the thirteenth day of the bright half of the lunar fortnight; and on this day, a Thursday, we see the powerful *taitala* conjunction of auspicious planets. There will come to pass an extraordinarily auspicious moment at the point of rising, a moment too powerful to be subverted: in late evening, during the thirteenth *daṇḍa*,[7] a shower of immortal star nectar will fall. Wherever those drops of nectar land, great things will spring into being. Should they fall on the head of an elephant, the fabled and enormous *gajamati* pearl will be shed; if they fall on bamboo, *tabasheer* will sprout up; when they fall into the oceans, magnificent pearls will be formed; when they fall on the head of a cow, it will issue forth that rich and valuable yellow pigment called *gorocanā*.[8] But should a drop fall on a woman hot in the throes of making love, she will bear a son of unprecedented nature. . . ."

From the mouth of this boy will issue pearls—this of course being all the merchant could hear, observes Kiṇkara.

The refined refuge of the sages' holy feet
the helmsman and crew had there for the taking;
    they slept easily on board that night,
all but the merchant,
who was still wide awake at dawn,
    the sages' predictions ringing in his ears.
The merchant was saddened
to hear talk of such an auspicious opportunity;
    if only he could find his way home in time.
"The sages' predictions are certain to come true—
Motilāl would have been born,
    a son would have graced my home."
He mulled over the prospects,
"How could I manage to return home

for I have already traveled some twenty days?"
With words like these did the merchant fret
while all the sages had long departed;
and so the good man wallowed in despair.
At just that moment Nārāyaṇa
was at repose in Mecca
and came to know of the merchant's anguish.
Wearing the clothes of a fakir,
he approached the good merchant
in order to impress him with his power.
He accosted the merchant with a query,
"Tell me what misery plagues your heart.
Speak frankly to me about it."
To hear this left the merchant dumbstruck,
but may Kiṅkara's wish be fulfilled
to land in the same presence of the fakir.

The merchant asked, "Who are you exactly? Where are you headed at this late hour, with only four *daṇḍa*s left of the night?"

"I am the Lord of the Universe. Listen carefully to my words. Now that you have encountered me directly, reveal that which ails you. May that which you desire be fulfilled. Anything you might want will come to pass if you but offer me *śirṇi*."

The merchant responded, "I have never known or worshiped any but Lord Śiva. By what virtue of yours should I proffer *śirṇi*?"

The fakir patiently countered, "Rāma and Rahim are but one. Why do you differentiate the Purāṇas from the Qur'ān? You clearly do not believe that I have told you the truth, but when you see it demonstrated before your very eyes, you will understand, my child!" And with these words Nārāyaṇa miraculously assumed the form of Śiva. He appeared replete with horn and drum, adorned with a necklace of bones; sitting on his bull, he played with deadly serpents.

When he beheld this spectacle, the merchant fainted and slumped to the boat deck. Casting off the form of Śiva, the fakir again stood before him, and the good merchant, when he regained consciousness, lost no time making his obeisance to the feet of the fakir. But the vision continued: At the foot of a *kadamba* on the banks of the Kālindī, Kṛṣṇa called out, "Rādhā, Rādhā!" and then played his flute, Muralī. Suddenly half of the fakir's body turned black, the other half a golden hue—Nityānanda and Gaura had landed up from Nadīyā.[9]

"By the mercy of the Lord have I seen, truly seen, his divine forms. It is no different from when Akrūra saw his form reflected in the waters of the Yamunā." The merchant continued, "I am not able to fathom anything of this divine play. But can you describe to me what burns my heart, you ascetic who aren't what you seem to be?"

The fakir replied, "You lay awake although you tried hard to sleep as the crew pushed back the boats. Earlier in the evening, when the sages had gathered, you came to know of the auspicious conjunction, the Māhendra Yoga, of which they all spoke. Today will bring a shower of nectar that makes everything fecund, producing riches—and a special child would be born if it fell when you were making love to your lover. All of this I divined from your thoughts, but most certainly that you would have gotten a son had you stayed at home."

The good merchant was utterly amazed when he heard this. "How can you read what is in my thoughts? Solemnly and truthfully do I vow to worship you as my Lord, O Shape-Changing Mendicant, if I am able to go home tonight."

When he heard the proposition, the Great Bestower and Lord, desiring to increase his prestige and position, immediately called to mind the king of all birds, a giant swan. As soon as he had been summoned by that mental call, the swan appeared and landed at the fakir's feet. "For what purpose, my Lord, have you called me?"

The Great Bestower said, "Listen, my child, king of birds. It is my desire that you dispatch quickly the needs of this merchant. . . ."

On his back will he take the good merchant away from that place and return him before night's end, predicts Kiṅkara.

That jewel among birds followed unquestioningly the command of the Great Bestower and carried the merchant on his back. By meditating on Lord Nārāyaṇa, it rose up into the sky, winging its way to the city of Āraṅga. He safely deposited the merchant there inside the house, then took roost on the roof to wait. The merchant was delighted to find everyone fast asleep, and so he entered his own quarters unmolested. To his attractive young wife the merchant called out, gently knocking on the door. "I have paid heed to the words of sages and so have returned home. Up! Up! Ruling goddess of my heart." But no matter how much the merchant called, his wife did not hear, although he did manage to disrupt her sleep.

When she finally woke up, she looked all around the room but did not see her merchant-husband. Melancholy crept back into her heart as she worried herself about this singularly odd voice. "Only one fortnight has passed since my husband left, but I do not recognize that voice at all. Perhaps it is some thief or amorous prankster who has come close by—but I don't understand his speech. He must be fearless to enter and call out my name, pretending to be my husband.[10] If my merchant-husband had come, he would have first called on his mother. Why would he come here in secret?"

Again the merchant called out as his wife stretched her ears, longing to hear, as the poet Kavi Kiṅkara tells it.

The merchant urged her, "Please open the door and be quick. I have deviated from my plan and come back, my beautiful. Once we are reunited I will explain everything.

But the night has nearly passed. How cruel the Fates! If I judge correctly, it would not be wrong to say that this fourth quarter of the night is fast slipping away. Yet when that auspicious conjunction has passed with no action there is bound to much suffering and regret over the missed opportunity."

The merchant's words finally penetrated the ear of this faithful housewife, who replied, "You cannot be my merchant-husband, because you have returned all alone. You left with untold numbers of boatmen, all in great spirits and cheer. Why do you now slink back alone in the middle of the night? Are you here to cause trouble? If you are really my husband, call on your mother. My husband took a vow and has gone on a trading voyage, not to come back until successful."

The merchant replied, "My beautiful woman, you do me an injustice in these matters. Please open the door quickly so that my mother does not come to know. Once I am inside your quarters I will satisfy your concerns. Light a candle of beeswax and look around. Let me start in the northeast corner and describe all the contents of your private room that only I could know. . . ."

Finally convinced, the beautiful woman accepted that only her husband would have this private knowledge, and so she lit a beeswax candle and threw open the door. The merchant quietly and quickly took his wife to bed. The love they made was radiant like that of Arjuna with Kṛṣṇa's sister Subhadrā. The love play between the two was prolonged and vigorous until all desires were sated during the alloted time of the *daṇḍa*. Then the wife demanded her own satisfaction, "Talk to me, my beloved, still my worries! Were you simply miserable without me and missed me? How could you return in the middle of your trip? . . ." And so the questions went.

The merchant replied, "My beautiful wife, listen carefully to all that I say. Upon arriving at the Triveṇī I anchored my boats. After spreading a great feast, the boatmen went to sleep; I alone sat awake on the boat. During that time the sages gathered en masse to perform their rituals. They sat all together and consulted, each adding his own calculations. 'Tonight will produce a particularly auspicious moment at the Māhendra Yoga planetary conjunction, and from the heavens a special shower will rain star-drops down on earth. From elephants will emerge the massive *gajamati* pearls, from bamboo its treasured immaculate eye, from the oceans gems of all sorts, and from a human a special son. This boy will spit perfect pearls from his mouth—but only from the couple who make love during the thirteenth *daṇḍa* of the night.' As I listened to these predictions, my heart grew weary, bereft of hope, when just at that low point a fakir magically came to grant me his grace. He told me in detail that which troubled me, then summoned a magnificent king of birds. On its back have I come and I have accomplished my goal. I must leave again before the night is over, but listen, this tale should remain secret for now, for if my mother hears of it she will see to it that I do not go back."

With this explanation, the couple fell back onto the bed for more pleasure, but as morning approached, the merchant was unaware, lost deep in his sleep. Then, reckoning their tardiness, that great lord of birds called out, "Come now, O merchantman, the night has nearly passed." Startled from his sleep, the merchant blinked his eyes awake and in a rush fled without saying a word to his still-sleeping wife. Before long the merchant seaman stood on his boat and the Great Bestower, Satya Pīr, instructed him to sail on. In the twinkling of an eye, the fakir was gone.

As the boats pushed off from the Triveṇī miles away, the merchant's mother chose that day to get up early. As she looked all around the old woman seemed a little agitated, in the way of those prone to suspicion, and she took herself to her daughter-in-law's door as she was wont to do. When she saw the door was ajar, she stepped right into her room. There in that bedroom the young wife was drowning in the deepest seas of sleep. Her ornaments, makeup, and other accoutrements still decorated her body. The old woman saw all the signs of a man having been in that bed. The beeswax candle burned fiercely like the inflamed passions of youth. "Someone must have plundered the riches of this fresh young woman last night. Someone must have planned this tryst well and in advance, for had it been a casual thief the jewelry that adorns her body would surely have been stolen. To see this is more than insufferable, her actions are audacious, her breasts are swollen with hubris. How will I ferret out the man who fulfilled her salacious desires?"

The old woman began to tremble with rage as a banana leaf in a light wind. Without hestitation she planted a violent kick square in her daughter-in-law's chest. The young bride was shocked instantly awake. The old crone demanded, "With whom did you go crazy and spend the night last night? As soon as the dark faded to dawn he must have fled. But you will suffer the full consequences of this abomination, you little whore! Hand over your fancy clothes and finery, every single ornament you own. I am only doing what your husband himself ordered; so don't blame me for your ills. Now find some rags and go as far away from here as you can!"

This beautiful young woman wept in her confused agitation, as is written by Kiṅkara.

At the scolding of the old woman, the faithful wife
looked but did not find her husband.
  The young beauty wept, beating her head with her hands.
She looked long at the empty bed
and cried out, "O, my husband and lord.
  Where have you gone, lord of my life?"
She wept like a child or one mad.
She made no attempt to fix her hair,
  but looked over and again at that empty bed.
"Why did you come in secret
but to drown me in a sea of misery?
  Why didn't you call your mother?

"Where have you, my lord and master, gone,
hurling me into this dismal disgrace?
  You have afflicted me with agony and torment.
"For what selfish pleasure did you make love
when it has cast your own wife into the depths of degradation?
  What did you hope to gain?
"It's no different from Śacī's own son,
who abandoned his own wife, Viṣṇupriyā;[11]
  that woman suffered immeasurably.
"That is my sad state.
No one will ever believe
  that it was my husband who returned. . . ."
With this lament the good merchant's wife
smashed her bangles against her forehead
  and then fainted, slumping to the floor.
"You left without saying even a single word to me;
consequently I did not make fast the door.
  What wrong did I ever do you?
"Listen, my dear mother-in-law,
to what your son said.
  He heard predictions from the mouths of sages.
"And he came here riding a great swan.
Many times he called out to me
  but I, a woman now with bad fortune, did not respond.
"He crept near and told me in a whisper
all the items that I kept here in the room—
  so convinced, I unbolted the door. . . ."
He went mad savoring the pure pleasures of love,
then he slipped away from the fateful bedroom.
  Kiṅkara intimates but the essentials of this private pleasure.

The old woman did not at all accept the young bride's explanation. She said, "I am going to throw you out of this house! . . ." And with promises like that she stripped off the bride of her "eight ornaments." Emboldened by her fury, she drove her away fiercely. The old woman forced her to wear tattered rags and then kicked her out. "Get out, you stinking wretch! Go! Right now, today! Go away from here, away from me!" And so the merchant's wife wept, heartbroken in her grief, just as the pure and chaste Sītā was cast out of the presence of her husband.

Reliving the events she thought, "When you returned, O lord of my life, to plunder me for sex, you placed me in mortal danger by not seeing your mother. She calls me unfaithful, and you alone are responsible for spreading this denigration. My lord, you put me into Viṣṇupriyā's sad state. When I was the respected wife of the merchant, what status and finery I enjoyed; now where will I go as a homeless waif, a *bāṅgāliṇī*?[12] And now I go with but a single worn sari and no jewelry, totally bereft. I must wander about in my weeping like some widow. Being the wife of a prominent merchant, I feel nothing but shame. I have no skills; what work can I even pretend to do? My randy husband went on a voyage to ply his trade as a merchant. Then at some strange predictions by a sage he comes flying back to my rooms on a swan! My lord made passionate love to me and left as quickly as he came, but he didn't alert his mother to his presence. First thing in the morning that ever-suspicious mother-in-law found my door ajar, unsecured. She took my standing, my eight ornaments, and drove me out. I am not defiled or guilty, so it can only be that I go now as the result of some past karma." And so it was that the merchant's good wife departed, leaving behind her one familiar kingdom to enter the unknown.

Not long after, the wife of the wazir of an adjacent land saw her and called her to her presence. The wazir's wife commanded her, "You must come to my house. I will fix everything and give you shelter." When she finally grasped these kind words, the now impoverished woman went along. The man of the house, the wazir, extended his protection as promised.

The days passed without event, but true to the sages' words, the merchant's wife had conceived. Day by day the women in the house watched her stomach grow to the point where the wazir's wife felt compelled to make inquiries among the female servants. No one knew how many days she had been pregnant, nor by whom. "How," they mused, "could this *bāṅgāliṇī* get pregnant while she has been sequestered in this house?" This of course got the wazir's wife to thinking: "I do not know whether or not the wazir is responsible for this, but when I see her bulging womb so radiant and effulgent my mind is confused, indeed troubled." Worrying along these lines the wife called her husband the wazir. "It appears that this wastrel *bāṅgāliṇī* has practically become my co-wife!" The wazir's wife, now worked up, continued, "This evil bitch has taken my place with the wazir and I am no longer desired. All of us will be shamed and our wealth and status dissipated by this. Drive her out! Rid us of this nuisance! Should the ruling *badshāh* come to know if it, we are surely ruined!"

The wazir calmly replied, "That would be an unjust pronouncement, contrary to righteous behavior. He who offers shelter to a woman like this makes her his own child of righteousness, a goddaughter. But you are certainly advising me to a contrary path of action!" And with these words he had the *bāṅgāliṇī* fetched to him. "I realize that Bidhātā, lord of fate, has turned his face away from you. Explain to me just exactly who did this to you, for this is undoubtedly the reason your mother-in-law drove you out."

The *bāṅgāliṇī* replied, "I am not of a stained character. I have known none other than my husband, not even in my dreams. My husband impregnated me and then went abroad. The old woman turned me out into the wilds of the jungle because of some past fault or bad deed. Please show me your favor and let me stay a few days longer. May the arbiter of justice, Dharma himself, witness whether my words are true or false." And thus she proclaimed her innocence.

The wazir considered carefully, "This is both inappropriate and infamous in our world. People will condemn us if we continue to shelter you. . . ." With these fateful words he quickly drove her out. So this afflicted woman went her way, crying convulsively with every step.

In the southern quarter of the village lived a poor brahmin. He was knowledgeable of the sacred Āgama scriptures and knew well the art of astrological calculation. He had no son, and no daughter either. He and his loving wife lived by themselves. It was at their door the *bāṅgāliṇī* landed. When he looked at her, the twice-born questioned, "Who are you? What has happened to put such a beauty as you into this pitiable condition? What is the reason for this?"

The *bāṅgāliṇī* then told him her tale from beginning to end. "My husband is responsible for my pregnant condition, but it was my mother-in-law who put me out."

As the brahmin listened he grew very troubled at these events, indeed dismayed. He divined the truth of it through yogic meditation that allowed him to see all. "I now can verify that it was indeed proper sexual union with your husband that made you pregnant, just as you say. The rumors people spread are all lies; you are not a fallen woman." The brahmin continued, "My dear young woman, you must live in our home. I am moved to compassion when I see you pregnant and suffering so."

The young woman gratefully replied, "You have shown mercy to this most unfortunate wretch. To be the wife of a fabulously wealthy merchant-husband, my misery is all the more extreme, for I used to live in luxury in a palace. . . ."

The young beauty's voice broke with emotion, according to Kiṅkara.

The brahmin advised her, "My dear woman, cast away your miseries. Listen with rapt attention and each bit of your suffering shall gradually be removed."[13]

> Lord Rāma, the son of Daśaratha of the Sun Dynasty, went into exile in the forest to honor the vow of his father. Lord Rāma, Lakṣmaṇa, and Sītā entered the Pañcāvatī Forest and there they built a small hut, where the three of them lived. Spurred by his demonic sister Sūparṇakhā, Rāvaṇa abducted Sītā to the isle of Laṅkā and kept her there in the Aśoka Grove. Grieving over Sītā, Lord Rāma befriended Sugrīva as an ally, and subsequently constructed a land bridge to Laṅkā, where he killed Rāvaṇa and rescued Sītā. He put Sītā through the fire to test her fidelity and then returned to Ayodhyā. There he was anointed king and ruled as the jewel of the Raghu Dynasty. Jānakī was one of three sisters born of Janaka. The other two were Alakā and Ujjvalā, each married to

a brother of Rāma. The sisters questioned Jānakī, "Can you tell us how Rāvaṇa looked?" Sītā replied, "I have never looked upon the ten-faced Rāvaṇa. I have never looked into the face of a man other than my husband. It is a fact that at the moment that horrible figure placed me on his chariot I saw only his reflection in the waters." Then she drew a picture to show them: ten heads, ten eyes, and twenty arms.

Just as the sisters of Jānakī were examining the picture, in walked that jewel of the Raghus, Rāma. When he saw the picture, Rāma grew instantly furious, "How can you draw that grotesque figure, Sītā, and still feel good? If Sītā, the moon-faced one, has never looked on him, how could she manage to draw him now that she is back home—this I'd like to hear! She has piously told everyone living that she never looked upon his face." Sarcastically he mocked her, "*I know no other man save my Rāma.* . . ." The great ruler of Ayodhyā seethed with rage.

Later that night Rāma ranted, venting bitter accusations. At that same time, a washerwoman passed by on her way to her father's house and overheard. There she reported, "I tell you truthfully, dear Father, her husband does not accept her. . . ." And so the rumors began as the old man cast aspersions on Rāma to his son-in-law: "Why has good King Rāma brought back a wife he has cast aside? For oh-so-many days was Sītā captured in the Aśoka Grove, but Rāma brought her home anyway. That in itself defies the imagination, is absurd. The king may find all this tolerable, but I will not stand for it. If this is going to be countenanced, then let Rāma hear of our feelings. . . ."

When Rāma did hear the rumors, he angrily ordered Lakṣmaṇa, "Exile Sītā to the forest under the pretext of procuring the special foods for her pregnancy ritual of *sādha*"—for she was then pregnant. The command hit Lakṣmaṇa like a bolt of lightning, but on the sixth month of her pregnancy he did as ordered and took her into the forest. He pretended that Sītā must desire to eat the wild fruits of the jungle according to the *sādha* ritual custom—and with this kind of argument he took her away. Once there Lakṣmaṇa told her, "Go anywhere you want. Because of the peoples' talk, my brother has abandoned you to exile." When she heard this, Sītā fainted straightaway, and Lakṣmaṇa made good his escape back to Rāma.

Sītā remained in the forest, weeping inconsolably, when Vālmikī found her. The great sage had already divined through his yogic techniques that Jānakī was completely without fault. And he kept the daughter of Janaka there in the Tāpovana hermitage. Deep in the Creeper Forest, Sītā gave birth to Lava, then Kuśa came forth fully formed, while the sage looked after Lava and took him away. The two sons were a treasure trove of fine qualities, and in time proved brilliant in the arts of war. Eventually in pitched battled with them, King Rāma himself would suffer defeat. . . .

Receiving this encouraging instruction, the impoverished *bāṅgāliṇī* moved into the brahmin's house. Out of great concern and affection, the brahmin fed her well. And so things went for ten lunar months and ten days—the typical gestation period—when the young woman told the brahmin of her labor pains. As soon as he heard, the brahmin fetched a midwife from the town; and as soon as others heard the news they too hurried forth. The young woman had no experience of childbirth and so was very much afraid, but even though one may not be aware of it, the power of the Pīr over the illusion of this world is always present. On an extremely auspicious moment, she gave birth to a son of unprecedented character. All the women gathered felt a thrill when they saw him. "Look at what an incredible son this vagabond *bāṅgāliṇī* has borne. The little boy glows like a rising moon dispelling the darkness."[14]

The midwife observed, "Had this boy arrived in the king's palace, the king would have lavished on me plates and vessels and fine clothes." And with this pronouncement, she clipped the umbilical cord and lit the ritual fire to incinerate the placenta. Then the old midwife gently placed the boy in the lap of the mother, the *bāṅgāliṇī*. Adjusting him on her lap, she placed her breast in his mouth. But as she gazed at his face her heart grew heavy in grief. Weeping now uncontrollably, the young woman told everyone there, "I would have stayed at home if I had known this boy would be born." As he snuggled in his mother's lap, the little boy made gurgling noises and from his mouth miraculously popped out a little pearl, perfectly formed. It fell to the floor; Śīlāvatī quickly moved to scoop it up. It glowed like the moon, casting a pinkish tint across the room. Then she wept as she recalled her husband's tale. As she looked at the pearl, a perfect *motilāl*, she rushed forward, joy racing in her heart. In that dark room, that beautiful woman was astonished.

Filled with loving affection, she rehearsed everything her husband had said as Kiṅkara narrates this divine message of the Pīr.

Recounting her miseries, the young woman was even more depressed. She gave the baby the name of Lālmohan.[15] The cheeky midwife said, "You used to be the wife of a successful merchant, but from the ugly consequences of some past karma you are now destitute, a vagabond. Now you are living in the home of a poor brahmin. Tell me now, what will you be able to give me as a proper fee for my services?" When she heard the request, the beautiful young woman handed over the *motilāl* pearl. "Wear this priceless bauble around your neck." The old woman greedily accepted the pearl and went her way, and soon reached her own house.

Before the midwife could settle at home, the wazir's wife, the *wazirāṇī*, went into an agonizing labor, so they quickly called for the town's only midwife and off she went again. Finally, in the middle of the night, the *wazirāṇī* delivered, but what dropped from her womb was a stillborn son. Grief gripped the faces of those present, and a general cry of sadness inexorably issued forth. Out of her own special unhappiness, the midwife cursed the situation, "May the womb of one like the *wazirāṇī* just burn in hell! What good is it for giving birth? What's its point for existing? Just last night that good-for-nothing *bāṅgāliṇī* gave birth to a robust and healthy son. His body was beautiful, perfectly formed. His name is Motilāl." The wazir's wife lay on the bed exhausted and nearly unconscious, but sat up when she heard the midwife's words. "From this day forward my fate has turned to ashes unless something is done. Please tell me all about the *bāṅgāliṇī*, dear midwife."

The midwife replied, "The *bāṅgāliṇī* is staying at the house of a brahmin. She gave me a pearl that came from her son. I hung it around my neck—see how dazzling it is! . . ." And when she looked at it, the wazir's wife was dumbfounded. Right then she left the birthing room and entered the house, where she counted out a sizeable amount of money to give to the midwife. The *wazirāṇī* instructed her, "Take this and go live comfortably in your home, but take my stillborn son with you—and be quick about it. Place this one in the lap of that useless *bāṅgāliṇī* and bring her son to me. She must be sleeping all alone in her room, exhausted and completely helpless."

The midwife protested, "*Wazirāṇī*, what you ask is out of the question. You want me to steal someone else's son? My mind is moved by my desire for riches, but in that act lies a great violation of what is proper, a sin. If someone finds out, then I will surely be killed—who then would get to enjoy my riches?" And so she protested with any number of arguments.

The *wazirāṇī* replied viciously, "If you do not honor my wishes, you can be sure that you will have your head lopped off in the cremation grounds. . . . The choice is yours."

When she heard this persuasive argument, the midwife was doubly grieved, but in her fear she spirited away the stillborn corpse as requested. Soon she landed up at the door of the poor brahmin, where inside the *bāṅgāliṇī* should be sleeping with her son. The door was unsecured, and inside the room was pitch black. There the destitute woman lay asleep with her own son cradled against her body. Taking a deep breath and holding it, the midwife entered. She quietly exchanged the stillborn for the living boy and took him away. In no time she was placing the handsome young boy into the waiting lap of the *wazirāṇī*, and instantly the pervasive gloom was illuminated by this child's brilliance. Everyone was happy and relieved to see the son alive after all, while the midwife slinked home carrying the blood money.

Back in the brahmin's house, the impoverished *bāṅgāliṇī* woke up with a start when she sensed that her baby was not moving or responding. She did not find in her arms her lively newborn son, who had been endowed with such extraordinary physical charms, but an inert lump, like a rock, a dead child. In spite of the brahmin's hospitality, she had grown thinner and weaker in her misery, and now, with the loss of her son, she collapsed into a heap on the ground. She beat her head over and over, expressing her agony, and the tears flowed like a river in spate. Grief-stricken, the beautiful young woman bewailed her lot. Any living soul who witnessed that lament would not have been able to bear it. The brahmin and his wife had been sleeping inside the house when they were awakened. The old woman muttered, "The *bāṅgāliṇī*'s son must have died." Cursing the lord of fate, Bidhātā, she commiserated in her grief and went to console her. "You pitiful woman, what wretched karma you have. But what now is the point of crying?"

The *bāṅgālinī* cried out, "O Lord, Gosā̃i, this is the horrible magic of Bidhātā, Destiny. Who could have taken my son and left a dead one in his place? My husband returned to our home in order to father this boy, and for that same child the old woman threw me out of the house. Knowing of my suffering, the Lord gave me the son named Lālmohan, and from his mouth he spat jewels worthy of a king, pearls of a radiant pink luster. Who could have stolen that boy?" Continuing her lament, she banged her head and wept until she lost her senses.

Sharing her grief, the brahmin woman consoled her, "You must take your dead child and go from here. . . ." Giving up all hope, Śīlāvatī dragged herself away. In her grief she contemplated drowning herself in the ocean. She abandoned the boy's corpse in the cremation ground, but along the way a flower vendor, a *mālinī*, saw her and began to ask her questions. "Who are you? Where are you going? Why do you weep so? You are so beautiful to look at—what has made you so miserable?"

Śīlāvatī called her by the affectionate address "Auntie," and then told her the entire tale of her woe. What a strange kind of blessing is this tale, comments the poet Kavi Kiṅkara.

"Listen, *mālinī*, to my tale of woe," the miserable woman began. "My grief for my son is so great that I shall go to the sea to drown myself. Please show me the way. This worldly existence is like a thief in the night who takes the riches of others, who takes one person's son for another. . . ."

The flower vendor listened attentively and then with a heartfelt compassion realized the truth of what she said. "Listen, my dear woman, please honor my request. You must come and stay with me. You are so aggrieved that you cannot possibly understand what has happened. Why do you try to blame others?"

The *bāṅgāliṇī* replied, "At the very low point of my suffering, fate chose to grant me the moon itself in my son. Who could be so heartless as to steal my son? Who could see fit to put me through such confusing turmoil? I was holding my son next to me. Who could slip in during the night to take him away and leave a dead child in his place?" The *bāṅgāliṇī* paused. "My heart and spirit have been broken. I shall kill myself by jumping into the waters. . . ."

Listening to her plaintive voice, the garland weaver consoled her, letting her know in various ways that she understood. "Stay here, my dear child. Your misery will soon give way—that I swear on my own head."[16] And with unexpected relief and no little surprise, the *bāṅgāliṇī* continued to talk until she took up the offer and went to live in the flower vendor's house.

Meanwhile the wazirāṇī *raised the young boy, as has been written by Kiṅkara.*

Elsewhere, the *wazirāṇī* had gotten a son not her own and she lavished him with all comforts, for he was dearer to her than life itself. If the tiniest thing, a beetle or some other insect, got after him, she would rush to protect him. In this pampered way he was raised. Everyone knew him as the wazir's son. The days went by, one much like the other, until the boy had reached the age of seven. It was time for the wazir's darling to undertake formal study in the school run by the scholar Ākṣuna, and into the able hands of Ākṣuna he was placed. Every day the four boys in this advanced school were escorted promptly by five young maidservants; on their way they always passed by the flower vendor's dwelling. By the grace of the Pīr, Lālmohan soon mastered the full range of subjects.

One day—and of course inevitably—as he passed the *mālinī*'s gate, he fell right into Śīlāvatī's line of sight. She could say nothing, but could not stop her heart from racing. It was impossible for her to approach him, for he was the son of the wazir. She found herself in a horrible predicament; she couldn't resist, but just to look at him broke her heart. Her food and water may as well have been poison; melancholy was etched on her face and she fell in tears at the feet of the garland weaver. "Listen to me, Auntie. Earlier I restrained my grief because of your kind words, and I have stayed in your house, figuring it was ordained by fate. The wazir's son goes to study every day. Just to look at him makes me lose my will to live. Had I my own son, he would have grown like this and been about his age. Now, my dear auntie, I beg you to save my life once again. You can cast a spell on anyone with your magical and bewitching words. Please indulge this capricious whim and fix it so that I might hold this boy in my lap at least once."

The *mālinī* replied, "You don't ask for much, do you? You're like the Dwarf Vāmana reaching for the moon.[17] I'm truly troubled when I see the depths of your agony, the way you burn so in your grief. It is as if you are the ram who wants the majesty and rich caparison of the king's elephant. You want to take the wazir's son to your lap, but should the wazir find out he will surely kill me."

The *bāṅgāliṇī* countered, "Auntie, you are experienced and wise. If you get him into my lap, my burning heart will be soothed. If you don't, I will kill myself. I will destroy this frail body. . . ." And with this promise she passed the night reliving her grief.

In the morning all the children went to school as usual, but the wazir's son straggled along behind the rest, alone. As soon as she saw him, the *bāṅgāliṇī* fell at the feet of the *mālinī*, "Look, see, there goes the wazir's son!" At that pathetic look, the old woman began to waver, then she prepared a special garland with a magical mix of flowers, and took it with her. She slipped the garland around the boy's neck and began to question him. "Tell me, why do you seem to be so distracted today, at such loose ends, tarrying behind the others?"

The boy respectfully replied, "The other boys have already made their way to school. If I stay and talk, I will be late. I really must go."

The garland weaver pressed on, "My child, I have something a bit unsual to say to you. My daughter wishes to cradle you in her lap. But before you respond to that, I have a vexing issue I need you to adjudicate based on your study: If one kills a woman, what sin accrues?"

"The killing of a woman is foremost among sins, violations of what is law," the well-schooled boy quickly answered. "In the end he will rot in hell and there will be no reprieve."

The *mālinī* seized the opportunity, "My dear child, go and see my daughter just once and avert this impending death sentence. Help her to bear up, for she has nearly lost her senses and her will to live out of grief for her lost son. Life for her is no longer worth living. . . ."

The young boy was moved, "Auntie, I will stay back from school for a while. Odd feelings of compassion stir my mind to meet her." With this bold pronouncement, the two of them went to see the hapless woman. When Śīlāvatī beheld the young man, she felt her heart could no longer bear up. Out of a genuine fear of the wazir, the still-beautiful woman did not embrace the boy, but the ground was showered by a torrent of tears.

The handsome young man inquired, "Tell me just who you are. Why do you stand there mute and weeping?"

The beautiful woman found her voice, "My child, I am the most unfortunate of women. At the sound of your sweet voice I felt I could no longer bear to live. I used to live in the city of Āraṅga as the wife of a prominent merchant. My husband had gone on a trading voyage when a certain truth was divined through yoga. Secretly my lord returned riding a *haṃsarājā*, the king of birds, made passionate love to me and then left. The next morning his old mother, not understanding at all the situation, threw me out of the house. I stayed at the house of the wazir, but when it was discovered that I was pregnant, I was once again thrown out. I eventually ended up at the place of a brahmin priest. It was there my son was born, illuminating the room with his brilliance. When the child murmured his first sound—cooing 'ooh' and 'aah'—a pearl dropped from his mouth. I settled with and dismissed the midwife by giving her that pearl for her services. But that night a thief stole my baby and left me with the corpse of another boy. Grief is the reason I am slowly dying here in the flower vendor's home."

This sacred story of the Pīr is narrated by Kiṅkara.

"To hear this causes no small consternation," the boy politely observed. "Our suffering and our joys are all ordained by destiny."

"What bad fortune I've had is past history," she rejoined, "but help salvage my life; come sit on my lap."

The child perceptively countered, "You seem to have a great love for me." To which the beautiful woman replied, "If you will but sit on my lap, I can live again."

And with these words, the woman sat down and spread wide her arms. The young man crawled onto her lap—but not without chanting the protective names of God, Hari. The effect was like that of the holy Bhāgīrathī River mingling with the waters of the Jāhnavī, or the virtue-minded Yaśodā holding the baby Kṛṣṇa on her lap. Such was the supreme bliss experienced by the woman when she hugged the boy to her body. It was as if a great fire had been extinguished by a flood of water. With great elation the *mālinī* muttered to herself, "What an extraordinary moon has risen from the lap of this downtrodden woman."

Śīlā prodded him, "Call me 'Mother,' my child. After that may the sins of my heart work themselves out in this worldly life." Humoring this distraught and wretched woman, the young boy called her "Mother," and suddenly a pearl, a perfectly formed *motilāl*, popped out of his mouth and fell to the earth. When she recovered her senses the woman cried, "Look, my dear *mālinī*, my auntie! This is my son!"

The *mālinī* was filled with an awful fear as soon as she heard this crazy talk. "The wazir will kill the both of us," she thought. "Why do you say such things? It will only bring your death. What used to be a good life has turned to rubbish by taking you in. My house and home are in danger because of you, a stranger. Thanks to the stupid declaration of a total stranger, I see no way out. I'm ruined!" Rebuking her vilely, the *mālinī* made the boy to understand: "Go, be off, now! Say nothing to the wazir about this."

The boy realized that for all kinds of reasons his own life was at risk, and so he took his leave and returned to his own house.

In the garb of a fakir, Satya Nārāyaṇa magically appeared and approached the boy to answer his questions. "Do not be afraid, my child, this woman really is your mother and you are the son of the merchant. Everything else is a sham. Knowing this, you will sit in the *badshāh*'s *durbār*, his public audience. It will be from the mouth of your birth-mother that the sweetened cream of truth will pour forth. You will end up marrying the *badshāh*'s own daughter, then you will settle down by the sea. You will intercept your father as he returns from a faraway land, and then you will establish the worship of Nārāyaṇa." The assurance delivered, the Pīr returned to his seat in Mecca, where he reigned in his majesty.

The young boy apparently listened, for he went back and told his mother to go to the court the next day to plead her case. With this instruction, the young lad returned to the wazir's house. For the rest of that day and night the boy could eat nothing. Śīlāvatī spent her last night in the *mālinī*'s house, and come morning bade her farewell and headed into the city. She entered the king's public audience and rolled on the ground to demonstrate her abject submission. Then she cried out, "The wazir is a common thief and I appeal to you, the great *badshāh*!" Over and over she babbled the same phrase, "The wazir is a thief; the *wazirāṇī* is a thief."

All those present were astounded to hear these vile accusations. They all cried for her to be beaten and dismissed. "Beat her, smack her! Send her flying! Out with her!" But the *badshāh*, wise as he was, intervened. "Wait. Let us find out the cause of this commotion."

Making deep salaams in obeisance, Śīlā paid her respects and petitioned him. "When my husband was off trading in another land, my mother-in-law summarily banished me to the jungle. I am unable to describe the suffering, the special suffering of a woman. What countless indignities the Fates bestowed on me. Expelled from Rāṅgpur I had at last arrived in this your jurisdiction. I had, just days before, become pregnant, and after wandering about aimlessly, I found a residence in the house of a brahmin. When the labor pains started, the brahmin sent for the midwife. After helping to deliver my son, the midwife returned to her home, but just at that time she had to help the wazir's wife, the *wazirāṇī* deliver. The *wazirāṇī* gave birth to a boy, but he was stillborn. She stole my son and put her own dead child in his place.

"In this great land, O King, you are the very incarnation of justice, *dharma*. Please apply the dictates of *dharma* and gauge your personal responsibility to the cause of this impoverished *bāṅgāliṇī*."

When he heard these remarkable charges, the *badshāh* detained the wazir right there in the court, and issued the command to the constable to fetch the wazir's wife. Of course anyone who defies the express command of the king is automatically beheaded before appearing in court! So the *wazirāṇī* climbed into her palanquin and rushed off. In a very short time indeed did she enter that *badshāh*'s august assembly. It gladdened her to see there the young boy, her "son," who was as handsome as he was well-formed. She made her salaam's and stretched out in full obeisance in the presence of His Majesty.

The *badshāh* spoke, "O wife of my wazir, you have at some point committed some grave offense. Because of this terrible misfortune, you were delivered of a stillborn baby boy. You have taken this *bāṅgāliṇī*'s son and replaced him with your own. He belongs to her who bore him. This deception is an abomination."

The *wazirāṇī* protested, "*Badshāh*, what kind of judgment is this? Is it a true *durbār* where only the complainant speaks? Everyone knows that I gave birth to a son. Why on earth would I take someone else's child?"

The king was not able to see his way clear to the truth of it, and was more than a little perplexed. Suddenly the young boy volunteered, "Allow me to sit on the throne to adjudicate the matter."

"Anyone who dares to sit on the throne will then and there have head removed!" bellowed the *badshāh* in response.

The boy confidently responded, "If I am not equal to the task, then you should cut off my head in front of the entire assembly."

When the king heard this proposition, he promptly stood up, took the handsome young man by the hand and seated him on the throne. Once properly ensconced the young man called the two women. "If you can squeeze milk from your breast and squirt it into my mouth from a distance, then the whole world will know you to be my real mother. The real mother will swell with the milk of supreme bliss simply because I am her son."

The courtiers saw the sense of the test and approved. The *wazirāṇī* was the first to be brought forward before the assembly. She massaged and pumped and finally managed to squeeze a little milk from her breast, but it squirted aimlessly on the floor. Everyone agreed, "This does not augur well. If the *bāṅgāliṇī* can pass this same test, then the truth is secure that this is boy is truly hers." And so they talked.

Listening to the challenge, the destitute bāṅgāliṇī *stood up and began to knead her breasts. This truly amazing tale has been written by Kiṅkara.*

Śīlāvatī made obeisance to the assembly and then, as she meditated intently on Nārāyaṇa, she began to knead her breasts. Everyone stood witness as the extra-sweet, thick milk shot into the open mouth of her son like an arrow tracing an arc, true toward its mark. The milk quickly filled up his mouth and began to flow down his chest in thick rivulets. It drenched his clothes and soon the flow was so great that he was choking on it and had to spit it out onto the ground. But not everyone was convinced that the *wazirāṇī* was not the mother. Some suggested that some strange magic, the net of Indra, had been cast.

The *bāṅgāliṇī* then proceeded to explain what had transpired. "My husband had struck out on a trading venture when along the way he heard a prophecy directly from the mouths of the sages who divined it: 'During the thirteenth *daṇḍa* of that night is to occur a special moment, a conjunction of planets called the Māhendra Yoga. The star Svāti will shower its auspicious drops all over. If one has intercourse during this special time, then a son will be born who produces perfectly formed *motilāl* pearls.' When he learned of this, my husband returned riding a great swan, the *haṃsarājā*. My husband made passionate love to me and then left. That is why my mother-in-law threw me out. But my lord had impregnated me and I bore a son. In the compound of a brahmin that boy was born. When he lay cradled in my arms cooing sounds of affection—'ooh', 'aah'—he produced a perfect *motilāl* pearl from his mouth. I placed it in the hands of the midwife for her fee and even now you can see it dangling around her neck. Call her and question her. Whether my story is true or not, she alone can witness. See for yourself right now who bore this boy. If the son sits in the lap of his own birth-mother, he will produce pearls when he calls her 'Mother.' "

The *badshāh* took up the challenge and immediately sent for the midwife. He questioned her about the whole affair. With hands pressed together in respect, the midwife confessed, her whole body trembling in fear. She revealed everything to the assembly. "You are a great ruler, O *Badhshāh*, you are my father. If you will grant me full pardon, I will tell the truth about the whole business." The *badshāh* gave his word of approval. The midwife began to speak deliberately, her conscience clearly deeply troubled all this time.

"This boy belongs to the destitute *bāṇgāliṇī*. It was from his mouth the pearl I wear around my neck issued forth. She had given it to me after the boy was born. As soon as the stillborn son of the *wazirāṇī* was delivered, everyone wept, no one could contain the sorrow. The wazir's wife threatened me: 'Take this dead baby and bring me the other one. If you don't bring it, I will have you killed.' When I heard this I was terrified. I swapped the dead baby for this one and delivered him to the *wazirāṇī*."

As he listened, the king began to understand. He ordered the *wazirāṇī*, "Take this boy on your lap and have him call you 'Mother.' "

At this command she took the boy and though he repeatedly called her "Mother," no pearls fell from his mouth. But the *wazirāṇī* was not giving up. "In all my life I've never heard of a human being who could spit up pearls. It's absurd."

The bāṅgāliṇī *only muttered under her breath, "Puzzling indeed!" Kiṅkara tells his tale, composed in the* pāñcālī *meter.*

"To imagine such adroit treachery! What can I say when it's none other than my own wazir? Come, you long-suffering *bāṅgāliṇī*. Sit and take your son to your lap. Your destiny will now be determined by whether or not pearls magically appear when he calls you 'Mother.' "

Śīlā listened and then called Nārāyaṇa into her mind: "Please bestow your grace this one final time so that all present in the court may witness. It was at your own encouragement that I came to the *durbār*. If I regain my dear child, I will undertake the *pūjā* to worship your holy feet." Now prepared, she said aloud, "Come, my child, crawl into my lap that my heart may be soothed at last."

The boy climbed into her lap in the presence and full view of the entire assembly. "Mother, Mother!" cried out the son of the merchant, with such force that *motilāls* spewed onto the ground like a monsoon cloudburst.

Everyone agreed that the woman had gotten back her long-lost son. Śīlā's heart finally gained the relief it had sought. Everyone said the name of Hari in jubilation. Śīlā prostrated herself in full obeisance before the king and presented the perfect *motilāls* to him. "O *Badshāh*, I present to you my son, whose name is Lālmohan."

When the king had managed to rein in his anger at his wazir, he issued his decision and decree. The wife of the wazir wept bitterly as she was sent back to her home.

The beauty and other fine qualities of this prince of a boy did not go unnoticed by the king. He too had a great treasure for a child, a world-bewitching beauty of a daughter. He had raised her with the name of Saṅgatulyā—She Who is without

Comparison. Her name fit, for she was incomparably beautiful, her figure always draped with ornaments and other finery. Around her neck hung a necklace set with a large diamond, flanked with strings of *motilāl* pearls. A hundred servant girls attended to the person of this girl, the king's daughter.

Soon Lālmohan was being dressed in the clothes of a bridegroom. The king gave his only daughter in marriage according to strict Vedic ritual. The *badshāh* formally made over his beloved daughter, and did so with a joyous heart. Afterward he presented them with all manner of fantastic riches. The bride and groom retired then to the traditional flower-strewn bedroom, where they consummated their marriage with a robust and loving passion.

Some time later, the young man spoke earnestly to his new father-in-law. "You are generous at heart, O great King, so I beg you grant me this: Let us build a house on the water's edge. After it is completed, please allow us to move in and reside there. From that lookout I can screen all the merchants returning home from trade." With a long face, the king reluctantly agreed. They passed the entire night talking about this and other things.

Then the young man focused his mind and thoughts on Satya Nārāyaṇa: "May it please you to build us a house on the banks of the wide river." Without hesitation Nārāyaṇa in turn called out to Viśvakarma: "Would you be so kind as to construct a house, a real home of distinction, for my devotee?" No sooner had Viśvakarma received the command of the Gāzī, that warrior of God, than he set about the task. And overnight a house, beautiful in all proportion, was raised at the desired spot.

The next morning the king hurried out to investigate, and there on the shores of the ocean sat a house extraordinary in every way. The good woman Śīlāvatī mounted the palanquin while the groom took the bride and and her hordes of escorts. Having safely installed them in this palatial new residence, the king retired to his own palace. The young man, his new wife, and Śīlāvatī, his mother, set up house there on the water's edge.

Meanwhile, Lāl had been worrying about his mother's physical appearance, which was thin and unadorned. He furnished her with all manner of ornaments, clothes, jewels, and bangles.

Now let us listen to Lālmohan's tale, says Kiṅkara.

Śīlāvatī began, "Listen, my dear child, listen to what I say. I beg you to please share some of your wealth with the poor brahmin who gave me shelter. . . ." Soon that twice-born brahmin and the flower vendor as well were fetched. Seats of honor were offered to both of them in turn. The merchant's son soon showed the highest honor to the twice-born. "You know all about this," Śīlāvatī said to her son. "I got you back while I was living in the home of the *mālinī*. I got you back, my son, through the power of Auntie. So please bestow riches on the both of them."

The young man listened to his mother and ceremonially offered an array of riches to the twice-born. To the *mālinī* he made gifts of rich clothes and an abundance of fine ornaments. He then bowed in respect to both of them and took his formal leave.

From his place there in the house the young man could keep a lookout and intercept any trading ships that came by. The Lord, Pīr Paigambar, showed his grace one evening, for he steered Raṅga the merchant, who was sailing back from his trading voyage, right by the place. The young man called out to the ship. "Hey, who are you? What fleet is this? By order of the *badshāh* I command you to heave to and anchor along this shore!"

Heeding the command, the merchant dropped anchor and came ashore. "Tell me about yourself, your voyage, your mission," ordered Lālmohan.

The merchant respectfully reported, "My home lies in the fair city of Āraṅga. My name, my good man, is Raṅga Sadāgar, a merchant. I left to do business in the trading city of Āṅgaja. Through the strange machinations of fate I have been away for a very long time."

"Since you have been gone on trade for such a long time, tell me truthfully how many are in your family now back home?" the young man queried him more directly. "How many sons and how many daughters do you have? Be honest, good trader, and tell me truthfully."

"I have my mother living there. When I left I had no sons, no daughters, only my wife Śīlāvatī," the merchant replied precisely. "But as I began my journey I made my way to the banks of the Triveṇī, where I received reliable information about an unusual conjunction of the planets called the Māhendra Yoga. When I heard about its effects, I began to think hard about it, in fact was obsessed over it, when suddenly a fakir showed up. At his command I mounted the back of a giant bird and returned home. While there I accomplished what I set out to do, and then returned to my trading venture. So after that brief conjugal visit, how can I possibly know whether I have a son or daughter now?"

"I have heard people say that that because of your stupid trick, your beautiful wife has suffered terribly," the young man chided him. "You left without telling anyone you were there and you left the door open, unsecured. When the ever-watchful old woman saw it, she wasted no time in kicking your wife out of the house. . . ."

Listening to this and remembering all he had done, the good merchant was struck dumb. He wept and he lamented his plight, as written by Kiṅkara.

Suddenly overwrought
the merchant began to cry,
  his hands flailing his head.
"This horrible omission was ordained.
I was not destined to be happy.

Lord Viśvanātha, Śiva, has turned against me.
"At the advice of the sages
did I return to my home,
hoping to father a pearl of a son.
"I failed to inform my mother
and so lost every thing I hold dear,
the result of my own foolish act.
"How can I blame my mother?
My life flees before me,
everything I wanted now slipped away.
"What hope remains in this life?
I have brought everything to ruin.
The lord of fate, Bidhātā, is hard on me. . . ."

Śīlāvatī heard the plaintive cry of the man who was her husband, and she ran to find out all she could about him. She ran weeping, then hugged her son tightly against her, and fell at her husband's feet. The good merchant was nonplussed, unable to fathom what was happening. As he watched he was even more confounded. "Who are these people? This attractive woman, so bewitching in beauty, has made my eyes go dark. I'm blind." And so he pondered.

"Who are you, falling at my feet? I cannot understand any of this. What's happening here?"

Kiṅkara observes: the good merchant does not recognize his own son and wife.

Struggling against the illusion-making power of the Pīr, the merchant cried out, "I am unable to understand why this child has come to me. From what great family do you descend? Why are you clasping my feet? It tears my heart to pieces to see the the two of you express such devotion."

When she heard this, Śīlā quickly stood up and touched her hands to her forehead. "Do you not recognize this miserable wretch of a woman, O you who are lord of my heart? By some questionable machination did you manage to make love to me while far away on your trading voyage—and for that, my lord, you made me suffer the same miserable fate as Jānakī. Stripped of all types of ornaments and finery—the eight ornaments marking my good fortune—I was cast into the jungle. It was because of your personal desire that I bore this son. His name is Lālmohan and from his mouth comes pearls, *motilāls*, pink and well formed. The wife of the wazir exchanged her stillborn son for my boy. . . ." Gradually the beautiful woman narrated the entire episode up to how she recovered her son in the royal *durbār*. "The king then gave his daughter in marriage to our son, showering us with much wealth. By the *pūjā* worship of Satya Pīr will all miseries be destroyed. Look at the ornaments that adorn my body. By the grace of the Great Provider I got these things and my son. But since I no longer possess the eight ornaments of prosperity, how could you be expected to recognize me, to know who I am for certain?"

In the words of that beautiful woman the good merchant found a veritable store of wisdom. He pulled the young man to him and smothered his face with kisses. He took the hand of his wife and expressed to her his profound contrition, the grief from his complicity. With his son and his son's new wife, his own wife, Śīlā, and members of the entire family and local retinue, the good merchant directed his attention to the Great Provider, Satya Pīr. He dedicated an entire boatload of goods to his worship.

Lālmohan then requested from his father permission to take formal leave of his father-in-law, the *badshāh*. The merchant remarked, "Anxiety and sorrow only increase when delayed. Take your leave with the *badshāh*'s blessings soon, for he may not be so inclined later."

Having avoided the possible complication, the merchant's heart soared in anticipation. "Prepare the ships to sail, O helmsman. We will head back soon to our own land." A short while later the prows of the boats cut through the waves like arrows. They navigated numerous rivers until they reached the Triveṇī. Father and son, Śīlāvatī and the *badshāh*'s daughter—all chanted the name of Hari when they touched the waters of the Gaṅgā. The merchant nostalgically recalled, "It was here I mounted the great swan and flew back to the house based on the sages' predictions. . . ." But pointing out the event was enough, for this time he did not drop anchor to take rest. With the deepest and most sincere devotion, he turned his mind to Satya Pīr.

Day and night the boatmen sailed the fleet of ships toward their destination. When they finally reached their home port it was in the evening, the close of the day, a good time to land. They tied up at the landing ghat and then dropped anchors, which were attached to sturdy wrought-iron chains.

The merchant's now much older mother was overjoyed when she got the news they had landed. She organized the married women of the city to ceremonially greet the boats with auspicious rituals of welcome. The merchant bowed deeply before his mother, paying his respects, before he finally asked her, "Mother, I do not see my wife among the women welcoming the boats. Where is she?" To which the old woman sadly replied, "At the time of your departure you had instructed: 'If you ever find the door to her private chambers open, then send her away from this house.' You hadn't been gone fifteen days when I found the door open and that hussy lying there exhausted, asleep after her long night of revelry. And I saw in the room that the expensive candles of beeswax had burned down completely—a sign she was up all night. So following your express orders, I banished your wife from our household."

The good merchant quietly replied, "It was I who came and went without informing anyone because of my foolish fear of being delayed. It was my own selfish action that caused my helpless wife to be censured and blamed. The sages told me when to make love to my wife and Satya Nārāyaṇa provided me with the means—the king of birds, the *haṃsarājā*."

When she heard the explanation of her son, the old mother swooned, overcome. Through the trickery of the Pīr she nearly lost her life. "Hāya! Cruel fate, you are so hard and unrelenting in this my life. I cast out and lost forever a daughter-in-law, beautiful as a golden moon, and who had a host of other fine qualities."

Listening to the old woman weep at her son's words, the young man and his still-charming wife could stand it no longer. They grasped her feet. Watching them, the aged woman was completely nonplussed. Then, in brief, Śīlā narrated the entire series of events—how Lālmohan gallantly discharged himself in the *badshāh*'s public assembly, and how the *badshāh* rewarded him in turn, and the way in which the merchant joined forces with the king. . . .

The poor old woman was stunned at the turn of events. But soon joy abounded everywhere as the fleet of ships was formally welcomed home with auspicious rituals. The helmsman and others off-loaded an fine array of goods, many of them treasures.

Then the whole family, with their retinue of servants, male and female, saw their way home. This divine message from the Pīr is narrated by Kiṅkara.

And so happiness reigned all around in the merchant's great house. Everyone was thrilled to meet the heir, Lālmohan. As before, pearls would emerge from the mouth of this prince of a boy, who was indeed now a prince, and everyone witnessed how the Pīr could manipulate in crazy ways this illusory world.

The following day the four beloveds of that family—father, son, wife, daughter-in-law—talked together, and began to assemble everything necessary to perform the worship of the Pīr. Musicians played instruments of all types in a dazzling array of songs. The merchant then publicly instructed everyone to worship the feet of the Pīr. Everyone who gathered there learned to worship the Pīr.

It was with an unmitigated pleasure that the merchant, Raṅga Sadāgar, gathered in his own house all the required ingredients, utensils, and other elements of worship. On all four sides—east, west, north, south—arrows were planted to demarcate the space, then the *āstānā*, that special ceremonial seat, was installed. A frame was erected and a beautiful canopy stretched above that now-hallowed ground.

Flower garlands of all types were woven, special clothing procured, and a machete made of gold fabricated as part of the ritual. One hundred twenty-five leaves of the areca plant were ceremonially placed on top of these offerings. One hundred twenty-five quids of prepared betel were offered as were one and one-quarter maunds of milk: "Please accept these offerings, O Bābā, Satya Pīr, and be placated." Then a brahmin performed a special *pūjā* to the five gods, conchs were blown, bells rung, and drums beaten, a cacophony to announce the gifts of worship.

At the end of the telling of the divine story of the Pīr, the *śirṇi* was divided. After it was portioned out, everyone ate the *śirṇi* of the Pīr. Young and old, everyone there together made salaams of obeisance. "May the jet-black Pīr, Ghanaśyāma, be gracious to those who make this offering."

May everyone chant the name of Hari as this drama comes to a close. The great episode detailing the exploits of the Pīr, this the twice-born Dvīja Kaṅka sings to its end.

The Erstwhile Bride and Her Winged Horse

Anonymous *Manohara Phāsarā Pālā*

I bow to the goddess of speech, Sarasvatī, by whose grace living beings are freed from delusion.

With pointed concentration I salute Brahmā, Viṣṇu, and Śiva. With great care I bow to all 333 million other gods.

I bow to the one more radiant than the moon, Durgā, princess of the realm of Dakṣa, the daughter who graces Dakṣa's realm; and to Gaṇeśa and Kārttika; so too to Mother Viṣaharī, Manasā, goddess of serpents. I praise Vāsukī and all the serpents of the netherworld.

I make obeisance to that accomplished seer Vyāsa, and to the other sages.

I single-mindedly bow to the feet of the Lord, Īśvara, by whose mercy I am witness to this mortal world.

With hands pressed together I pay my deepest respects to my father and my mother. And with lowered head, I bow to my teachers.

I have made these few salutations to begin my book, but what do I truly know? For I am ignorant and foolish! Everyone should listen intently to the song that tells the qualities of the Pīr. Should you listen, your miseries will come to an abrupt end.

Satya Pīr Sāheb and all the many *pīrs* of the world who had come to God sat together in Mecca.

It happened that in the citadel of Maheśvarī stood the house of King Bhojapati. He suffered deeply that both of his sons were absent from his home, for soon after their births, each had mysteriously disappeared in the forest. The king and his queen were given to loud bouts of weeping out of grief for their issue. Each time the king was given over to these weeping fits, he would promise in his prayer to Satya Pīr: "Should my sons return home, I will give you a suitable dwelling—an *āstānā* composed of a heavily decorated raised platform seat, a ritual object made of pure gold!"

And so the days and nights passed in terrible misery, until one day, quite unexpectedly, divine words wafted down to the king from heaven: "I shall return your sons from the bosom of the forest!" The king's heart leaped in joy at what he heard. He called his queen and said, "Our desires have been fulfilled! I shall now have that golden *āstānā* made for Satya Pīr." Reiterating his promise, the king voiced his pleasure and then called his courtiers. "Pay close attention, my messengers, to what I am about to make public to one and all. Carry my royal command to Kaliṅga! There in that land dwells a merchant named Śaṅkhadatta, whose name appropriately means 'Purveyor of Conchs.' And he has a handsome son named Vidyādhara, named after a celestial figure who 'possesses spells.' Fetch him!"

As soon as the prefect of police heard the command, he sallied forth and after a short while arrived in the Kaliṅga country. The policeman sought out the merchant and made his formal greetings of salaam. Then, by systematic questioning, he ascertained the name and particulars of the merchant's son. "Your Excellency, may I introduce myself by the name of Raṇasiṅgh. The king has issued instruction to fetch you."

No sooner had he heard this than Vidyādhara equipped himself to travel. They departed, accompanied in a long procession of elephants and horses. They finally reached the citadel of Maheśvarī, where they prostrated themselves at the feet of the king. Looking on the merchant, the king spoke directly. "Listen carefully, merchant's son, to what I have to say! Your father has on many occasions complied with my wish and whim. This time it is necessary to undertake a special commercial venture. You are the seventh man I have sent to this country. And by virtue of your presence now, no other merchant will be allowed to trade here; you have exclusive trading privileges. My dear son, please go to that famous mercantile center and acquire for me a finely crafted *āstānā* of pure gold! Take six hundred rupees for the *āstānā* and take another hundred rupees to cover your expenses!"

What transpired was just like the time when the demon King Kaṃsa in Mathurā city bade farewell to Akrūra and sent him to Gopapura, Kṛṣṇa's home. At the command of Kaṃsa, the sage Akrūra happily made the trip to the Vṛndā Forest, site of the round dance, the *rāsa*. In a similar fashion the merchant begged his leave of the king, collected his seven hundred rupees, and returned to his home. His mother lived as a widow there in his house, and Vidyādhara sought her out directly. Just as Rāma begged leave to retire to the forest because of the treachery of Kaikeyī regarding the king's promise,[1] and just as the five-year-old Dhruva went to Madhuvana, taking leave of his mother,[2] so did Vidyādhara present himself to beg his own leave. His mother, Subhadrā, stricken with grief, rolled on the ground. "Please grant me permission to leave, Mother!" pleaded Vidyādhara, "I will return to your house after six months!" And so he consoled his mother, but it was only with great pain and much distress that she finally acquiesced and gave her permission.

The merchant immediately called a pair of servants. "Outfit a chariot with proper equipment—and be quick about it!" As soon as they heard, they complied, and quickly brought around to him the fully rigged chariot. The chariot was replete with six sandalwood wheels, and a combination of pleated silk and tufted jute, decorated with stylish taste. On the elevated floor of this fine wagon they spread a padded pallet, and on all sides they installed decorative bolsters. Jutting above it all, a white mushroom-shaped parasol spread magnificently, while from it hung multicolored jute streamers, which swayed gently back and forth.

The merchant prostrated himself at his mother's feet. With tear-suffused eyes, his mother pronounced her blessings. Taking the dust of his mother's feet to his head in that time-honored gesture of humility and respect, the merchant mounted his chariot and settled in comfortably. To his right sat a spouted waterpot of gold, beautiful beyond compare; to his left gleamed a box of betel with a matching gold trimming knife. The chariot was spurred forward along the road he indicated, and so the charioteer of the merchant Vidyādhara headed for the southern land of Rukmiṇī.

Soon the merchant left his own country far behind and entered the kingdom of Maṅgalapura. Leaving behind the land of Rājā Candana—the Sandal King—he came into Kuraṅgī Maheśapura, the Citadel of the Lord of Does. The merchant passed through the Land of the Bears, whereupon he suddenly found himself in a country notable for its highwaymen. And it was in this region that Manohara Phāsarā—the Beguiling Cutthroat—made his home. He had six sons, but a single daughter. These six brothers, highwaymen all, were exceedingly shrewd and clever. In the twinkling of an eye could they traverse the triple worlds of the heavens, the middle regions, and the earth. The solitary daughter was like a tiny jewel, the facet of a gem, and that was precisely her name: Ratnakalā. She would always dress in clothes of the most attractive color and style, and sixteen times in the course of a single day would she dress and adjust her hair!

Listen, one and all, with a pointed mind to the saga of Satya Pīr. He who heeds this song suffers misery no more.

The beautiful young daughter of that highwayman went by the name of Ratnakalā, and appropriately enough, for she was always adorned with a great variety of jewels and gems, a fine line of gold stringing across her throat. In the first blush of her youth, her form proved more radiant and attractive than a digit of the moon. With a string of pearls round her neck, she was the very image of Bāsavara, the twenty-third star in traditional astronomy, favoring Indrāṇī, or any of the legendary beauties Ahalyā, Draupadī, Madana's Rati, or Kṛṣṇa's beloved wife, Jāmbuvatī. In a previous life, this young woman had been a servant to Vāgvādinī or Sarasvatī, the goddess of speech. But as a result of a curse, she was condemned to be born into the family of a highwayman. She could easily calculate the number of grains of sand in the ocean or count the stars in the heavens, but better yet, her knowledge extended to allow her to divine the essential matters concealed within ordinary appearances, that is, she saw things invisible to others.

When a man laden with wealth would arrive in their part of the world, this beautiful young thing would quickly calculate his worth and inform her father. The highwayman would then make himself known to that stranger and lure him into his home by calling him by the affectionate term "son-in-law." Then, casting suggestive sidelong glances and employing other subtle tricks, this rare beauty would enchant the hapless man and bring him totally under her spell. Then he would be fed, sumptuously of course, on curds, sweetened milk, rice, milk sweets, and so forth, and when fully sated, made to lie down. The room of honor was where they would slit his throat. He would lie down to sleep, happy in the knowledge that he was in the home of his newfound father-in-law. The old man would then send in his daughter finely arrayed and seductively adorned—and seduce she did. This wickedly delectable slayer of men knew all the tricks of her trade. She would enter the room and slide into bed beside him—only to treat him to a lacerated gullet. And precisely in this fashion had she coldly murdered untold hundreds of unsuspecting traders—and of course their riches soon filled the highwayman's own stores. So incalculable was the family's wealth that they burned lamps during the day when they were not even needed. Always the highwayman wore the very finest of clothes. He and his six sons all wore shawls of the best Persian weave. And by the grace of his daughter, they lived in a compound that offered no fewer than three tiers of walls. With the money provided by his daughter, the old man would feast like a king.

Listen now with special attention to the tale of Satya Pīr.

As the merchant Vidyādhara moved down the highway, the beautiful young woman calculated his wealth from a distance and passed on the information: "A solitary merchant has arrived from Kaliṅga. He is trading in gemstones in order to purchase an elaborate gold *āstānā*. If we can lure the merchant into our compound, by morning we can realize a gain of at least six hundred rupees!"

When he heard what Ratnakalā had to say, Monohara Phāsarā praised her, "Thanks and praise be to you, Ratnakalā, for your extraordinary skill in reading the stars. If I clear a substantial sum of money from this merchant after I bring him here, then I will give you in marriage to the most suitable groom I can find—nothing less than an ideal match. I shall furnish you with a dowry of male and female servants, and veritable mounds of wealth. I shall give jewelry of such variety as to be beyond count and measure."

Now the ablest son of the highwayman was Govinda Phāsarā, and as a highwayman he was no less accomplished than his father. All six sons, as a matter of fact, were adroit in the arts of deception and fraud, and so they readily, indeed eagerly, agreed to entrap the merchant. Just as the lion roars when it sights some prey, so these highwaymen descended on the unsuspecting merchant, quickly encircling him.

The merchant Vidyādhara was idly driving his chariot down the road, while the six brothers nervously lay in wait all around. At the appropriate moment they accosted the trader and queried him closely. "What is your name? From which land do you hail? And who are your parents?" they asked.

"My mother's name is Subhadrā, a dweller in Kaliṅga. My own name is Vidyādhara and I am a Gandhabene, the traditional calling of unguent- and spice-trader, but now a simple merchant."

As soon as they heard this, all six brothers feigned excitement as they spoke animatedly. "In truth, this must be our merchant brother-in-law; it must be so! When our sister was but two and one-half years old, and you, O merchantman, were a mere seven, you were married. But you left after the wedding and twelve long years passed, yet you never returned . . . until now."

The merchant objected. "How can you intimate such a thing? To the best of my knowledge, I have never been married!"

All six brothers—Govinda, Jayanta, Gopāla, Mohana, Hari, and Janārddana—swore it was so. And in this simple fashion did they argue. "Since it happened when you were but a child, you simply do not remember it."

The merchant quickly countered, "If I did get married, why did my mother never once mention it?"

The six young highwaymen continued their clever deception undeterred. "Your mother never said anything because this land is so far from your own. We received news that you had died, so our sister tried to immolate herself in the purifying flames. We have endeavored to console her, having her live with us. Since then we have been searching out news of you. Only by the strange workings of fate have we found you today. After so many bad days has happiness been written into her fortune. Now that we have found you, we will never let you out of our sights; we shall take you home no matter what excuse you might conjure."

By now the Pīr's magic had begun to work on the defenseless merchant Vidyādhara, so much so that this trader actually began to believe that it was not only possible, but was in fact true. Just as the bee is intoxicated by the discovery of the day-blooming lotus, so the merchant went with them mesmerized and totally unafraid. In exactly the manner that Aniruddha was kidnapped by Uṣā's beauty,[3] so was this handsome merchant disposed to be ensorcelled. Held in their sway, the merchant proceeded to the highwaymen's home, where the aged Manohara Phāsarā awaited them, sitting in the doorway. The six brothers advised him, "There in that doorway sits our honorable and respected father. You know the proprieties—both incidental and serious—to be observed in the family. Go and prostrate yourself before him when you declare him to be your father-in-law."

The cutthroat's six sons accompanied the merchant—front and back, in case he had a change of heart—and entered into the outer apartments of the extensive housing complex. When the old highwayman caught sight of the merchant, his joy knew no bounds.

Listen further to the divine play of the Pīr.

The merchant offered his salutations to the cutthroat's feet. The old highwayman wept openly and placed his arms expectantly around the trader's fine neck. The old man expressed astonishment and kissed him on the lips, exclaiming all the while, "We have all suffered through the fires of sorrow on your account! When my daughter was a mere two and one-half years old, you, my dear boy, were only seven. As soon as you had married, you left her far behind. For twelve years you failed to return or even inquire of her. You never came back here, which caused us great shame. No more could we bear the public humiliation and insult. When my beautiful daughter reached puberty, our embarrassment grew even greater! We could no longer eat or socialize with friends or even relatives. Tell me of my daughter's father-in-law, your sire. Speak to me of your household weal, and the blessed woman who gave you birth, your dear mother. Speak so that we may hear how things are for you!"

The merchant listened respectfully and responded. "My honorable father passed on to the heavens some six months ago, but I have not yet had the opportunity to perform the customary *śrāddha* or obsequies. My widowed mother lives with me at my home. At the express command of the king, I have come this way on a jewel-trading expedition."

When he heard this story, the old highwayman smacked his forehead in regret. "Alas, I failed to meet my daughter's father-in-law." Weeping for a moment, the old man managed to instruct his sons. "Take my son-in-law to the inner apartments of the house. This good merchant-son must be exhausted from his time on the road. But before anything, take him and feed him properly!"

At this, the young trader suddenly fell into a panic; "I have not performed the obsequies for my father these six months. How can I take food in your house?"

The old man artfully replied, "You can take sweets and other acceptable foods. Do not worry yourself with this idle talk right now. Go on inside the house, for your mother-in-law is waiting expectantly to meet you."

Heeding these words, the merchant lowered his head in humility and went inside. But the highwayman's massive housing complex proved labyrinthine. The golden Laṅkā was the citadel of Rāvaṇa, around which even the deities found it difficult to tread. Likewise was the merchant struck with wonder to find himself in just that kind of palace, and it was dawning on him that his father-in-law was not only a respectable man but a very rich one, too.

Now the daughters-in-law of this old highwayman were an exceedingly mischievous lot, as one would expect from dacoits. They caused no small amount of embarrassment for the young merchant as they impeded his progress with various delaying, and quite feminine, subterfuges. One in particular baited him accusingly: "Merchant, you don't have the wherewithal to support a wife. So why did you marry her and make her suffer so much shame?"

The merchant defended himself, "You accuse me unjustly, for I never even realized I was married." Then all six daughters-in-law chided him, "It never even entered your head? Perhaps it was your wife who reminded you in a dream! Now you have come seeking her out for some ulterior and obviously dishonorable motive." And so they mercilessly cajoled him. And it worked! The merchant did not dare to raise his head for the shame of it all!

The highwayman's youngest son took the trader and led him into the private apartments of the house. There they found Ratnakalā, stunning as ever, brimming with joy. She quickly proffered a golden stool and seated the merchant on it. This enchanting young woman greeted him with a pot overflowing with cool water, just as Satyabhāmā used to bring for her husband, Govinda. The merchant was instantly captivated by her seductive sidelong glance. Aided by the Pīr's magic, he completely forgot himself, losing entirely what was left of his already beleaguered wits. When he finished bathing, this well-bred son of a merchant sat down to eat, and eat he did—sweetmeats of all shapes and sizes, all to his heart's content. When he had finished eating, the merchant cleansed his mouth and hands. Then he was given camphor-laced betel to freshen his mouth. The youngest son of the highwayman then escorted the merchant to that special room where they slit throats—and bade him lie down to a peaceful sleep.

A bed was spread, appearing rich and elegant, with tufts of jute and silk in different colors. All around it gaily patterned bolsters were laid down. Draped above this pallet hung a mosquito net woven of the finest muslin. A colorful silk fringe of neatly tailored tassels gently swayed in mesmerizing, undulating lines. Sleep began to beckon this sacrifical victim, contented there in his father-in-law's house. Then the old man dispatched his daughter, made up in her finest and most attractive dress.

Listen in rapt attention to the lyric beauty of this gleaming gem, Ratnakalā. And may the sound of Hari's name pour joyously from your mouth.

This gorgeous lady did not formally forgive her foreign merchant; she simply entered his presence, dressed fit to kill. She personally prepared her own coiffure in a particularly elegant style. Vermilion dotted her forehead like a moon shining full. Through her locks she braided strands of jasmines—each one different—the sight of which would daze the wits of austere sages and the heart of Śiva himself, that lord of ascetics. The vermilion in her hair's part she painted in a crescent bow; from her ears dangled ornamented orbs, radiant like iridescent moons. She blackened with collyrium her darting birdlike eyes, eyes that would steal the heart of any man bereft of his lover. She wore a fancy bustier purfled in elaborate gold, across whose strategic points were draped delicate strings of pearls. This woman, apparently simple and helpless, was anything but: she was sly and cold and exceedingly hard at heart. She secreted on her person a razor intended for murder. Bells in a string settled in clinks atop her broad hips, while above her feet, which were like beautiful lotuses springing up from the mud of the earth, jangled elegant anklets. Her perfume was wonderfully redolent of sandal. For betel, she collected camphor and lime, and the nut of areca and its leaves; and arranging them on a tray for the purpose, this lovely damsel carried them nonchalantly into the room. She entered confident and dignified, swaying with the graceful gait of an elephant. The tassels that hung from the cloth over her breasts swayed in the breeze with each jiggling step. The sight was enough to dazzle the minds of the gods and stop mere mortal men dead in their tracks. The comely beauty moved her body with elegance and grace. Any man who glimpsed her imposing form surrendered readily and without a fight.

Dressed to enchant the world,
in she strutted, set to beguile
  this man she planned to kill.
Ensconced in the firmament, Satya Pīr
was aware of everything, by virtue of meditation.
  He prepared the merchant to be fully alert.

Stretched out in sleep on his bed,
this merchant looked for the all world
  like Indra's very own son, the prince of heaven.
While at that very moment, Ratnakalā
glided toward him, fully composed, smiling sweetly,
  carrying a tray of fragrant sandalwood.

As she entered through the sliding door
she wore a sweet, reassuring smile,
  while her steely eyes remained fixed on the trader.
Moving with a practiced grace, this handsomely endowed damsel
exuded the freshness of her newfound youth
  just as cold creamy butter weeps under a blazing sun.

When she looked on the merchant's extraordinary physique,
emotions she could not check swelled in her bosom
  and tears soon flowed, torrents from her eyes.

She lowered her head and wept.
Addressing no one in pariticular, she cried,
"What has fate contrived for me?

"Wasted and abortive has this birth become
for I have perpetrated countless heinous acts;
I have murdered merchants in cold blood.
I have never served the feet of a husband.
My life passes in futility;
people call me scandalous and disgraceful.

"The wealth earned by one is enjoyed by another,
while I have never worshiped any lord as husband.
The days of my life aimlessly waste away.
A merchant from some strange and faraway place
has landed at my door—
His slave will I become; his feet will I ever serve!"

When she declared her change of heart, Ratnakalā
took her prepared garland and sandalwood paste
and adorned the merchant's feet.
Startled by the touch of this seductive woman,
the merchant, who had been deep in sleep,
sat bolt upright in bed.

Roused from his sleep, the merchant became quickly alert. Opening his eyes to the beauty of Ratnkalā, his heart was in an instant smitten. With growing affection did the merchant speak, "Listen carefully to what I say. After so many long days fate has seen fit to reunite us. Open your heart and speak frankly, you who are the goddess of my life! When I look on your melancholy, it finds mirror image deep in my heart."

When she heard this, the attractive young Ratnakalā smiled and queried him. "What are you thinking, merchant, as you lie here on the bed? You probably believe that this is your father-in-law's house, but listen to me, merchant, it is all lies, a concocted story. Each of my six brothers has the heart of a lion. Everyone knows how incredibily merciless and cruel they are. My father, Manohara, driven by greed, lures home foreign traders by calling them 'son-in-law.' He feeds them milk and cream and ghee and then shows them to this apartment to sleep. My father is devoid of compassion when wealth is involved. He dispatches me to do the killing for him. The three realms are heaven, earth, and netherworld; when their signs are properly read through the esoteric and magical knowledge of the Āgama and Nigama scriptures, he sends me. Untold numbers of merchants, sons of kings, and other casual visitors I have put to death with a swift pull of the razor. But as soon as I saw you, my heart fluttered and my breath grew short. I felt a sudden responsibility for your well-being, and I wept involuntarily. I am smitten when I catch you looking suggestively out of the corner of your eye. I weep simply to see you, a wonderful puppet dancing in my eyes. During those brief moments I forget my own youthful desires and wish only to mold myself to your body. . . ."

Meanwhile, the old man started to grow uneasy and then angry as he noted the unusual delay. He seated himself in the doorway and cast aspersions on the character of his daughter. "I swear I will have that little wench Ratnakalā flogged. Why has she taken so long to kill that merchant?" He yelled at the closed door, "Now you have turned on me and become my personal Kāli Karāli—the frightfully fanged goddess Kālī who has become an indelible and dark stain on my lineage.[4] You must have lost yourself when you looked into his face. You are talking too much to this merchant. Please come on outside, for the night is fast passing away!"

Ratnakalā whispered through the closed door, "You are getting upset over nothing! This handsome merchant's son has not yet fallen off to sleep. Restrain yourself a little longer. As soon as the merchant goes to sleep, I will make cool and quick work of him!"

The old man admonished his daughter, then repaired to his own quarters. Then Ratnakalā turned to speak to the trader Vidyādhara. "You have witnessed yourself, O merchant, how my father rebuked me. Will I manage to escape this time with my life?"

When he heard this plea, the merchant's heart seemed to melt away just as the hot rays of the sun dissolve butter into a formless liquid. The merchant's throat was dry; no words could form in his mouth. He sat transfixed, eyes staring into space, his arms wrapped tightly around his heaving chest. After a seeming eternity, the merchant spoke to her. "There is no one here to back me up. First you come on strong with love and affection. Why now do you plot to kill me? You brought me into your private chamber and treated me as your husband. Now, should you murder me, you will be doing an evil, a violation of the laws of *dharma*, with much greater personal ramifications. Camphor, betel, scent, and sandalwood paste you brought and carefully prepared for my personal pleasure. You have received me with such kindnesses, how now could you bring yourself to slay me? . . ." And so the bewildered merchant continued his queries. "I am the only son of my mother. There is no other in my lineage to perform the *tarpaṇa* rites to sustain my forefathers. O my beautiful lady love, why did you not murder me when I was asleep? Now forced awake, I come to the end of my days suffering a broken heart. I have neither chariot nor charioteer to aid me, so I have no choice but to place all my hopes on your feeble promise, my beautiful! Go ahead, love of my life, put the knife to my throat! Do not rend my heart with false hope only to kill me later!"

As he spoke, the merchant's gaze searched deep into the heart of this beautiful damsel, unleashing a torrent of tears. This simple act completely destroyed Ratnakalā's composure. She cried out, threw her arms around this merchant-son's neck, and wept, clinging tightly. Ensnared in the noose of her love, she protested between sobs. "I am powerless to raise my knife against you!"

Ratnakalā spoke. "My lord, put your mind at ease. There is no reason whatsoever for your body to go weak. One look at you dashed my career as a thief, and from that very moment I have desired only to be your servant. Being a woman, I am most unfortunate, dependent on others throughout this life. My days have passed in the murder of countless hundreds of mercantile venturers. I have never known any man as my very own lord and husband. But now I am your slave and you my master!" The dacoit's daughter urged him, "Do not despise me! Here. Take my razor and kill me instead! . . .

"Remember carefully what I am about to tell you, my beloved, for it shall be the way by which we both escape. When you return home from your trading venture, come back this way and stop in my vicinity. Then you can take me back to your own abode. Please fulfill the heartfelt desire of this poor miserable wretch!"

The merchant replied, "In truth and by the gods do I promise to take you back with me. I have taken the solemn vow with you as my witness. Now tell me truthfully and in detail your plan to save me!"

Ratnakalā then spoke. "As soon as the dawn breaks, beg leave of my father to continue your trading journey. Say 'On my successful return from trade to purchase the *āstānā*, I shall collect your daughter and take her with me.' In precisely this manner you must beg leave, and go. It will be my job to reassure him should he object in any way."

No sooner had they spoken of their plan than dawn crept in and the Lord of Night sank into the western sky. All who would question, listen to these divine words, for the churning of Satya Pīr's story produces a satisfying stream of frothy cream at the end.

As soon as the light of dawn emerged, the merchant got up from his bed. He took himself to the dacoit with palms pressed together in respect. "On my way back from my commercial journey I shall return bearing the golden *āstānā*. Then the two of us—your daughter and I—will go back to my own home." And with the carefully rehearsed words, he departed.

The old man seethed with anger, which soon blazed like a roaring fire. He screamed for Ratnakalā in his rage. "For so many days you have floated and bobbed safely in the waters of our family undertakings. But when you dallied so long in the so-called 'bridal chamber,' I realized that you had finally been swept under by the mighty undertow of love!"

Listening patiently, Ratnakalā skillfully offered her reply. "Your pleasure has been in others' sorrow. You have grown old craving only filthy lucre. Even though you learned a little astrology from the Āgama scriptures, you completely miss their point. In vain have your hair and beard turned grey. You have learned nothing. The trader goes out on his mercantile venture because he has little of value on him now. But when he completes his savvy trading, he will return bearing riches for our treasury. He will carry back a solid gold *āstānā*. Then you can kill him! Where can he escape? By merely sitting in this doorway you will come to possess an *āstānā* of solid gold. When it is melted down, you can give your daughters-in-law thick golden bangles to encircle their arms."

This impassioned argument managed to impress and console everyone, and they could not but agree that what Ratnakalā said made plenty of sense.

By then, having managed to get well away, the merchant Vidyādhara began to breathe easily and turn his thoughts to God. "Only by the benevolent power of my personal God did I escape a sure and certain death by this quick-witted dissimulation." Thinking along these lines, the merchant continued his journey to the commercial trading center. He announced his arrival with the usual gifts of tribute and honor. He tarried for many long days in the city, waiting to have the *āstānā* made to carry home. The *āstānā* was solid gold, with a gold column standing on each of its four corners, supporting in the middle a platform seat for the worship of Satya Pīr.

When the *āstānā* was completed, the merchant paid his respects to the local king and took his leave. Having accomplished the goal of his trading expedition, he departed for his own homeland. With a deeply troubled heart, the trader declared that he would never grace the door of the dacoit again, should his life depend on it. "My mind is constantly locked on thoughts of home, and I am reminded of the story of King Śṛṅgadhara's trust of a woman. Dhanvantari likewise depended on a woman for the knowledge of *mantras* used to subdue Viṣaharī, Manasā the goddess of snakes.[5] It is undoubtedly true that if I do not return, I will break my solemn promise; but when I return home safely, I will summon the destitute and offer them gifts. I will not go back to that place even if it ensures my demise. I will expiate my fault, my breach of *dharma*, through lavish gifts of charity."

The merchant then left behind the land where he traded, keeping that fateful house in the land of the dacoits well to the south. Meanwhile, speaking with the voice of agamic astrological authority, Ratnakalā called her brothers. "The merchant is trying to flee his new home. Tell him to remember our conversation, then escort the trader back here before he manages to get away!"

Her six brothers took note of what she said. "Your mind seems to be wavering, sister, but now you are making sense. When we brought him to the house before, you failed to kill him, but now. . . ." So off they went to position themselves along the path of the merchant's flight.

The highwaymen soon surrounded him on all sides and as soon as he saw them, the merchant figured that doom was falling around him. The six brothers derided him, "Merchant, shame on you! Where are you going, leaving behind your wife? If you do not have wealth sufficient to support your wife, then you can jolly well stay in our house till you grow old."

The merchant stammered. "I got completely confused on the way and had inadvertently come along this route to reach your house. It is my good fortune that I have stumbled across the lot of you. Come brothers, show me the way to your home." Thus did the merchant proceed to the house of the old highwayman, walking right in the middle of the brothers, with some carefully staying in front, some in back.

They escorted the merchant into the confines of the estate, where he made salutations to his father-in-law. The old man addressed him with a rude anger. "Merchant-boy, you are of such paltry intellect. It is your good fortune that you were not born one of my sons![6] You are the son of a respected merchant, yet you do such dastardly deeds. Feel you no shame in abandoning your wife once again? If you are not in a position to support my daughter properly, then I insist that you stay here in my house until you grow old."

Standing behind a screened partition, Ratnakalā spoke. "Father, you are talking too much! Calm down!"

Interceding like this, Ratnakalā came out and grabbed the merchant's hand. Saying, "Come!" this image of beauty led him inside the house. She had sweets and other delectable morsels brought to feed him, just as the women of Gokula used to feed Kānu, the child Kṛṣṇa. After the merchant ate, he settled into a deep depression and reflected: "The Fates have not been beguiled by my paltry actions these last few days." Then this prize of a woman filled a tray with camphor and betel and served him. When she moved she cast an aura in all directions. Then she went and stationed herself in the doorway, keeping her guard. The merchant, however, had no idea that Ratnakalā was even there. But when she would move her body, her bangles would clink. As soon as he heard the noise, the distraught merchant jumped upright. A great fear pumped through his heart when he saw this enchanting beauty, fully resplendent, come and seat herself on his bed.

Brothers, listen to the play captured in these divine words, the grace granted to the merchant Vidyādhara and Ratnakalā.

The merchant broke the silence. "Recall, my beloved, what I said before. Please forgive me my offense! Raise your head and look at me!"

"You need have no fear of me, honorable one, for you are a clever man—even though I could easily break your pride this very moment. With the sun and the moon and the guardians of the ten directions as my witness, I have committed no offense. It is but the workings of your own fate. Knowingly and willfully did you break your promise to me. I do not know what your Fates now portend. My six brothers are dangerously powerful and violent. In strength each and every one is the son of the Wind himself. You stay put and I will return in the morning. You have seriously endangered yourself by your own volition with respect to your vow. He who honors the law, *dharma*, never conducts himself like this. Your actions impel you to unrighteousness. The man who truly knows and revels in the experience of love would always uphold and respect *dharma*; he would never act as you do. You have heaped shame on me by your attempt to flee. Over and over again my mother and father call me 'whore'!"

The merchant could only reply sheepishly. "I fled to save my life. I have committed a terrible offense against your person. Now take up your razor and kill me with your own hand. How could you hand me over to your brothers?"

When she heard what the merchant said, she was secretly pleased. And so in this kind of pointed exchange did half the night pass. Finally Ratnakalā pleaded with him, her palms pressed together in submission. "Come! Let the two of us run away and disappear in some faraway place! There is no more need to talk. Let us move quickly and fly from here!"

The merchant replied. "When we escape from the danger of this fortified citadel, have you no fear that I will abandon you, my beauty?"

Ratnakalā ignored him and suggested her plan. "We will slip out disguised as armed sentries." No sooner had she proposed it than the couple were putting on pants and tunics. They rounded up from the stable two of the fleetest of horses, each a winged horse, the famed *pakṣirāja*. When these two valiant "soldiers" then took their swords and shields, they were just like Sundara when he headed for the kingdom of Bardhamān. It was late, toward the end of the night's second watch, when the two made good their escape.

To ease the tension, the merchant cracked jokes with the beautiful woman as they made their way. They carefully kept the kingdom of Maheśapurī on their left. There lay the ghat at Mathurā where Nārāyaṇa met the hunchback,[7] and to their left they passed the beautiful citadel of Lakṣmī's abode. Lest anyone following anticipate that they might go to Ayodhyā, Rāma's citadel, they followed another route much farther to the north. The son of the merchant was mulling all kinds of alternatives, when finally he looked Ratnakalā straight in the face and spoke.

"Listen, my beloved, for I have something to say that worries me greatly. It is going to be virtually impossible for me to take you along the road during daylight hours. You should stretch out and take rest here on the bank of the river, while I go into the local bazaar to fetch some food. We shall proceed at night and no one will recognize us. Rest awhile here at the foot of this tree. I shall go do the necessary shopping and return quickly. In the meanwhile, you stay here and do not worry yourself further, just relax and rest." Imparting this instruction, the merchant headed for the bazaar.

On the banks of the local pond lived a woman everyone knew as Auntie. She was the local flower vendor. Now this woman, who went by the name of Hīrā, which means "Diamond," was a character. Her cheeks bulged red with betel and she was given to suggestive, even bawdy, talk of love play, but with a comical rolling of eyes and exaggerated expressions. She wore a red outfit to match her mouth, and carried a small wicker basket on her left arm. And when she looked up at the merchant who was coming her way, this woman actually swooned. When she could finally collect her wits, she inquired politely, "Where are you from? Where do you call home?" Then she generously offered a string of *campaka* magnolia blossoms to place on his neck.

Catching the drift of her line, the merchant was quick to reply. "Listen, sweetheart, you cannot engender love in this heart with a simple garland. I am not inclined to wear the garland you offer, but it would be truly beautiful gracing your own lovely neck."

As soon as she heard this witty reply, the garland weaver hung her head and cried loudly, "Why are the Fates so hard?" Then she thought to herself, "How might I bewitch this fine trading man? If I do not use something powerful, he might well give me the slip." So she sprang up and slipped the garland around his neck before he could react, and as the string of flowers slid over the merchant's head, she rubbed a little magic into it.

And so it was that the Fates arranged more misadventures for the merchant, for he was now ensnared like a hapless bird in the net of a fowler. In a flash, the handsome merchant Vidyādhara metamorphosed into a jet-black ram. And that old flower lady gleefully escorted him home. She kept her ram secure with a tether around his neck, sequestered, hidden deep inside her house. She fed him only tender *durbbā* grass.

And so it came to pass that the flower vendor managed to kidnap the merchant.

Listen, all good brothers, to the divine story of the Pīr. Just as Sītā lost Rāma in the Pañcavaṭī Forest, and Cintā lost King Srivatsa, so did Ratnakalā lose her merchant.

A few minutes soon stretched to eventide, and Ratnakalā wailed, "I have been cursed to bad fortune, to become a widow!" In great agitation, Ratnakalā sought to call up her extensive knowledge of agamic *mantras* and spells, but thanks to the Pīr's own deluding magic, she could remember none of it. Galvanized to action, she moved out with the two horses. No one could tell that she was not a man.

The king of that land was one Bhojapati Rāya, and at his court Ratnakalā soon arrived. She dismounted and paid her deepest respects.[8] The king politely inquired, "What, my good man, is your name?" To which this soldier replied,[9] "Listen to my particulars, O King. I was born in a clan of warriors and my residence is in the Malla country. My father is the well-known Vīrasiṅgh. I am Ranasiṅgh Rāya, the fighting son of that venerable man. I have four brothers, with whom I do not get along, so I have come to this land seeking employment in your personal service. You are the supreme lord among the many lords of this earth. I present myself as a servant at your palace door."

As soon as he heard this elegantly stated explanation, the king accepted the offer of service and appointed her with a salary of fifty rupees. He also provided over twenty-five hundred cowries for expenses and furnished her with a splendidly appointed residence. She took the opportunity to announce that she had taken a vow to fast when the sun was up and never to bathe and perform any sacred rituals and so forth during the daylight hours—a convenient vow, thereby protecting her identity. Late at night, during the second watch, she would perform her daily ablutions so that come sunrise she would be ready, dressed in her soldier's trousers and tunic. In just this routine did she pass many days, until one fine day the kingdom was swamped in paroxysms of fear from a marauding rhinoceros.

There were, of course, any number of truly brave and valiant soldiers living in the kingdom, but the fear of this rhino paralyzed every single heart. The king finally proclaimed that anyone who could slay this rhinoceros with arrows, or any other weapon, would win the hand of his daughter in marriage. But, alas, being sorely afraid, no one stepped forward to lay claim to this wonderful prize, until finally the courageous Ranasiṅgh stood up to be counted.

Everyone held his breath as "he"—they still had no idea who she was—set out to subdue the rhino, whose destruction was made possible by the grace of the Pīr. Listen with wonder and delight to the clever machinations of the Pīr.

The king's warriors were outfitted and resolute in their commitment to this battle. The hero, Ranasiṅgh, sped forth like a shooting star, and in the twinkling of an eye came upon that ferocious rhinoceros. The rhino was right then deep, deep in sleep. With a solitary raging blow, she slew the beast. She cut off its horn, its tail, and its tongue and quickly mounted her horse, the same way that Śyāmārāya or Kālī would kill from her fearsome tiger-mount.

Immediately thereafter the other soldiers fell on the rhino's carcass with a fury, and, having reduced it to tiny strips of meat, each offered his piece to the king to claim the reward. Watching this strange and confusing event unfold, the king worried just how he could possibly choose one ordinary soldier from among these to make his son-in-law!

"To which one shall I have my daughter submit? Please advise me the proper way of discriminating, my good minister!"

The savvy minister quickly replied. "Listen to my advice, O King. That warrior who produces the horn, the tail, and the tongue is the true slayer. To him you should award your daughter. This you must publicly proclaim, O King!"

The great king acknowledged the sense of it. "This really was what I had intended." And about that same time, the heroic warrior Ranasiṅgh arrived in court.

Making a deep and formal obeisance, she offered the horn, the tail, and the tongue; and in return, the king proffered his own royal raiment and announced: "To this man shall I award my daughter!" But the soldier quickly countered, "Please consider my earnest request. For twelve years have I faithfully observed the Uṣā vow, honoring the daybreak. When I have completed this devotional observance, I shall ask of you a boon. This is how I worship Hara-Gaurī. Only when my vow is completely fulfilled am I free to marry. I bid you to construct for me a special temple that I may do good acts, honoring brahmins and the gods."

The king, of course, was extremely gratified and relieved at Ranasiṅgh's plea, and he wasted no time in having the special temple constructed. This lovely young woman, still believed a man, then devoted herself to serving brahmins and Vaiṣṇavas, but her thoughts were far away with the critical question: "How long will it take to recover my husband? Alas, I am wasting away. Into what strange place and circumstance has the lord of my life disappeared? . . ."

By the divine decree of the Pīr, this woman shall in the end get what she desires. Listen, Brothers, to the holy tale of the Pīr, whom I circumambulate and to whose feet I make a thousand joyous salutations. Shrewd and threatening plots are circumvented and obstacles to success torn asunder by this Pīr who is replete with mercy, and who is friend to all of his devoted servants.

With pointed intention did Ratnakalā worship Hara-Gaurī. This lovely woman thought only this: "When will I get back my lost treasure, my husband?"

Just as Jambuvatī, daughter of Jambara, in the netherworld propitiated Hara-Gaurī for the sake of Kṛṣṇa, and Satyabhāmā, the daughter of King Satrājit, worshiped the three-eyed goddess in her desire for Kṛṣṇa, so too did this beautiful woman regularly and systematically serve brahmins and deities on account of her merchant-husband.

One month passed in this way, and Ratnakalā began to worry because she had not located her husband. "When I sleep, when I eat—I never forget him. I continue to worship Hara-Gauri, but I wonder how much longer it will take," this image of beauty worried. "My luck has turned sour, just as when Bhānu's young daughter Rādhā was estranged from Kṛṣṇa." And in this way did wild thoughts begin to tumble through her head by the hundreds, for she had found no trace of his whereabouts nor any clue to his condition. "O my fate! When will I get back my treasure? What can I do? When can I have my husband?"

The suffering that unsettled the mind of this beauty quickly multiplied to the point that she gave up food and water and could only sit with her head hanging in despair.

Listen, my brethren one and all, to the divine story of the Pīr. This woman found her heart and mind inconsolable at the loss of her husband; and through such suffering few if any can surive. Listen now to the merchant's claim to misery.

In the private abode of the flower vendor, the good merchant Vidyādhara passed his days as a ram, but his nights as a man. The merchant had been transformed into a ram by the garland weaver's powerful magic in a manner not dissimilar to the way King Nala suffered from his curse.[10] After many blurry days, the flower vendor wanted the merchant for intimate companionship and conversation, so she granted him a new body—somehow different from the old—which sent ripples of pleasure through the merchant's heart. The merchant spoke. "Talk to me, my beautiful! For twelve years I have been worshiping Hara-Gauri. I have vowed that so long as my wish remains unfulfilled, I will never suffer the touch of a woman. But be neither anxious nor worried when you hear this, for in the end I will fulfill your heart's craving. But first, tell me the story behind these loud noises I am hearing. Why do the royal kettle-drums boom from the temple grounds? Everyone has been carrying on with obvious excitement and great commotion, so much so that my heart constantly yearns to visit there."

The garland weaver replied, "If you go, what will you be able to see? How will you eat? And what can you learn? You will still be a ram!"

The merchant readily countered, "Take me as a man! I will never forget your kindness, even at the cost of my life!"

As she listened to the merchant's plaintive cry, a little compassion welled in her, so she transformed him into a man and off together they went. They moved in tandem, the end of her garment tied to the end of his. She seated them in the northeast corner of the temple compound, where they attracted no attention.

While the flower vendor's mind was absorbed in the acting and singing onstage, the fire of separation seared the heart of this merchant's son. With his mind thus agitated, his thoughts were directed to the Supreme Lord, Īśvara: "Woe is me, for my lady love and wife has completely forgotten me! What more can I say about this cruel misery? By the writing on my forehead, God has decreed this fate of separation."

As his thoughts mounted, his grief intensified all the more. He sat transfixed in this abject condition, his head down, refusing food and drink. Then the Pīr said to him in benevolent and consoling tones: "Why do you worry so? May your mind be patient and endure, for you will get what you want in the end. Misery graces my own brow on account of you!" Then Satya Pīr concluded, "Never turn your face from me again!"

Listen, dear brothers, to the divine tale. The merchant's heart was distraught at the loss of his wife.

Ceaselessly did his mind survey the seemingly endless possibilities. "How long must I wait to find you out?" he wondered. Ingeniously, he surreptitiously wrote of his experience on the wall of the temple compound. "Listen, my beloved, to what the Fates have inscribed on my forehead. I had you stop and wait for me while I went to the bazaar. A flower lady transformed me into a ram by some powerful magic concoction. Bearing the body of a black ram, my soul knows only humiliation and torment. That misery burns my heart like a flame. I have been given only water from an earthen pot to drink. Take note, my lovely, of the fruits of my fate! That you live comfortably in the palace compound redoubles the intensity of my affliction, to the point of breaking my will to live. You have not even tried to use that fabulous knowledge of the magical Āgamas to save me. Why and how could you have heaped such misery on me when I am not at fault? One time I lied, laying waste my promise and undermining your trust. Now I imagine that perhaps you are getting even. Is your personal conduct becoming to you if, by dwelling on that, you fail to rescue me? . . ." And so the merchant managed to write these and other anguished words that struck straight to the heart. But soon again he was forced to return to the flower vendor's house.

Meanwhile, Ratnakalā had returned to her own quarters to sleep. She got up before the crack of dawn as was her custom. Inspecting all four sides of the temple, as she always did, she noticed the special notations that had been scribbled on the wall of the northeast corner. When she deciphered their meaning, a thrill raced through this good woman, just as Sītā Devī had felt upon picking up the first trace of Rāma! The same excitement that electrified Rādhā's heart when she received news of Kṛṣṇa from the hand of Uddhāva elated even more the mind of Ratnakalā.[11] It was as if a corpse long inanimate had been suddenly revived.

This brilliant woman read the handwriting on the wall and understood completely. "It kills me to imagine what suffering my good merchant has endured!" she cried. "Even if I could have resurrected my memory of the Āgamas, he would still have suffered in the house of the garland weaver. Would I give you such affliction on purpose? It is God, Fate, who has bedeviled you! How else could such suffering be written into our destiny?" With this kind of reasoning, the fair woman immediately departed and betook herself to the king, whom she approached with hands pressed together in supplication.

"My vow of greeting the daybreak, Uṣā, has at last been fulfilled. Be pleased, O King, to procure for me a particular black ram that I fancy!"

Listen everyone with rapt attention to the play of Satya Pīr, wherein the fair woman Ratnakalā saves her merchant-husband.

"Just as Yudhiṣṭhira long ago lost everything in a dicing match and was imprisoned to servitude in the court, only to have the situation salvaged by Draupadī's action—as Vyāsa has made famous in the ancient epic *Mahābhārata*—so too shall I, living here in the king's court, rescue my merchant, who is trapped in the flower vendor's house." For the sake of a ram, then, did this woman have an anxious heart and come to entreat the king to her aid.

The king promptly summoned the prefect of police and ordered him to retrieve the jet-black ram. As soon as he received the king's order, the policeman wasted no time in departing. He scoured the countryside from top to bottom. Just as in that age long ago King Duryodhana dispatched his couriers to search out news of the Pāṇḍavas, so too did the king send out his own messengers, who pried into every house in every village of the land. Nowhere was the jet-black ram to be found, and this unfortunate news they duly reported back to the king.

The king fretted when he got the story, but he promptly called Ratnakalā and informed her. Ratnakalā listened, and then said with a knowing smile, "Go and fetch that goat that the flower vendor keeps penned up in her house!"

The policeman jumped at the suggestion and straightaway arrived at the garland weaver's house. Imitating the havoc raised at Laṅkā, they ransacked the house of the flower vendor in their raid. They apprehended both the flower vendor and her ram, and quickly returned to the august presence of the king. Ratnakalā angrily and directly charged her: "If you value your life, transform this goat into a man, into my merchant!"

Everyone present was stunned to hear such a crazy demand. No one had ever heard of a goat becoming a man! But Ranasiṅgh pleaded. "O King, do not be hasty here! Rest assured that this goat can and will be made into a man!"

Searing blows then rained down on the garland weaver as a form of subtle encouragement. Hīrā fell to the ground, thrashing about in her agony. Hoping finally to save her life, she magically transformed the goat into a man. The head dropped off and the form of the goat completely dissolved. The handsome young merchant emerged, resuming his own prior bodily form. Ratnakalā was overjoyed.

No one there had yet realized that she was a woman in the dress of a soldier, in a manner not unlike the Pāṇḍava brothers hiding in the palace of Virāṭa. Gazing upon the face of Vidyādhara, the great but incredulous king questioned him, "How did you mange to get turned into a jet-black goat?" To which the good merchant replied, "Hear, O King, my tale of woe. . . ."

Only by the grace of the Pīr has this misery come to an end.

The merchant said, "Hear, O King, a tale of great suffering. I have appeared at your feet only by the merit of my father. At your behest did I go to collect the *āstānā*, but I soon found myself imprisoned in the house of one Manohara Phāsarā, the so-called Beguiling Cutthroat. I fell in love with his daughter, and this lovely woman—dressed now as a solider—kept me alive. Hauling the gold *āstānā* from the city of my trade, I came to my own country with her in my company. I made her stay at the foot of a tree, while I ventured into the bazaar. Using a magical potion, this garland weaver caused me to be metamorphosed into a ram."

Hearing this story, this jewel among men was overcome with anger and issued a hasty command: the garland weaver was to be beaten until she died. Just as Kṛṣṇa had sucked the life from the demon Pūtanā's breast, so these king's warriors dragged her back to the bank of the river. Having had the flower vendor slain, the king took the good merchant and escorted him into the palace, both quite pleased with the outcome of events. He furnished cooking gear to the merchant, then they retired into the private apartments of the palace to eat. Purifying himself by properly completing his prescribed daily ritual, the king sat to eat with the merchant. Ratnakalā sat together with Citrāvatī, the king's daughter, in her specially reserved spot. When the king was about halfway through his meal, this second woman—Ratnakalā—approached him with her palms pressed together in respect.

"Hear my petition, O King! You are my godfather, my protector in the law, and you will always know me as your daughter. Be merciful to me as you would to your own daughter. Bestow both your daughter and me on this merchant. Heed well my request, for this is the way to preserve the proper order of things, your *dharma*. You have learned the complete truth from the merchant himself."

When he heard this, the enormity of it all dumbfounded the king, but he promptly initiated the sequence of events to marry the two women to the merchant. With proper invitations, the king summoned brahmin *paṇḍitas*, who executed the appropriate purification rituals and arranged matters at the auspicious times. They promptly erected mango shoots in the four cardinal directions, installed waterpots, and demarcated the ritual space, in the middle of which the two daughters were properly committed to the custody of the merchant. As he gave away his now two daughters, the king's elation grew, and he offered a dowry of coral, ruby, and other fabulous gems. Then he escorted the groom and his brides into the living apartments of his citadel where, deep in the private chambers, the women performed rituals appropriate to their gender.

After they completed the women's rituals, they ate, then camphor and betel were passed around to the cleanse the palate. This ménage à trois then mounted the flowered bed in the bridal chamber, but Citrāvatī was soon drowned in a deep sleep.

Gazing hard at Vidyādhara's face, Ratnakalā spoke. "I never dreamed deep in my heart that I would be with you again. Tell me, my lord, everything of your suffering, from beginning to end."

When one takes the name of Nārāyaṇa, the god of death has no hold.

Slipping her arms gently around her merchant's neck, Ratnakalā prodded him. "What kind of terrible agony did you suffer when you were a goat?"

The merchant replied, "I simply got what my fate dictated. What more can I say, my beauty? When I left you and went over to the bazaar, the garland weaver ensorcelled me with a magic potion that transformed me into a goat. Each day until night I was kept tied under a wooden deck. I knew nothing of regular food and rice, and I ate only *durbbā* grass. Listen, my dearly beloved, to the fruit of my destiny. She dug a hole in the ground and filled it with water for me to drink. Because I broke my sacred promise to you, I suffered this ignominious fate in the house of the flower vendor!"

Ratnakalā responded emotionally, "Alas, woe is me! Even at the cost of my life, I could never believe that to be the case. No one carries the blame for what is written in my own karma!" And then the couple made love. . . .

And so they reveled in their love until night gave way to dawn. After they arose, the merchant met with the king. He made over the gold *āstānā* and then begged his leave. The king outfitted his son-in-law with great pleasure. This king then adorned his two daughters and his new son with fine raiment and assorted costly pieces of jewelry. Then King Bhojapati Rāya granted leave to the merchant; he accepted the golden *āstānā* and promptly offered worship to God, Khodā. All of the brahmin *paṇḍitas*, their aides, and others present performed the worship in the eight-chambered shrine with great joy. From its raw and cooked ingredients the *śirṇi* offering was assembled in the living quarters and used to perform the worship of the Pīr, which delighted the hearts of all. With magnificent pomp and show, war trumpets blared and double-ended drums echoed their call, while untold numbers of women blasted conchs and trilled the auspicious *hulāhuli* sound with their tongues. The Pīr and Prophet were venerated in the king's palace, which received in turn the tiniest glance of favor from the corner of the Pīr's eye.

Whoever might sing of, and whoever might listen to, the divine story of the Pīr will have his heart's secret wishes accomplished and his desires fulfilled. Everyone be pleased to say, "Hari, Hari!" for pleasure ensues. The poet records that at this point the story is coming to a close.

The merchant finally arrived at his own home, where he made obeisance to the feet of his mother. The old woman was thrilled to meet her daughters-in-law, whom she quickly seated on a fine blanket spread especially for them. The young merchant sat on the right side of the two brides. The trader then ate rich foods—all the delicacies, including smooth cream, clotted cream, and curds. And in this way the family passed the night. When they arose in the morning they formally remembered Hari in ritual. The merchant said, "Pay special heed to what I have to say, my dear wives! We shall routinely offer the worship of the Pīr in our house."

Milk, jaggery, the finest wheat flour, betel, flowers, perfumes, sugar, sweet drops, and *sandeśa* milk sweets were made ready—each in measures of one and one quarter maunds. He sent for the brahmin *paṇḍitas*, and invitations were issued to good friends, close associates, and those especially cherished by the family. The participants were assembled and seated properly. The worship of Satya Pīr was executed in strict adherance to the Vedic ritual prescription. The altar or *vedi* was demarcated, spread on the ground, with a wooden platform erected and covered to be the object of worship. Inside was deposited a knife, a large hooked machete, a curved broadsword, and a discus. Betel leaves and betel nuts were distributed in measures of one and one quarter maunds.

And so the merchant offered *pūjā* to the Pīr and honored God. Lifting their faces, they worshiped Satya Nārāyaṇa. Special friends and loved ones were seated in the honorary positions to the east. Everyone made his obeisance at the conclusion of the *pūjā*. The *prasāda*, that special sanctified food left over from the *pūjā*, was distributed to all present. After the last of the *prasāda* was parceled out, they consumed the *śirṇi*, and the crown jewel of *pīrs* showered his grace on the merchant. When people finished eating the *prasāda*, they went home, and Satya Pīr returned to his own city of residence.

May all dedicate themselves in joy to make the sound of "Hari," whence beneficence will redound everywhere by the good grace of God!

The Bloodthirsty Ogress Who Would Be Queen

Kiṅkara Dāsa's *Śaśīdhara Pālā*

May everyone listen and with attention,
you can sidestep the snare of Yama, the god of death,
by simply taking the name of Satya Pīr Sāheb.
All goals and objectives are successful,
while disease, persecution, even fear of snakes,
every imaginable misery flees by virtue of the name.

Dwelling in Maga in the old land of Burma,
there was a great king named Mayūrdhvaja, the Peacock Banner,
who had a son named Śaśīdhara, Beautiful Moon.
He was a great devotee of Nārāyaṇa,
and was born to this world
to the business of destroying *rākṣasa* demons.
Greater than that of the celestial nymphs, even greater than the gods,
was the sheer physical beauty of this young man,
giving the king an unfathomable joy to behold.
The child could always be found crawling in the lap of the king,
who looked upon him with an affection dearer than life.
So day by day did this Śaśīdhara grow.

Like any five-year-old, Śaśīdhara could be found playing in the dirt and dust with his dearest companions. He would sing the names of God, of Hari, along with the other children, clapping hands and clanging small finger cymbals; the tenor of his voice rivaled that of the fabled *kokil* or cuckoo. Soon thereafter this king had augured the most auspicious day to begin the boy's education, and so he ritually placed the chalk in the boy's hand, as was the custom. And so in this fashion Śaśīdhara was made over to his teachers, which pleased his mother and father. At the end of his fifth year, he was deemed competent in all phases of education taught at the local school. After this the young prince learned a set of eighteen classical arts, and then mastered spelling and orthography. The child read the ancient *Bhāgavata Purāṇa*, in which one finds the stories of Kṛṣṇa's activities, and he studied Tantra, *mantra*, and other ancient texts. He studied the rules of euphonic combination, case-endings, but left for later the study of the science of declinables in Sanskrit grammar. A veritable treasure of virtues was he in his study of a full range of texts. Any number of sacred texts fell under his gaze, and then he undertook various philosophies, and their advanced *ṭīkā* and *ṭippanī* commentaries. In the company of learned *paṇḍitas* did Śaśīdhara expound the ancient texts and render sophisticated interpretations of astrology and astronomy. In the manner of the sun illuminating the world, Śaśīdhara aspired to poetry and composed any number of verses in the *śloka*, that is the standard couplet, and in other meters.

On the feet of Lord Nārāyaṇa Śaśīdhara kept his mind firmly fixed and so saw Nārāyaṇa in all things.

Seated in Mecca, the pleasant and entertaining Pīr consulted his adviser, the wazir. "To what land should I go, in order to receive my proper worship—this has been worrying me day and night."

The wazir listened attentively, then, placing the palms of his hands together in a gesture of respect, replied, "Listen, O great treasure trove of virtues, there is in the land of Maga a great house, that of Mayūrdhvaja, king and foremost among men. He has a son named Śaśīdhara. Take yourself to his palace and that crown prince will offer you worship accompanied by other devotees who will do the same. He is the dear *badshāh* of Sāheb, the Pīr, and was born to this world specifically to slay demons. As his name suggests, the beauty of his form is more radiant than the moon's, and the king is filled with affection when he sees him. He keeps him close by all the time, seeing in him his own life; he feeds the young man clotted cream and milk with his own hand. At the age of seven years the boy has successfully completed the course of study in his local teacher's school. With his many companions does he go around; day and night he reads the *Bhāgavata Purāṇa*."

After this consultation, Nārāyaṇa assumed the form of a fakir and traveled to that capital city. Taking a seat on a low cot, he appeared to the young prince in a dream and gave him a *mantra* of initiation. Then the venerable Hazrat Pīr spoke, "Pay attention, child, for in truth you are a great devotee of mine. My desires have yet to be fulfilled. Take yourself to the citadel of Gayā, my child, decamping from the king and his castle. In the Tretā Age, Raghunātha, at the command of his father, took Sītā as his companion to dwell in the forest. Proceeding to Pañcavaṭī, Rāma constructed a small hut in the midst of the jungle. It was there that Sītā fell into Rāvaṇa's grasp. Crossing over ranges of towering mountains, then constructing the land bridge Setubandha, Hanumān bounded across to the isle of Laṅkā. When he crossed over, Raghuvīra hacked off the heads of Rāvaṇa, then picked up Sītā and escaped Laṅkā. Taking along Hanumān and Sītā, Raghunātha roamed back through the forests to his own encampment. Hauling two demonesses, called *rākṣasakās*, back along the Setubandha land bridge, he cast them out into the wilds of the jungle." The Pīr said, "Listen to me carefully. When those two had safely traversed the embankment they took up residence in the forests. Śaśīdhara, you have been born to slay these moronic good-for-nothings with your own hands and to spread goodness in the world." Revealing this to Śaśīdhara in his dreams, then imparting a *mantra* into his ear, the Pīr vanished.

The Pīr disappeared into thin air, and the entire depths of the night passed before Śaśīdhara got up. When he did, he was uneasy and restless, so taking his three companions he went to a quiet place to sit, a solitary place where he could calm himself. "I must slay the demons in the forest"—this idea began to consume him, though he knew not why. He wanted desperately to escape the palace to effect it.

Recognizing some remorseful malady on the part of her son, the queen, Madanā, inquired of him, "Why, my little child, are you suffering so, why does your body waste away? Go and play mindlessly with the other children all covered with dust. I think I am beginning to understand something of the nature of this mendicant stoicism you are projecting. I have heard in the *Bhāgavata Purāṇa* that to sing the qualities of Śrī Kṛṣṇa in *bhajana* leads one to search for an appropriate manner of striving for religious perfection. And on many occasions have you recited the sacred *Bhāgavata* text with arms upraised, calling out the names of Rādhā and Kṛṣṇa. It was Bhagavān who liberated Prahlāda from the flaming weapon and from under the foot of the elephant. He showered favor and compassion on Prahlāda, and as Indra strode through the heavens, Prahlāda slew Hiraṇya on the limen of the doorway. In a manner such as this do I sense that you wish to abandon your home, casting off your mother and father."

This the queen respectfully reported back to the king, and so it has been written by Kiṅkara Dāsa.

The queen addressed the king, "O King, I humbly submit to you that I am not able to fathom the heart and mind of Śaśīdhara. Śaśī plays with his friends and never returns home. When I call for him, he never answers." At these words of the queen, the king reflected, indeed began to worry, and so took himself to find Śaśīdhara. "Come into the house and sit on my lap, my little darling. Let us hear once again you calling out for your mother and father. With my own eyes I wish to see you once again playing in the house. To see again your face like the moon would soothe and cool our burning hearts."

Śaśī gave no reply, but kept his own counsel in his heart of hearts. Just as Rāma had resolved to destroy the demon Rāvaṇa, so too did Śaśīdhara mull over deeply his need to leave home in order to destroy the *rākṣasī* demonesses. About this time, the son of a courtier, the son of the finance minister, and the son of the chief of police all arrived, having slipped away from their houses. Śaśī made obeisance at the feet of his mother and expressed his desire to go into the gardens with his friends. Though just a child of seven years, Śaśī desired to renounce the world and enter the forest, and it was for this that he sought the blessing for his departure at his mother's feet. When Nandarānī heard that Kṛṣṇa desired to go to Madhupurī, she broke down, weeping bitterly and rolling in the dust in her grief. It was just as Queen Kauśālyā wept for Rāma, just as Śacī Ṭhākurāṇi wept for Gaurāṅga.[1] All the good citizens of this king's realm wept in the extremes of their grief, just as the citizens of Ayodhyā were loath to let Rāma depart. There was only one dear son, not the usual five or six. And when that child is not visible in the house, it falls into darkness. "Do not go, do not go, my child, stay a while longer. When I drink this poison and die, only then may you go," pleaded the queen.

Śaśīdhara finally spoke to the larger assembly that had gathered. "May the responsibility for my mother be shared by all. Please honor my promise, my playmates and companions: all of you must call my mother 'Mother' as your own. . . ." And speaking like this, Śaśī and his three companions made themselves scarce, after making obeisance to the feet of Satya Nārāyaṇa. They departed for and eventually arrived at the land of Śaśī's maternal uncle. Meanwhile the queen alternately wept and fainted out of grief for her only son.

Kiṅkara Dāsa composed the auspicious song of the Pīr, while the king and queen remain distraught in their grief for their son.

Keeping Tripura's Kallārapura at a distance, Śaśī and his companions finally gained sight of the land of the Mallas. The king of Mallabhūma, one Daṇḍarāya—whose name means "Lord of Justice"—was out hunting in his forests and there he spotted Śaśīdhara. King Daṇḍa greeted them with affection and took them along, feeding them sweets as is customary for honored guests. Offering scented betel quids and seating them on a palanquin, the great king began to inquire of them, "Even though you are but mere children, you have abandoned your mothers and fathers and left your own country. For what possible reason did you, the son of a king, bring your three companions and give up your palaces?"

Śaśīdhara replied, "My dear uncle, listen carefully to what I have to say. We are planning to visit five different pilgrimage centers. This is all I have ever planned. When that is done, I will return once again to my father." Thus easing his uncle's understandable concern, Śaśīdhara departed with his three companions. Seeing Candramukhī in the town of Jājapura, they caught sight of Viṣṇu Nārāyaṇa, and then visited Vaidyanātha. Day and night did they journey along their path, fulfilling their secret desires, until eventually they entered the land of Gayā. As a great adept, a *siddha*, Rāma had sat there at that spot in meditation, deeply absorbed, in the yogic position, and brought the ancestral manes, the *pitṛloka*, down to earth to pay his respects. The fortunate and blessed Lord Raghunātha, acting together with Jānakī, offered the riceball obsequies of *piṇḍadāna* at the pilgrimage center of Gayā. Rāma auspiciously proceeded with his divine yoga, and Sītā took her seat right there when the manes of *pitṛloka* appeared. With Jānakī made to stand in front, the ancestors begged the offering of riceballs when they saw Rāma's reflection. Sītā offered the *bālī piṇḍa*. When they were sated, the manes returned to heaven and the ancestors were satisfied. So blessed is Gayā, a place of great merit, dear to holy mendicants and devotees, and at whose simple sight one's heart is purified. The four friends moved as one, traversing the byways of Gayā. All of them were thrilled.

Seeking refuge at the feet of the Pīr, Kiṅkara Dāsa writes. May Satya Nārāyaṇa grant you his grace. Your servant seeks your protection. My Lord, please save this wretched evil one, and may your favor be turned toward this unfortunate soul.

After visiting Gayā, then the Gaṅgā and Godāvarī rivers, they arrived at the holy ford of Kāśī, where they took sight of Annapūrṇā. At Prayāga, where the three sacred rivers meet,[2] they visited the sacred banyan tree called Bācchāvaṭa. Eventually this crown prince entered the land of Kurukṣetra, the fabled battlefield described in the *Mahābhārata*. Śaśīdhara then announced, "My friends, let us now return to our own land, for I wonder how our mothers and fathers are back home." With this pronouncement, the crown prince began the journey.

After some time they found themselves right in the middle of a thick forest grove. After triumphing in Laṅkā, Rāma, the sage of the Raghus, had returned this same way. And even now the two *rākṣasīs*, Jaṭīlā and Kuṭīlā, terrorized the area. One ogress, Kuṭīlā, saw Rāma on the banks of the Surnadhī River, while Jaṭīlā remained deep in the forest. The two *rākṣasīs* exercised various forms of magic and used numerous subterfuges to trap their prey. They would sit here and there along the river at various landing ghats, with beautiful garlands hanging from their necks. Pots smeared with auspicious marks of vermilion and decorated plates right and left, and before them were lined up row upon row of offerings made of sugar and banana. The prince found the place extremely charming. When they beheld the feast, each wanted to eat and slake his thirst. The four of them decided to get some water to drink. So they made their way to a small lake to bathe. The minister's son was dispatched to procure proper food for offerings, and so that innocent child went straight to the ogress. With a happy heart did he go to collect the necessary ingredients, but suddenly the *rākṣasī* assumed her own form and grabbed the boy's legs. In this fashion was the first boy quickly swallowed into her ravenous stomach. Then, exercising her magic, the *rākṣasī* resumed her position of sitting quietly on the landing ghat. Śaśīdhara commented, "Now that our good friend has filled his stomach with sweets, he must be sated from his meal and has decided to lie down for a nap." The finance minister's son, whose name was Sanatāna, was then sent to procure the necessary items for worship. He soon found all the articles right before him and as he looked around, he surmised that his friend had lost his way along the forest path and had ended up who knows where. Thinking this, he went to collect the ingredients for offering when the ogress snatched him by the neck and swallowed him up. Then the son of the chief of police was finally sent, and the *rākṣasī* witch ate him like the rest and resumed her position.

By this time Śaśīdhara had begun to worry. Kiṅkara Dāsa tells how all three were eaten alive.

Famished and thirsty, Śaśīdhara finally went himself. And what he got was sight of the *rākṣasī,* who was sitting hunched like a vulture, belly distended. Her eyes were shot through with blood, and her fangs appeared hideously long. The crown prince's heart was paralyzed by fear. Witnessing this sight, the prince grew terrified and fled as far away as possible, but the ogress with gangly arms and legs rolled along right behind him. "My Lord, please protect me!" he thought as panic filled his heart, and in that panic he bounded up a nearby wood apple tree. The *rākṣasī* thought over the problem, "I have already consumed three young men. How can I climb the tree with such a full stomach?" Contemplating her plight along these lines, the demoness circled the tree restlessly, over and again, then settled in to keep watch over it, holding it fast.

Śaśīdhara began to worry, "Must I die after so few days of life? Save me, O Protecter of Devotees." In order to save Śaśīdhara's life, Satya Pīr produced a *marmelos* fruit that grew on the tree right then and there. Having fallen into such dire straits, Śaśī wept. He kept crying out, "Satya Pīr! Save my life, grant me your protection!" Satya Pīr responded and granted his mercy. The *marmelos* or wood apple split open and Śaśīdhara was able to crawl inside it. Even as Śaśīdhara was ensconced inside the wood apple, the *rākṣasī* stared at it intently. The ogress pondered, "Where on earth can he have got to? He must have taken refuge inside the wood apple!"

At the feet of the Pīr and in desperation does Kiṅkara petition, "Nārāyaṇa, please save this sinner!"

But the *rākṣasī* eventually climbed up the branches, causing the wood apple to drop from its perch into the water, where a giant sheatfish swallowed it in one big gulp. From the heights of that tree did the ogress too fall straight into the waters. Fearful for its life, the giant sheatfish sought refuge in the nasty muck at the bottom. Burrowed deep into the sludge, the fish went undetected. Jaṭilā the ogress then resumed the form of a bewitchingly beautiful woman.

May both Hindus and Muslims listen carefully with a single-minded devotion.

At this time King Mayūrdhvaja undertook a hunting expedition. Escorted by great numbers of foot soldiers, and accompanied by elephants and horses, this great king entered into the forest. Eventually the king stumbled across this charming and beautiful young woman and the effect was the same as when Aniruddha fainted upon first beholding Ūṣā.[3] The king spoke, "My beautiful young lady, why and how have you come to be here? Whose wife and lover are you? And to whom are you daughter?"

Listening to this string of inquiries directly from the king, the enchanting ogress artfully replied, "I am the daughter of a king. In my father's palace I was the elder unmarried daughter and, in conflict over that humiliation, I have now fled deep into this forest. I had constant bickering encounters with my sister and now I have come into the forest to abandon my life."

To this the king replied, "Ah, my beautiful woman, please come home with me instead. I shall make you the chief queen of my palace."

The *rākṣasī* countered, "I will come with you only if you catch and give to me all of the untold numbers of fishes that populate this lake. When I was bathing, my necklace dropped into the water and a large sheatfish swallowed it, imagining it to be food. Please catch all the fishes in this lake and I promise you truly that I will accompany you."

The king replied, "I will catch the fish just by indicating with my finger that it should be done." Then the king ordered the minister to comb the lake for fish. The minister in turn ordered all of the coolies who were gathered there, "Cast your nets all over the lake and catch the fish now!" No sooner had the command been given than they jumped to, sifting the lake's waters. Eventually they caught all of the fish and brought them forward. The fish were stacked in heaps before the enchantingly beautiful young woman. All the fish were gutted, their stomachs emptied, but not one yielded the wood apple. Contemplating the situation, the *rākṣasī* reasoned, "The sheatfish must have already digested it. So why should I continue to live here all alone? I will go and take up residence in the king's palace as the chief queen. And there I will be able to procure countless numbers of elephants, horses, goats, and other animals, while here in the forest I find very little if anything to eat. . . ."

The king then pressed her, "My beautiful woman, come still to my house."

And off went that alluring woman to the king's palace.

About the time the beguiling demoness was accompanying the king to his palace, a young and very poor cowherd boy who lived in the capital city was crying out in anguish, "O Mother, give me some food, some rice, I'm hungry!" To which his mother replied, "Come my child, eat some rice, but that is all there is." The cowherd boy rejoined, "Then I shall go and catch a fish." His mother responded, "Don't go, for that is the king's private lake." The young cowherd replied, "Let me see what I can find that can be roasted or fried. I shall snare something from down in the muck among the scavenging bottom-feeders—what will the king do about that, for he would never eat such a catch." And so the cowherd went off to catch fish, and just at the wrong time that sheatfish raised its head out of the slimy mud in which it had burrowed. It was landed. Its grizzly face was puffed out like some blacksmith's bellows, a fisherman's line looped over its head and snagging two or three of its fins. It was so big it had to be dragged to the old woman. "Please fry up this fish, but it has a large batch of eggs in its belly." The poor cowherd went off to bathe, while his mother looked at the fish, her heart abounding in joy. As soon as the knife sliced into the fish to gut it, the wood apple popped out of the fish's stomach. "When he went out he told me there would be eggs inside. When he returns I'll have to have a word with him for there are no eggs, only the wood apple." But the wood apple, being intact, the old woman kept safely aside in her room. She cleaned the fish and cut it into pieces to make a rich fish curry and a savory accompaniment.

When the cowherd returned to the house the old woman served him his rice. He ordered her, "Please fry up the eggs first, then I will eat the rice." The old woman retorted, "There were no eggs, only a wood apple stuck in its stomach." Hearing this the young cowherd got up from his meal, leaving his food untouched. When he found the wood apple, the cowherd decided to break it open to eat it. Still inside, Śaśīdhara cried out, "The cowherd is rescuing me!" Just as Śukadeva had spoken angrily from inside the womb of his mother,[4] so could a young man be heard from within the wood apple. Carefully the cowherd cut open the wood apple with his machete and out popped Śaśīdhara. As soon as he saw the prince, the cowherd fell down in full prostration at his feet. "How on earth did a young man like you end up inside a wood apple?" And so Śaśīdhara narrated to this cowherd his strange tale. After he heard it, all the cowherd could do was prostrate himself again at his feet.

Kiṅkara Dāsa says, "Listen to the magic spread by the Pīr. O Lord, full of mercy, please shower your grace on your humble devotees.

The cowherd offered a full salutation with hands pressed together in respect, and then spoke, "Hear what I have to say, my lord. Bidhātā, the god of fate, has prescribed for me nothing but misery. Only by tending the expensive herds of other people's cattle am I able to eke out a living. Whether he be a god or mere mortal, what difference is it to me for I what else can I do but serve? I am totally and completely bereft of wealth, I'm broke. I manage to earn a pittance by husking rice on the side. I am apprehensive about my mother's health. Such is the misery and pain that hangs over my head."

Hearing out the cowherd, Śaśīdhara offered in reply, "Listen, my child, do not feel so downtrodden, things are not that bad. Do your best to take care of me and I promise I will save you from your miseries."

The old woman interrupted, "My adorable young child, I am an incredibly miserable wretch, come look at my humble room, which is in utter shambles. And in the evening things only go from bad to worse, with hordes of mosquitoes buzzing in your ears. How can one keep it together in surroundings such as these? I have but this simple thatched hut. Go find the house of someone who is better off. With unswerving devotion will such a one serve you day and night. My humble abode can offer you nothing you need."

The young lad quickly responded, "Why do you speak like this, as if to drive me away? I have no illusions that you truly are impoverished in every way. But whatever wealth you desire you must take until your mind is put at ease. But apart from riches, what else do you desire?"

The old woman let out cries of "Hari, Hari!" in regret. "I am about to die, subsisting as I do solely on the dregs of husked rice. I have no idea whatsoever what wealth and riches mean. If you are an honorable and forthright gentleman, grant us your favor and bestow wealth upon us, and I will always treat and care for you as my own son."

Śaśīdhara was deeply pleased and produced the astronomical sum of two hundred rupees, which he handed over to the cowherd. That miserable woman was suddenly freed from her misery, having finally seen the face of wealth. She fell down completely prostrate at his feet. The old woman spoke, "My dear child, my pleasure knows no bounds. I must go and get cleaned up as is appropriate. But how did you manage to live inside the wood apple with nothing whatsoever to eat? And then how did you manage to produce such prodigious wealth?"

The prince humbly replied, "Mother, he who bestows boons is but the Pīr. It is only his wealth that one carries. I keep my heart and soul centered on the feet of the Pīr and miraculously I receive the riches, and so it will always be as long as I reside in Bhārata, the land of India."

The old woman couldn't have been happier, and she took this son of a king and cherished his very life as if he were in his own palace. More than a few times did she mull over the prospects. "Now that I have gained such a treasure trove, is there anything or anyone whom I should fear?" Banishing her hesitation, she spent five rupees and proceeded on a buying spree in the market, purchasing a wide assortment of items. She bought the rare *martamān* banana, special sweets, betel nut, and fully matured betel leaves—these and many more things did she collect from the market. Gathering them all together, she hauled them back to her house, where she put her wares on display for Śaśīdhara. Then she prepared and fed him, finishing the meal with sweetmeats. Then she offered camphor and betel slaked with lime. She spread out some bedding and put him down to sleep. Only then did the mother and son cook and eat.

The cowherd served Śaśīdhara to the very best of his ability, and day by day his prosperity grew. But about the night-stalking demoness ensconced in the king's palace, please listen carefully to what I submit to you, appeals Kiṅkara Dāsa. Hindus and Muslims alike should listen to this adventure.

The alluring young witch took up with the king and exercised a full range of pleasurable erotic pastimes. But when at night the lord among men, exhausted, would fall into a deep sleep, the demon woman would venture into the royal stable and gorge herself on a horse and an elephant. Whatever animals happened to be in the stable—elephants, horses, goats, and so forth—the ogress would consume as her nightly repast.

One day the king remarked, "It is odd that since about the time you arrived, any number of horses, goats, and buffaloes have somewhere disappeared; it is all very puzzling. . . ." The beguiling demoness slyly replied, "Do listen carefully to what I am about to submit to you. There is a *ḍākinī*—a female goblin of a particularly voracious sort—ensconced here in your own quarters. Do not be too quick to blame others from outside. Since you procured me, you have completely ignored your other queen. But tomorrow night, my king, I shall expose it all and show you."

After contemplating the enchantress' explanation, the king seemed satisfied. And, mesmerized by the pastimes of night, the king went fast asleep. The demon woman went as usual to consume the horses and elephants, then slipped into the other queen's apartments and pressed her bloody mouth firmly against the queen's and vomited blood, then silently slipped away. That queen, who was deep in sleep, continued in that state unperturbed, while blood oozed from her mouth down onto her breasts. Suddenly the ogress sounded the alarm, "Get up, get up! my king! Come quickly and see for yourself what is on your other queen's face! Listen carefully to the story of my co-wife. It is utterly without purpose to have two wives in this river of life. The woman who is displaced and becomes the second wife inevitably seethes, my lord, even though no one may notice. King Daśāratha sent Rāma into the forest for this. If one is foolish enough to procure two wives, there is no end to the misery and suffering, and he ends in the citadel of death, Yama's abode. Trusting in his dear wife, Rājā Satrājit, who enchanted the heavens and the earth, died. Believing in his attractive wife, Dhanvantarī lost his own life while the goddess of poisons, Viṣaharī Manasā, was victorious. It was this same error that exterminated the lineage of Rāvaṇa: for the sake of Sītā was Rāvaṇa slain at the hands of Rāghava." As the demon woman continued her tirade, the king looked in disbelief at the blood-stained clothes of his now second queen, the blood still dripping from her mouth.

At the suggestion of the demonic witch, the king moved to slay his now displaced queen, but Satya Pīr intervened by taking a seat in the throat of the chief minister, who then spoke. "The demoted queen has turned out to be an ogress. But killing a woman of any sort is a venal sin; banish her to the forest instead. The slaughter of cows and the killing of brahmins are both incredibly serious, but ultimately remediable offenses. For the killing of a woman there is no reprieve. . . ."

At the minister's wise counsel, the king relented and approved the course of action. "Chief of Police, take her into the forest and be quick about it!"

And no sooner had the chief of police received the king's command than he took the queen and abandoned her deep inside the forest, returning as quickly as possible.

Meanwhile, the cowherd's mother had gone out to collect firewood, and before long she heard the plaintive weeping of the abandoned queen. Moving toward the sound, she gradually reached her, and then the old woman began to question this jewel among seductive women. "Whose daughter are you? Why are you here? Why are you crying? Here in this forest tigers and bears make their home. Tell me what on earth landed you here? Why must you continue to weep, sitting here all alone? My heart trembles and aches to see you like this."

At the old woman's solicitations, the queen began to settle down. Weeping quietly, she hugged the old woman's neck. "The king went on a big-game-hunting trip and brought back some unknown but beautiful woman as his queen. Then the king tossed me aside and accused me of being a goblin, a bloodthirsty ogress." The queen continued, "Listen to my particulars, Mother. I am the wife and queen of Rājā Mayūradhvaja." Then she added, "Apparently through some fault in my karma I have ended up here in the forest. But when I look at you, my very soul is soothed. You are my mother and father, you are my life breath. Protect me from this misfortune and give me the gift of life!"

When she heard this, the old woman drew her close and hugged her tightly, the tears flowing uncontrollably. "Sit right here and wait for me to return," she consoled the queen, and then slipped away. In about the time it takes to catch your breath, the old woman had managed to run all the way home. She burst into the hut and breathlessly filled in the young prince about her adventure. The crone cried out, "Listen, my child, to the words of the *rākṣasī*. Branding her an ogress, the king turned her out. Now that he has found the other woman he is quite satisfied, indeed bewitched, and so he has banished the first queen to the forest."

When he heard this news, tears began to roll quietly down the prince's cheek. Then Śaśīdhara interrupted her, "My aunt, please go and fetch her here." But before he could finish, the old woman objected, placing her hands over her ears as if to say she couldn't believe what she was hearing. "If I fetch the *rākṣasī* here, she will eat all three of us!" The prince cut her off, "My aunt, do not be afraid. That good woman is none other than my mother; she is no demoness." Instantly convinced, the old woman headed straight back to the queen and presented herself to her.

The old woman then spoke, "Come, Mother, to this old woman's humble shack. At least for the next few days, please stay in our simple hut." As soon as she heard this, the queen burst into tears, and the old woman tried to comfort her with soothing words. "Please don't cry, O Queen, and calm yourself. It breaks my heart to see you in such misery." Even though she could not stop weeping, the queen went and soon they found themselves staring at the entryway to the cowherd's shed. Śaśīdhara made respectful obeisance to his mother's feet. Tenderly holding her feet as refuge, Śaśīdhara began to weep. The queen was nonplussed, "Who are you? Whose son are you? Why do you hang onto this miserable woman and cry so?"

When he heard this opening, his spirits lifted, and he narrated to his dear mother his many adventures. "Please stay here in the cowherd's house at least for a few days, Mother, and I will provide you with the details of everything that has happened." Then Śaśīdhara handed over some two hundred more rupees to the cowherd to cover expenses, while the young prince prepared to leave for the royal palace. Donning his suit of armor and arming himself with a scimitar and shield of royal authority, the crown prince mounted a spirited steed. Keeping the Pīr constantly in mind, the child departed and soon presented himself in the king's court in disguise. With hands pressed together in respect, he made salutations to his father.

May Satya Pīr grant his mercy, writes Kiṅkara.

His physical form was of exceeding beauty, surpassing that of a full moon. Everyone who saw him in court was pleased at the sight. "Tell me your name. From what country do you hail? Tell us forthrightly, whose son are you? . . ." and so it went. Śaśīdhara replied with these words: "Hear me, O jewel among men, my name is Jayasiṃha. Śikhidhvaja is my father's given name,[5] of a *kṣatra* clan, he is successful in all he does. He makes his home in the west in Magadha. So hear me out, O great lord, I can do all manner of dirty work such as catching thieves, and so forth. He who pays me the sum of two hundred rupees will retain my services, and I do not return until and unless I am successful."

The king replied, "My dear young man, please alleviate a great misery that has befallen us and fulfill my wish. I will pay double that to the one who can vouchsafe my protection and guard my life. Please apprehend the thief that resides here in this house. Everything from soldiers and their officers to elephants disappears mysteriously during the night, yet no one ever seems to apprehend the culprit. The chief of police is on the scene during the night yet never manages to catch the perpetrator, and by morning there is no trace."

The prince-in-disguise then replied, "If the criminal is to be apprehended, no one must hear anything about my plan. Repeat to me your promise as follows: 'I will neither visit nor even enter the inner quarters where I normally reside.' "

The king quickly agreed, "Hear me well, I give my sovereign word. You must come and live in my abode from today foward. If you are able to discover and expose the criminal who steals my soldiers, then I will bestow wealth and half of my kingdom on you." The king then turned to his sumptuous meal spread out neatly before him, and a short while later that night retired to sleep. The young prince stationed himself at the king's door.

Meanwhile that ogress, posing as the glamorous wife of the king, joined him on the bed for a variety of amorous pastimes. One of her close companions, however, expressed concern about her going out. Outside, the young prince stood guard, pacing back and forth during the night by the steady light of beeswax candles so as to miss nothing. The *rākṣasī* watched patiently for her opportunity, keeping an eye out for her accomplice Yama, the god of death. But when morning arrived she was still trapped, unable to budge. The scene was repeated night after night, and gradually the *rākṣasī* ogress began to grow thin, denied as she was her steady diet of blood and flesh. Deprived in this manner of her infusions of meat and blood, her body began to waste away. Her physique, once so sexy and enticing, withered. Even the king observed, "My dear lover and companion, when I look at your face my heart aches for you. I have watched as your body grows ever more emaciated. What disease has gotten hold of you? Why do you not speak up and say what is going on?"

The queen replied, "What can I say? Fate itself has turned against me and I will forfeit my very life. The strength in my body has dissipated. Food and water have become like poison. I am watching my own death draw near. But if you would do me the kindness, please honor my request. To treat my condition I wish to smear my body with mud from the Gaṅgā River at that place where it is known by the name of Suradhanī. Send only that individual who can guarantee to deliver it, then I am certain my illness will be cured."

The king replied, "My beautiful woman, you say such impossible things. Who is there who can manage the trip to the Suradhanī?" The demoness, growing ever more bilious and agitated, berated him, "Is there really no one at all who can reach there? No one with the virility and fortitude to pull this off?" But as she spoke she had been piecing things together: "Why is this person camped permanently at my door? He was there in the forest and then was secreted inside the fruit of the wood apple tree. I think I am beginning to see what is going on. If he can be the one sent, my second older sister will be certain to snatch him and eat him up. Then and only then will I be able to eat freely here in the king's confines, and my mortal enemy will go to perdition." Plotting along these lines, the nefarious night-stalker gently suggested, "Indulge me, O great ruler of men. Why not send that stout young man stationed outside my door?"

Kiṅkara offers this scenario with fear and trepidation.

The king spoke directly to Śaśīdhara, "My good young man, the brave Jayasiṃha. Please fetch mud from the Suradhanī River and bring it back to me." As soon as the command was given, the child quickly made ready to go. "I will venture out to the

Suradhanī River and retrieve the precious mud." The young man made formal obeisance and took his leave. But as he traveled along the byways he called out to his Lord Nārāyaṇa. "As Kṛṣṇa, who ever nurtures his devotees as a parent would a child, you saved the Pāṇḍavas in the war against the Kauravas, and all for the sake of those devotees. You saved Prahlāda, my Lord, when you ripped apart Hiraṇya, and you protected Gokula when you lifted Mount Govārddhana with your finger. To the first form of your descent to earth, the *avatāra* Matsya, do I make obeisance. Obeisance be to the Kūrma *avatāra*, which descended as a tortoise to uphold the world. Respects to Varāha, the enchantingly attractive form of the boar. And to that crown jewel of all incarnations, the Lord of the Universe or Jagatpati, Lord Jagannātha, I make obeisance. You are Indra, lord of the gods; you are the moon; you are the Supreme Spirit of all humanity as Agni the Vaiṣvānara fire. O Lord Gadādhara, Who Wields the Club, you are the heavens above and the worlds below. Your plenipotentiary power pervades every atom of this universe, your eternal soul plays in every nook and cranny. You stand first and foremost among males, the Nārāyaṇa who was there from the beginning. I beseech you to rescue me from this grave peril, a truly life-threatening predicament. . . ." And so in this way did the handsome young man sing praise. Seated in Mecca, the Pīr would finally hear it.

For the sake of his devoted servant, Nārāyaṇa became a fakir, and soon he drew near the young man and showed him his auspicious visage. The fakir spoke, "My young boy, why have you called me? I have come here from Mecca just for you. Take a look, O son of a king, at the fruit of your ascetic privations, for the son of Nanda, Kṛṣṇa, is there at the foot of the *kadamba* tree."

The young man replied, "I wish to see you, my Lord and Master, in the very same form that Akrūra glimpsed in the waters of the Yamunā River." Accordingly, the crown prince beheld that form. "Save me from the bloody maw of that demon woman, the *rākṣasī*, O Nārāyaṇa. For your sake alone did I leave my mother and father behind, and for your sake, three of my close companions were given into the mouth of the ogress. My dear mother has been exiled to the forest through false testimony and now the meat-eating bitch Jaṭilā has requested mud from the Surayū, the Suradhanī River. . . ."

Satya Nārāyaṇa reassured him, "Your earnest wishes will be fulfilled. The power over the demon woman's very life will fall into your hands. . . ." But no sooner had that been promised than the second ogress picked up the scent of human flesh.

May Satya Pīr shower down his mercy and grace, sings Kiṅkara Dāsa.

At the whiff of fresh human flesh, the *rākṣasī* landed on Śaśīdhara in a flash in order to eat him. The crown prince grieved for himself as he shamelessly hurled himself to the ground, grabbed the feet of the demoness, and groveled. The night-stalking monster roared angrily, "Now that I've got you, why all the fuss? No matter how much you cry and whine I am not going to let you go. Only after a long, long wait has fate brought you to me, and I have every intention of eating you up, count on it."

"First let me tell you a little story so that the fear that grips my heart might be turned to something more salutary. I am the son the of your own sister. My mother, too, is a night-stalking carnivore. She entered the forest and was sitting on the edge of a small lake. The king was out big-game hunting when he suddenly caught sight of my mother and wasted no time in taking her back to his own palace. She had taken on the appearance of a charming lady of the court and lived in the king's palace as queen. From her union with the king I was born. When my mother was stricken with a grave illness and no appropriate medicines could be located, she said to me—and now I tell you—'Go right this minute to the only place where the medicine is located and bring it right away.' And so it was that my mother dispatched me with great haste. 'Take yourself to the banks of the Suradhanī where lives my youngest sister. . . .' My mother has taken up residence in a proper home, while you continue to live in the wilds of the forest. Nonetheless I am still your sister's son, your nephew."

The demon woman found herself torn by indecision, but finally threw her arms around the neck of the young man and wept as she muttered, "This is truly my good fortune." Then the ogress listened a little longer to what he said and she suggested, "My child, my darling nephew, you must come and stay with me in my house. You can have anything you desire, just stay here as my own son, stay here beside me always."

Śaśīdhara pleaded, "O Mother, listen carefully to what I say. I must at least return and inform my own mother. Give me the special mud and water from Suradhanī so that my dear mother might get well. After that I will explain everything to her and return."

"When I look upon him I am enthralled with the sense of motherhood and my eyes drip with the blood of affection. How then can I let him return home just like that? Yet if I do not give him a proper gift, what will my sister say? In the end she will cast aspersions on my character and blame me for ill conduct. . . ." And so debating back and forth, the *rākṣasī* picked out a beautiful gold necklace and presented it to Śaśīdhara. In the same manner that King Satrājit received the gemstone after making offerings to the sun god, Divākara, and then singing his praises,[6] Śaśīdhara received the gold necklace, found the desired mud, and headed back on his return journey. He moved like the wind, and on the evening of the full moon—a very auspicious time—he entered the august presence of the king.

When the king espied Śaśīdhara, his heart raced, his body rippled with gooseflesh, and his eyes were riveted on the Suranadhī water. The king was overjoyed. He scooped up a handful of the water and when he looked, he saw that it was a beautiful golden mud color. The huge pot was whisked away and taken directly to the enchanting witch, who was still in disguise. When she saw it, her heart sank. "My sister did not eat him up. Where can I send him this time? It seems that he holds my life in his hands. . . ." And so with this agitated thought the night-stalking carnivore decided, "I shall send him to the citadel of Laṅkā and then my life will be safe again. There reside any number of flesh-eating ogresses. When I send him to them, they will tear him apart and feast on his flesh." Settling on this course of action, the night-stalking monster put her plan to work, approaching the king, "Please, O great-souled protector, indulge me. I have an insatiable desire. In the citadel of Laṅkā can be found a special cucumber. If you could have that fetched for me, then my craving could be sated. . . ."

At the feet of the Pīr the brahmin Kiṅkara speaks, "Lord Satya Nārāyaṇa, please bestow your grace. You always remember your faithful servitors, so grant your indulgence to the one subservient to you. May you show special favor to our young hero.

The king commanded, "Jayasiṃha, give me your full attention. I want you to go to the isle of Laṅkā and fetch me a special cucumber called a *śaśā* which is some thirteen cubits in length."[7]

"Your wish is my command. . . ." And so Śaśī headed off again. Every step of the journey he kept his mind firmly fixed on his Lord, Satya Nārāyaṇa. "O my Lord, friend of the downtrodden, may you grant the protection of your holy feet. You protected the righteous Pāṇḍava Arjuna in the pit of fire, you saved the innocent elephant when you killed the crocodile with your discus, and in the densest, darkest forest you rescued the trapped antelope doe. I have fallen into a similarly grave danger and I call out to you, beseeching you to extend the protection of your holy feet, just as you protected Dhruva when he marched through the Madhuvana Forest."

This earnest and distressed plea of his devotee reached the attention of the Pīr during his meditation. Once again he assumed the guise of a fakir and entered the forest. The fakir spoke lovingly, "My child, why did you call me? I have come to directly from Mecca."

"I am headed to the isle of Laṅkā because the king has commanded me. But I am heading directly into the gaping maw of the *rākṣasīs* who live there. My Lord, I beg you to vouchsafe my life." Śaśīdhara continued, "Listen, O Lord Nārāyaṇa, how will I ever manage even to reach Laṅkā for the sake of this ostensible cucumber?"

Hari protects his devotees as his own children, so for the sake of this one devotee the Pīr called Hanumān and commanded him, "Go now to the isle of Laṅkā. Convey Śaśīdhara to the *rākṣasī* demonesses. After you deliver him, take up station in the grove of *aśoka* trees." Following explicitly the command of the Pīr, Hanumān came and appeared before Śaśīdhara. Śaśīdhara took a seat on Hanumān's back, just as Govinda rode the back of his winged mount, Garuḍa. Like Kārttika on his peacock mount and Gaṇeśa on his rat did the crown prince sit in the freshness of youth. In the manner of Brahmā riding on his swan, Śaṅkara on his bull, or the king of the gods, Indra, riding on the back of his bull elephant, did Śaśīdhara sit majestically on Hanumān's back. In the twinkling of an eye, Hanumān had traversed the distance to Laṅkā.

Śaśīdhara entered directly into the citadel of Laṅkā, while Hanumān hid himself in the *aśoka* grove. All of the *rākṣasī* carnivores instantly picked up the scent of human flesh, and they all wondered why a man had so suddenly appeared there in their midst. The demon women spotted Śaśīdhara in no time, and hundreds of these bloodthirsty monsters descended on him in a feeding frenzy. They were fixated on the idea that after such a long time they had the opportunity for human flesh. "For twelve long years have we been bereft of this sight and now the Lord has delivered to us this most succulent of human meat." Some of them urged, "Don't get so carried away in your passions," while others screamed, "Tear him into tiny little pieces now!" They soon surrounded him on all sides, trapping him in the middle. Standing in their midst, the crown prince lost the ability to think rationally. Just as Nala, put under a spell by the god Kali, lost all normal sense in a trancelike state, so did Śaśīdhara stand there dumbly rooted to the spot. In unmitigated fear the young boy wept uncontrollably and called out for Bhagavān, the Lord: "Snatch me from the mouths of these bloodthirsty monsters, O Lord! Once you protected the Pāṇḍavas through the conflagration of the house of burning lac, and to Prahlāda you extended your mercy, pulling him into the protection of your lap. . . ." And seeing him in such dire straits, the Pīr overflowed with grace and Lord Nārāyaṇa descended and sat in Śaśīdhara's throat.

Firmly ensconced in the crown prince's voice, Nārāyaṇa then spoke, "Is there any one of you who wish to eat me, for you will be eating the son of another *rākṣasī* like yourselves. Look and see that I have the mark on my forehead. When Lord Rāma constructed the Setubandha land bridge to invade Laṅkā, he returned only after destroying Rāvaṇa and his clan. Jaṭilā and Kuṭilā were brought back with Rāma and Sītā, then Lakṣmaṇa destroyed that land link with his mighty bow. Kuṭilā settled on the banks of the Suradhanī River, while Jaṭilā took up residence deep inside the forest. Jaṭilā assumed the disguise of a seductive woman and kept regular watch on the bank of a local lake. A local king came big-game hunting one day and took her away instead, and this is how Jaṭilā became the number-one queen, which she remains to this day. My birth was the result of their union."

When they heard this tale, the monster women were uniformly struck with wonder. An ogress named Śaṅkāsurā said, "I will look after my cousin-sister's son. I went to visit Jagannātha some time ago and now my wish has been granted. . . ." And so they jabbered. Some hugged him warmly, some fondled him lovingly, others pulled him onto their laps, some smothered him with kisses, and a few even carried him around on their shoulders. One especially aged demon woman named Hiḍimbi had given birth to more than seven hundred demonesses during her lifetime. She addressed Śaśīdhara as "grandson," and pulling him onto her lap, inquired of him, "My young sire, just how is your birth-mother these days?"

Śaśīdhara replied, "Granny, how can I put this delicately? My mother is suffering an extended and acute ailment of the stomach. Mother said to me, 'Look at my condition, my young child. Go to the citadel of Laṅkā and fetch back a special cucumber that grows there to a size of thirteen cubits. . . ."

Kiṅkara Dāsa says, "Grant to your earnest devotees the protection and grace of your holy feet so that lives can be saved."

All of the night-stalking monsters—and their numbers were legion—took Śaśīdhara in tow back to their own abodes. The haggard old Hiḍimbi kept him close, showering him with a grandmotherly affection, "You just come and live here with me in my house. . . ." To which Śaśīdhara replied, "Granny, I beseech you to allow me return to ask a proper permission from my mother before doing so. Please supply me with the special cucumber of thirteen cubits so that her heart's desire might be fulfilled. Grant me leave so that I might go."

Hiḍimbi responded, "That is both good and proper. Let's go so that I can give you one of those cucumbers." And so she led the young man away. They saw there the cucumber vine, more like a tree actually, that had on it cucumbers of at least thirteen cubits' dimension. She plucked one and placed it into Śaśidhara's outstretched arms. As the young man looked around, he espied any number of pumpkins hanging from the branches of another large vine, and smiling mischievously he inquired, "Tell me granny, what on earth is the story behind those?"

Hiḍimbi replied solemnly, "My child, these contain the energizing life force of the entire community. Each pumpkin is attached to one particular individual. . . ." And as she prattled on, Śaśīdhara began to worry and to plot: "I will have to stay awake all night tonight, for if I simply abandon this place, calamity is sure to follow. The irrepressible demons cannot be defeated, but if I can manage to destroy their pumpkins, then the entire lineage would be wiped out. . . ." And the old woman confirmed it, as she continued her lecture, "Should anyone discover this secret connection, and then cut these pumpkins, all of us would find ourselves headed through the door of death into Yama's domain."

The young man replied, "Granny, since you are sharing so openly, where is the pumpkin that holds my mother's life force?" The old hag monster led him away and pointed to the very top of a large tree, "Your mother's life hangs there in that tree." The crown prince then marked the tree by tying a thread around it, as he thought, "I shall take this back and give it to the king."

As he ate the fruits of the fabled isle of Laṇkā that night, Śaśīdhara was invigorated, infused with new strength. He meditated constantly on Lord Satya Nārāyaṇa. The untold numbers of night-stalking monsters consumed their food in massive quantities, then, as the deep night approached, took themselves off to sleep. By the time of the night's third watch, this son of a king realized that all of the night-faring demons were fast asleep. Śaśīdhara began to move, slowly, holding his broadsword tight in both hands, his strength and stamina building. Śaśīdhara went to the trees that bore the pumpkins and braced himself, then with terrible blows began to hack them to death. Each time he sliced through a pumpkin, the head of another demon woman would fly off. He cut his way through hundreds upon hundreds, each beheaded. Fortunate was the king's son, for he slew all of the *rākṣasīs* without giving up a drop of his own blood. Then he plucked out the seeds from one of the thirteen-cubit cucumbers, shouldered another, picked up the pumpkin that held the life of his "mother," and began to meditate on Hanumān.

The valiant Hanumān appeared before him in an instant and said to him admiringly, "Well done, my child, well done indeed. No one can destroy these demonic beings except by the express command and help of the gods. It's as if Rāma himself has triumphed over Laṅkā again." Māruti, the lord of the winds, then swept them up on his back and whisked them out of Laṅkā across to their own lands. Bearing the thirteen-cubit cucumber on his shoulder and the pumpkin in his hand, sweat flying off his body from the exertion, he soon arrived in the august presence of the king. The retainers and ministers of the king all witnessed his arrival and they were uniformly pleased. The king greeted him with the ceremonial gift of a golden necklace. It tickled the king to no end when he took the thirteen-cubit cucumber and entered into the sanctum of his palace. The king was so happy to see the extraordinary fruit from Laṅkā that he could barely contain himself as he presented it to his *rākṣasī*-wife. The woman, who rivaled even the moon in her beauty, was riveted in her seat. As soon as she saw the thirteen-cubit cucumber, this demon-witch's heart went into palpitations: "I have reached the point of my death. That the special cucumber from Laṅkā has been fetched can only mean that all of my relatives and friends have been slain."

Opines Kiṅkara Dāsa, "You have indeed reached the end of the line, your death comes if not today then tomorrow."

The king spoke, "Now you can eat the special cucumber to assuage the symptoms of your disease," to which the demon woman thought, "I feel I am about to depart this existence." The beguiling one added, "What kind of a god is he? Otherwise, how could he possibly know how I might be killed? I am responsible for the deaths of my friends and family. Now I am bereft of siblings and I am dying here in the king's palace all alone." Worried and anxious, her body showed the effects, gradually wasting away to skin and bones. The raging fever of her anxiety reached such a pitch that she was approaching death. As she was denied any food, her body became increasingly emaciated; day by day her frame withered and became arthritic and desiccated. It was painful to watch her, for she could no longer walk. The king pleaded with her, "Please, my lovely bride, won't you talk to me? I will provide you whatever treasures or other items you may crave. Should you not survive, my life too is lost."

Jayasiṃha then interrupted, "O King, please do not worry. When I visited the citadel of Laṅkā I learned there a special *mantra*. Have the queen taken outside on a cot. Then have your retainers and advisers stationed around her on all sides. From behind the cover will I recite the *mantra* aloud. All those who are stationed around her should take careful note of what transpires."

As soon as he heard the advice, the king spoke to his enchantress directly, "My beautiful sweetheart, please go outside and take your place on the cot. . . ."

"How can I, the chief queen of this palace, go out there? What kind of place is that for me to sit when I venture outdoors? . . ." she objected.

The king replied, "Why, my beautiful companion, would you throw away the chance at life? This is neither wrong nor inappropriate, for the physician prescribing this course is none other than Lord Nārāyaṇa Hari." The king then took her by the hand and seated her on the cot. The *rākṣasī* could only remonstrate, "This time my life is surely lost."

The young prince came out and stationed himself on the cot, where he kept her life-pumpkin concealed close at hand. Behind the veil of the curtain, the youth squeezed the pumpkin tightly, and the demon woman let out a horrendous cry, "Aiyee! The life is being squeezed out of me!" Then, behind the curtain, the young man tossed the pumpkin up and down, making it dance, and though reduced to a bucket of phlegm and bile, the wizened old hag herself began to dance around the area. Again the king's son tossed the pumpkin into the air and this time the old demon-woman landed in a disheveled heap on the ground. The demoness cried out in desperation, "Please release me from your grip. I have hidden all kinds of treasures in the jungle, which I will go and get for you."

Śaśīdhara rejoined, "First, restore all the horses and elephants you consumed." To which the demon-hag responded, "Okay, okay, just quit manhandling the pumpkin." And so the son let it rest against his chest while the *rākṣasī* began to vomit and out came all the soldiers, then untold numbers of horses, elephants, goats, and other animals she had devoured. Then the demon-woman pleaded, "I have regurgitated everything, there is nothing left." But Śaśīdhara pressed on, "Restore my three dear companions who were among the first victims you ate in the forest." Hearing this command, the old demon-hag strained and vomited them out, after which Śaśīdhara invoked the Pīr, "Please grant us your grace! Please come here into the court of this good king and restore all the soldiers and others to life so that all may witness this event!"

It may as well have been Bhīma raising his face and calling out for Kṛṣṇa on the battlefield, such was the compelling call of the young boy. Who can fathom the magical mystery of Kṛṣṇa as Ananta, the endless support of the universe, for he suddenly appeared there at the palace of this king. Casting off his outer garment, the fakir once again stood, enveloping the young man in an aura of lustrous glory, proper and appropriate for one who restrains the appetite with only bread and a small pot of Ganges water. The young man grasped the feet of the mendicant and issued his plaintive appeal, "Please triumph over this death that grips the court of our king. At your holy feet, my Lord, I make this humble plea. Please restore the lives of the king's good soldiers."

Nārāyaṇa judged Śaśīdhara's grief to be genuine, so as the fakir he replied, "I will revive the soldiers now." Nārāyaṇa handed his small waterpot to the son of the king and bestowed upon him the special *mantra* to bring the dead back to life. When he received the *mantra*, the prince returned to the king's public assembly and then sprinkled the water from the pot over the dead bodies of the soldiers. With the uttering of the revivification *mantra*, new life breath coursed through them, and not only the soldiers, but the horses, elephants, all who had died were breathing again.

The king eagerly queried, "Jayasiṃha, please reveal to me how we are going to manage to kill this unkillable demon-hag."

The young man replied, "May everyone in this assembly watch closely." And there in the royal court he split the pumpkin in two. The young prince ceremoniously raised the pumpkin and with his broadsword sliced it apart, letting it fall, whereupon the demon-woman's head likewise fell to the ground. The king and all his courtiers stood transfixed, watching the death of the demon-hag, then the retainers, minister, and soliders all together let fly the joyous sound of Lord Hari's name. Grasping the feet of the king in humility, Jayasiṃha petitioned him, "For too long have I served here, please grant me your permission to leave. I have exterminated the entire lineage of the old demon-hag as promised. . . ." And so he wept as he continued to hold the feet of the king in supplication. The king asked him, "Where do you wish to go after you leave me?"

"Now," opines Kiṅkara Dāsa, "is the time for him to tell his tale."

The young prince spoke, "O great ruler, to your illustrious person have I humbly narrated the true story of the demon-hag's slaying. With no more fear in your heart, please mount your lion-throne, while I go to my own humble abode."

The king promised, "When you leave I will turn away from things of this world in my grief. You must stay and take control of my kingdom and affairs. My son has been long gone on sacred pilgrimage; my wife, the first queen, I exiled to the forest, and my home has become a house of darkness. The full extent of my wealth and domain I will make over to your custody." And the king confirmed his words by making a gift of his own royal necklace. "My son has gone, to what strange land I do not know. My wife dwells deep in the forest. You must act to save my pitiful life. Who knows what was eating at me at that moment when I went took my ministers and courtiers big-game hunting in the forest, for I brought back to my own house nothing other than a *rākṣasī* in disguise. Then I banished the first queen to the wild and in so doing cast away the only true love of my life. My life breath seeps away in grief for my son as surely as a the fatal strike of a warrior's missile of molten lead hitting my chest. Divorced from my queen, everything has gone dark. . . ." The king collapsed in a paroxysm of tears, paying no attention to his baronial appearance or royal apparel. The young prince added his own tears to the flood.

Seeing his father weep, the young man was himself moved to tears, both eyes welling, then he pressed the palms of his hands together in a gesture of respect. "Don't cry, please don't cry, Father. Let your troubles fly far away for I, who stand before you, am your son Śaśīdhara." He went on to say, "O King, let me explain everything to your august presence. Together with my three close companions, I went on a pilgrimage with a happy and carefree heart, and Lord Satya Nārāyaṇa showered us with mercy. With those three companions I ventured forth to the country of my uncle, and eventually reached the entrance to my mother's brother's world. He is the king of Mallabhūma, and he showered us with all manner of affections and seated us royally on an elevated palanquin. After enjoying my uncle's hospitality, the four of us sallied forth to visit and receive the auspicious sight of a string of holy pilgrimage places. After we had completed our pilgrimage circuit, we spotted a woman of exceeding beauty seated along the pathways through the forest. I espied beside her a wide range of assorted goods—mostly scrumptious foods—and we were heartened and felt a keen affection for her. And each of us went in turn to bathe farther down the banks of the lake beside which she sat. One by one, she grabbed my companions and ate them, then innocently resumed her seat on the landing ghat. When they were all delayed in returning from the forest, I went there myself and the demon-hag sneaked up behind me. Startled, then terrified, I scrambled into the branches of a wood apple tree. The demon-woman resorted to a brilliant and patient subterfuge: she stretched her arms completely around the trunk of the tree and then in that position lay down to sleep, knowing I could not descend without waking her. But Satya Pīr was favorably disposed toward me and cracked open a wood apple, into which magically I could crawl. Then suddenly, sensing something amiss, the old hag ogress let fly a bloodcurdling scream, scampering up the tree, scouring each and every branch. This night-stalker wanted to eat me! The wood apple, now having grown much heavier with me inside, was loosed and suddenly dropped into the waters of the lake. When the wood apple fell into the lake, the *rākṣasī* herself deliberately followed, diving into the lake. Spotting the oversized wood apple deep in the waters, a giant sheatfish—a monstrous bottom-feeder—gobbled it up and then buried itself back in the muddy floor of the lake. The night-stalker systematically searched the lake, her arms snaking back and forth through its waters. When she failed to catch sight of me, she smartly resumed her enchanting appearance and seated herself. About this time you came along, and she made sure you saw her. After your departure, a particularly destitute cowherd came along to try to catch some fish and just then the old sheatfish raised its head and was snared. He took the fish home, where his mother discovered the wood apple as she was gutting and cleaning it. The cowherd came into the room, carefully split open the wood apple, and I was able to emerge unscathed from my imprisonment."

Kiṅkara Dāsa writes, "All this takes place while the demon-hag lies comfortably at your side, gorging herself on a steady diet of horses and elephants."

Śaśīdhara continued, "You, Father, took a bloodthirsty demon under your protection, while exiling your queen, my mother, into the forest on trumped-up charges. The cowherd's mother had gone to fetch wood when she stumbled across my mother and reported back to me. Hear me well, O great king. I have been keeping my mother all along in the humble abode of the cowherd. She lives."

When he heard this astounding tale, the king threw himself on Śaśīdhara's neck and announced, "My son lives no longer as the epitome of misfortune; come here to my side and be restored." Śaśīdhara replied, "Come, let us go to the house of the cowherd and fetch the good woman back here to our own palace." And so Śaśīdhara went in the company of his father and found the dear woman. It was exactly like the time Lord Kṛṣṇacandra left Mathurā after slaying King Kaṃsa and then called Devakī his mother. "Whatever ill fortune you have endured, Mother, was only the fate inscribed on your forehead at birth. But know now that I am your own Śaśīdhara. Please come and be reunited with me." The king then said, "My chief queen, please listen to my tale. Try to put aside all your suffering and misery and come back home. During one incredibly inauspicious moment, I lost all sensibility and carted home a *rākṣasī*. I was unable to discern the truth of the situation and so ordered you into the wilds of the forest." He could go no further before breaking down in a flood of tears as the ever-faithful and devoted wife witnessed her husband's humiliation and distress.

When she had heard him out, the queen fell at the feet of her husband, made obeisance to him, and then hugged her son. All kinds of riches were showered down on the poor cowherd, and the king took his wife and son back. Now properly dressed in regal attire, the queen returned to her apartments. Śāśīdhara, however, reminded his father to worship Satya Pīr. When he heard this reminder, the king promptly made offerings to Satya Nārāyaṇa, preparing the *śirṇi*—mixture of banana, rice flour, sugar, and milk—according to the most exacting prescriptions. The blessed leftover offerings of *śirṇi* were then distributed to all relatives and friends. The remainder was then distributed to all subjects in the realm.

After they ate the offerings, everyone went their separate ways, bringing this tale to an end.

May everyone cry loudly the name of Lord Hari. Kiṅkara Dāsa sings at the auspicious feet of Satya Pīr, "O Pīr, Lord of the Universe, may you be merciful to all your devotees.

The Princess Who Nursed Her Own Husband

Gayārāma Dāsa's *Madanamañjarī Pālā*

First I bow to Nirañjana, the Stainless One, the Lord God, who lies on the serpent Ananta, the Endless One, on the ocean of Milk, and who annihilates all that is untruth. Then I pay my respects to Brahmā, Viṣṇu, and Śiva, respectively mounted on the swan, on Khagapati Garuḍa lord of birds, and on the bull. I bow to the Goddess, Śiva's mate, the primordial power, and I praise lords Ganeśa and Kārttika, and the goddesses Lakṣmī and Sarasvatī.

I praise Brahmā's Sāvatrī, and Śacī, queen of gods. I bow to Chāyā, wife of the Sun, and the Moon's mate Rohiṇī. I make obeisance to the ten who descended to earth: Matsya the Fish, Kūrma the Tortoise, Varāha the Boar, Vāmana the Dwarf, Narasiṃha the Man-Lion, Paraśurāma the Ax-Wielder, Śrī Rāma, Balarāma, who holds the plow, the Buddha, and Kalkī the horse of the future—these are the names of the ten avatāras.

I bow to the Vedic gods: Indra, king of the gods; Yama, lord of death; Kubera, lord of wealth; Varuṇa, lord of moral order; and Agni, god who is fire.

Likwise do I bow to the four clouds and the forty-nine winds, the eight Vasu divinities, the nine planets, the Aśvins who are the twins of dawn, the deities of the ten directions. At the feet of all of these gods I make a untold numbers of salutations. I bow to the moon and the sun and the stars, to demons, ogres, ghosts, spirits, heavenly musicians, and other demigods.

I praise Jayā and Vijayā, Bhairavas, vampires, the sixty-four Yoginī witches, and Nandī and Mahākāla, the Great Death, Time grown old.

I salute the ten manifestations of the goddess on earth: Kālī, Durgā, Bhuvanā, Kamalā, Bhīmā, Mātaṅgī, Bagalāmukhī, Tārā, Dhumāvatī, and Tripurā. At their feet I prostrate myself. I bow to her who is the sacred Mandākinī River in heaven and the holy Bhāgīrathī River on earth; and I extend my prostration to the goddess Gaṅgā when she flows into and through the netherworld as Bhogavatī, the Giver of Sustenance.

I praise Śyāma Rāya, the Dark Lord, gem of Vṛndāvana, and I salute Vrajeśvarī, the Queen of Vraja, and her sixteen thousand cowherd companions, the gopīs.

I seek shelter at the feet of Manasā Devī, goddess of snakes, and I hail the serpent Vāsukī, lord of the underworld and all his serpent Nāgas. I praise the Cool One, Śītalā, goddess of smallpox and dread diseases, perched on her donkey, and I make obeisance to her fever-demon, Jvara, and to Śītalā's bloodthirsty servant of dread diseases, Dāsī Raktāvatī.

I bow to the sages and seers, with my palms pressed together in respect. I honor the rivers and streams and the seven seas. I praise high the months, the years, and day and night. And I honor the six seasons and the fifteen days of each lunar cycle.

But most of all, I concentrate pointedly in praise of Satya Nārāyaṇa, the mere reflection on whose name relieves all suffering.

I pay my profound respects to the feet of my first guru, *to my mother, and to my father. I seek the protection of my initiatory guru and my instructional* gurus.

To anyone I may have inadvertently omitted in my repeated offerings of respect and salutation, I prostrate myself a hundred times over at their feet.

And so Gayārāma has sung these praises with hands pressed together in obeisance. Now that the invocation has come to an auspicious end, may everyone rejoice, crying, "Hari, Hari!"

Vinoda Vihārī ruled as king over the city of Vijaya by virtue of the power of Satya Pīr. He could be favorably compared to that famous world ruler, the mighty Raghuvīra of the Solar Dynasty, or Yudhiṣṭhira in the city of Hastinā. He protected his subjects like Rāma; in physical beauty he bested even Kāma; and in his resolve he was the young Śāntanu. His generosity was equal to Karṇa's; his skill in the warring arts that of Arjuna; and he was keenly devoted to the gods, brahmins, and his guru. His chief minister was Dharmadhvaja and, as the name implies, he held high the banner of righteousness. At the mere suggestion of an unrighteous act, he would cover his ears. Through the great strength of his guidance and advice, neither lawlessness nor anarchy ever held sway in the kingdom.

This king, who was by any standard blessed with good fortune, still maintained a healthy respect for Indra and Yama, lords of war and death. So he manned the entrances to his citadel with untold numbers of guards to guarantee his protection.

Horses and elephants he possessed by the hundreds of thousands. Deer and wild game he owned herd upon herd. Who could even count the number of camels and asses?

His queen was Citrāṅginī—She of Picturesque Frame—whose beauty sparkled brighter than a flash of lightning. In fortune she was blessed like the faithful and exemplary Śacī. She was deeply cherished by her husband. She was Sāvitrī in her commitment to virtue, and Ramā in knowledge and discrimination. Her nose was as fine as Śuka's pointed beak, her voice more enchanting than a cuckoo's, and her gait more elegant than that of a swan. Her complexion made bright yellow turmeric appear mottled and stained; it outshone even the gold ornament that encircled her waist. Her pleasing face rivaled that of Lakṣmī herself . . . she was perfect in every respect.

This youthful woman and man lived together quite happily and comfortably with their many servants, male and female. And so for some time did they live uneventfully until, through the direct power of Satya Pīr's grace, the queen became pregnant.

Two months passed without anyone realizing her condition. In month three, however, she took to sleeping on the floor. After the fourth and fifth months passed, her pregnancy was obvious to the whole world. During the sixth month, as is customary with pregnant women, she began to eat dirt. By the seventh month her belly protruded noticeably and her head bent forward for balance. After eight months she experienced great difficulty in walking. And after nine months had expired, milk still swelled her breasts. The king then performed the *sādha* ceremony, feeding her special foods according to her whims.

At the end of ten lunar months was Citrāṅginī's gestation period complete, and she began to suffer the pains of labor. She had to place her hand on the shoulders of a friend in order to move anywhere in the palace.

The king, like expectant fathers everywhere, grew nervous. He had the chief of his guard fetched. Then this gem among men commanded, "Go out now quickly and search for a midwife who resides in the area! Bring back one who knows well the science of bringing forth a child."

The guard executed the command and promptly produced a midwife, who immediately set about massaging the queen with all the appropriate oils. From the back she wrapped her arms around the queen's body, chest-high, and squeezed, putting a downward pressure on her abdomen. The queen, for her part, only dropped to the ground, writhing, crying out in an excruciating pain.

At that critical moment, who should arrive but the Progenitor of the Universe himself, Lord Nārāyaṇa, in the guise of a Muslim fakir. Going straight into the presence of the king, he extended his blessings and announced, "I am skilled in the arcane arts of parturition. . . ."

How can I capture in words the profundity of merit that warrants a meeting with Lord Nārāyaṇa?

The king, distraught and desperate, pleaded with him. "Please do me a favor, my dear friend. Divulge some appropriate remedy—an herb or anything—to save the life of my Citrāṅginī!"

The Father of the Universe was moved to compassion, and so explained how to deliver the child. He proffered sanctified water and, without warning, magically disappeared.

Citrāṅginī drank the water, made available as the direct result of her exquisite merit, and quickly dropped a baby girl to the ground. "Wah, Wah!" cried that healthy newborn—the sound of which brought an undeniable thrill to the queen. The king in time heard the good news. This gem of men then bathed and distributed vast sums to the twice-born, all for the exclusive benefit of his new daughter.

A wick of straw was fashioned from the thatched roof and brought into the delivery room to cauterize the unbilical cord and incinerate the placenta. For three days special foods were prepared and fed the new mother. On the ninth day they celebrated the dance of the newborn, in which everyone joined the fun. On the thirty-first day they worshiped Ṣaṣṭhī, goddess of children's welfare.[1]

After two or three months had passed, the princess could roll herself over. She was formally presented, dressed as the king's daughter, a princess. After five or six months had elapsed, she could smile and chatter in that delightful baby talk. She was then fed her first rice, thickened with heaviest of creams. Sometime after the seventh or eighth month, two tiny teeth pushed through her gums. With each day her body grew and with each day her beauty increased. Sometimes she would laugh and sometimes she would cry. But by ten months, she was trying to walk on her own, away from her mother's protective embrace.

When the princess was but one year old, she could clap her hands in time with her nurses'. The anklets riding above her lotus feet glittered with each tiny step, and from time to time she would slap her hands together in sheer delight. Often she would be dressed in a tiny loincloth or skirt, and sometimes an added turban or headdress. Her golden hue was reminiscent of the fine glow of pollen.

Her first year passed quickly, and hard on its heels the second. Soon the king's daughter was three years old. By the time she was four, the king and queen were both enchanted, content just to gaze at their daughter's fine distinguishing marks. It seemed that a Vidyādharī, one of heaven's musicians so renowned for beauty and skill in the arts, had abandoned a life of immortality in Indra's abode, and had been born to this earth through the king's semen. The girl's waist was a slender as a lion's, gently rolling at the touch, causing myriads of gods to forget themselves and stopping men dead in their tracks. Her body glowed with the five arrows of Kāma, the god of love. To look into her eyes would distract even the firm minds of sages. Her two ears were proportioned perfectly to the size of her eyes. And her face was naturally radiant like the full moon. Her lotus-bud breasts bounced suggestively under the cloth stretched tautly across them, while at her throat the Sarasvatī necklace bobbed as she moved.

Noting her extraordinary beauty, her mother and father considered many possibilities, but in the end, they bestowed on her the affectionate name Madanamañjarī—the Blossom of Madana the Enchanter, the god of love. And so this lovely young girl grew up happily in the palace of her father, accompanied everywhere by a bevy of delightful female companions.

Now the king was deeply immersed in the affairs of state and for this reason never visited the inner quarters of his palace; this went on for a long time.

No one can imagine the inscrutable play of the Pīr.

After twelve such years, Madanamañjarī had surpassed in beauty the heavenly Vidyādharī, Tillottamā herself. One day the *mahārāja*, escorted by female attendants, visited his queen, arriving amidst much gaiety. He was highly animated. The king, who seemed to be in rather a strange mood, sat on the bed. So Citrāṅginī sat herself down right in front of him. The king shared all kinds of news with his queen, for he had been busy during his last twelve years of rule, and they seldom talked. "I can only frequent the women's quarters for brief periods of relaxation. Were I to come more often, the affairs of state would inevitably suffer. When a king fails to discharge his royal duties, he is for that sin destined for hell. When a teacher fails to educate his students, the scriptures say that he is no different from a dumb beast of burden. When a trained warrior flees the battlefield in fear, the Veda classifies him in the category of coward. . . ." In this way did the great wielder of the rod of justice talk, until Madanamañjarī came in to see her mother.

She caught the king's eye as would a flash of lightning descending from the heavens to touch the earth. The king was stunned. He asked his wife, "Whose daughter is this living in my palace?"

The queen could not help but laugh. "O great upholder of the law! She is none other than your own daughter, Madanamañjarī. While you have been so deeply engrossed, indeed intoxicated with the business of running the country, your ministers never thought to remind you of your daughter and her need for marriage. You must see to her wedding arrangements now. O my king, you must find a suitable groom to whom you can give her!"

The king responded quickly, as he was wont to do. "Listen, my beloved. I will pledge my daughter in marriage to the first eligible man I see tomorrow morning. Social rank, caste, occupation—none of these will matter! I vow to give my daughter to the first man I see." And having made such a momentous vow, the king, exhausted, lay down.

In the heavens, however, Satya Pīr began to worry. "Why, O great king, did you make such a cruel and hard vow? If her lot falls to an unsuitable man, then that beautiful young girl will be utterly humiliated and dishonored, a disgrace to the kingdom." Mulling this over, Pīr Bhagavān took pity and conjured his magic.

Gayārāma sings his new song of Satya Pīr.

Listen to the story of the king's chief minister, whose name was Dharmadhvaja. His wife was Saudāminī—Brilliant like Lightning—a woman completely adoring of her husband. And from her womb she produced his son. That boy's beauty and physical presence, much like his mother's, exhibited a burning splendor not unlike the jewel of the daytime sky, totally illuminating in the way a lamp hurls back the thick darkness by its flame. In the same manner that Devakī gave birth from her womb the lord of the Yadus, Kṛṣṇa, while deep in the dungeons of King Kaṃsa, so did Saudāminī, in the house of the king's minister. It was as if by some strange twist of fate a full moon had returned to be born on earth. He was truly beautiful to behold, his body rivaling Gaṇapati, as if Indra himself had somehow descended.

The astrologers calculated the time this child should be fed his first food, rice. They set it for an auspicious sunrise, to take place the following morning. On the day set aside for the formal ritual feeding of the male child its first food, he was by custom displayed before the king. When the auspicious moment neared early that morning, the minister instructed his maidservant. "Listen carefully to my directions. Take the child quickly and put him on view before the king. Then bring him back right at the crack of dawn!"

The servant took sweets and other items in amounts that were fitting for the king, and cradled the child in the crook of her arm. Following the minister's exact orders, she hurried and found her way into the king's quarters. The watchmen at the gate recognized her as the chief minister's servant woman, and immediately opened the gates for her. Much relieved, the servant reached the four level of apartments and waited by the main entrance.

The *mahārāja* got up that morning and was walking out, carrying in his hand a small waterpot; he was muttering, "Rāma, Rāma" over and again in simple meditation. He looked up and saw the servant woman stationed patiently by the main portal, cradling the son of the minister in her arms. The king politely inquired of her, "Tell me, just exactly who are you? And what is your reason for coming here?"

At this cue, the servant woman pressed her hands together as best she could while holding the child, and answered the king, "Please allow me to introduce myself. This is the son of your chief minister, who goes by the name of Dharmadhvaja, and I am the maidservant to the minister. I have brought his son so that he may get *darśana* of you.[2] The honorable minister has sent along these items for the pleasure of the king. Please grant him your blessing, my lord of justice. This morning, as soon as the sun rises, marks the auspicious time calculated for the ritual first feeding of solid food for the boy. I must get him back quickly."

As he was listening, the king suddenly remembered that he must fulfill his vow of the previous day. "I will give the hand of my daughter to this minister's baby boy. This chance of the Fates has turned out well!" With his sudden announcement, this bull among men took the child from the servant woman and cradled it against his own massive chest. He was rewarded with the tiniest of smiles and a nearly imperceptible laugh. He turned to the servant and said, "Convey the following to the minister. Your son's rice-eating ceremony will take place as scheduled in my private residence, for to him I will have my daughter betrothed. The minister should not worry nor suffer about it, for this has brought me great happiness. Now go quickly and explain it all to him!"

Gathering it all in, the maidservant rushed home and in a bubble of excitement informed the minister of the event. The minister could only respond in disbelief, thoroughly nonplussed. "This is utterly amazing! How can they hope to marry my six-month-old son to his twelve-year-old daughter? This a public embarrassment! What can this king, that erstwhile 'wielder of justice,' possibly be thinking? How can I show my face there? Let the king do what he wishes. I will never return to his service. How can I even appear in public?" His lament pains the heart.

King Vinoda Vihārī was truly elated, very pleased with himself. He entered his private chambers carrying the minister's son. The queen, fearing the worst, promptly inquired, "Please explain, O great king, just whose child have you found this morning?" The king responded, "My dear queen. By my great good fortune I have found this morning the son of my own chief minister. His rice-eating ritual is slated for this morning. The minister's maidservant had brought him to show him to me, as is the local custom. Then I suddenly remembered my vow of yesterday, so I decided that I would give my daughter in marriage to this son of my minister!"

The queen protested. "The minister's son is only six months old! How can you give our daughter to him in marriage? Our daughter is twelve years old, and in beauty she outstrips even Tilottamā in the prime of her youth. This news will produce a terrible scandal, and our daughter will gain nothing but grief and shame. Only after her youth has come and gone will her husband be old enough to mate with her! We will be marked with disgrace by everyone everywhere in this world. We shall suffer a terrible burden of indignities on behalf of our daughter!"

The king reassured her, "My beloved, you know what has happened. I took a vow yesterday in your presence. My promise was that I would give my daughter in marriage to the first male I saw when I got up this morning. It was my daughter's fate that I saw this particular fellow. Who is able to counter what fate decrees? Should a king fail to honor a vow he has solemnly made, then according to the scriptures he is headed for hell. Bhīmasena, the son of Pāṇḍu, took a solemn vow and later drank the blood of Duḥśāsana on the battlefield. King Duryodhana had also taken a vow, so he refused to grant a kingdom as small as the point of a needle to the sons of Pāṇḍu. He met his death along with eleven divisions of soldiers,[3] but faced with war, he begrudged them any piece of the kingdom. The great king Haṃsadhvaja took a binding oath and as a result was compelled to throw his own son into a vat of boiling oil. The mighty Śikhidhvaja made a promise that forced him to saw his son's body in two. King Raghu, in order to honor a pledge he had made for the sake of the world, fed flesh cut from his own body to a hawk. And listen to the tale of events that transpired even earlier. In ancient time, a war was waged between the gods and the antigods called *asuras*. In a battle with the antigods, Indra was soundly defeated, so he beat a hasty retreat to the hermitage of the sage Dadhicī. Covering his neck and shoulders with a bright yellow cloth in his humility, Indra pressed his hands together in respect and entreated the sage. 'Please give me, O holy man, a bone, the sternum, from your very chest! If you would be so gracious as to provide me with this bone, O great ascetic, I shall fashion a lightning-bolt weapon to vanquish the legions of antigods." To Indra's audacious request, the sage gave his promise, and in the act of offering the bone, he gave up his own life.

"He who honors and fulfills his vows automatically attains Vaikuṇṭha heaven. Explain to me how I can break my vow, knowing that by abrogating that vow I shall certainly go to hell!"

As the words struck home, the queen bowed her head and wept. She then knew for certain that this fate had been truly etched on her forehead.

With great haste the king summoned the astrologers, who after consulting the stars and planets, determined a proper name for the boy. Since his beauty radiated more than moonbeams themselves, the name Candrasena—Moon Warrior—was bestowed on him. Observing the auspicious moment, he was fed his first solid food, according to the ritual. That evening the young girl was formally betrothed. The brahmin *paṇḍitas* blessed the union and the couple was joined in matrimony in the king's quarters in accordance with scriptural injunction. The bride and groom were ushered to the bridal chamber. Just as the moon climbed into the sky, the groom was carried into the room in the arms of a maidservant. The daughter of the king went with head bared. She was accompanied by a number of her close companions. Then the groom was laid on the traditional bed of flowers. The young woman stared intently at him and then wept bitterly.

Meditating day and night on the honeyed feet of the Pīr, Gayārāma composes his song, which is incomparably sweet.

The bride and groom, surrounded by her many companions, were installed in the bridal chamber of flowers. The daughter of the king sat and stared straight ahead, her heart broken. This pure and dedicated girl, a true *satī*, Madanamañjarī, wept bitterly. She could not bear to look at anyone. For comfort she could but silently repeat the name of Rāma. "What madness has befallen me? My father has married me to a baby boy who still sucks milk from his mother's breast! Fate has thwarted my simplest aspirations." This way Madanamañjarī cried, banging her bangles hard against her forehead, while her companions tried to console the distraught girl by telling her a story.

"This story comes from the ancient past, before the period of the recorded histories. Listen to its moral. Madana, the god of love, was commissioned to interrupt Śiva's yogic austerities, but Śiva incinerated Madana for his trouble by the fire of his wrath, turning him into a heap of charred flesh. Madana's wife, Rati, was a *pativratā*, devoted to her husband. She was virtuous and chaste, *sādhvī*, and totally faithful, *satī*. After Madana's misfortune, she took birth in the lineage of a tribal hunter. Long before this, the lord of the Yadus took birth on earth in a warrior caste to alleviate the terrible burden of evil crushing the earth. After enjoying himself in Gokula, he slew the demon King Kaṃsa in Mathurā and moved into the citadel of Dvāraka. According to the scriptures, Hari eventually married eight women, with Rukmiṇī being chief among them. Similarly, it was to counter Śiva's terrible anger that Mīnaketu—He Whose Banner Displays the Fish—or Madana the Enchanter descended to earth, taking birth in her womb. At the time of Madana's debacle with Śiva, there was an antigod, an *asura*, named Savara. It was he who carried Madana's corpse and threw it into the deep waters of the river. A monstrous sheatfish lurked below and, as Madana's remains floated down, the fish swallowed them whole in a single awesome bite. But this very fish was soon caught by one of the hunting community. Of all the fish he had landed, this one he gave to Rati, who immediately started to gut and clean it for cooking. When she sliced open the stomach of this fish, Rati was startled to find a tiny baby boy. She began to raise the child, going to great lengths to care for it. But every time she spoke to the baby as a mother, the child quickly covered its ears. Rati finally realized: 'This is my husband—I now know it for certain. Eventually he will grow into a handsome youth. . . .[4] Always remembering this, Rati, the faithful wife, raised her husband in a strange yet wonderful way.

"And this same situation, Madanamañjarī, befalls you. You too must raise your husband with the same trouble and care as Rati. Your desires will be fulfilled later."

After her friends had consoled her with their tale—as much consolation as such a tale could offer—they headed for their own homes, while the beautiful little woman simply worried. "What will happen now? When the night gives way to morning, all the women will return. How can I show my face?" When she looked again at her husband's tiny face, this king's daughter's eyes were again awash with tears; she stretched out on her bed in what can only be described as agony.

Meditating on the feet of the Pīr, Gayārāma Dasa sings: "This tragic young lady is on the verge of becoming a heroine!"

Madanamañjarī wept hard in her flowered bridal chamber. "Why did you write such a terrible fate for me, my Lord Hari?" It was just like this that she addressed the Fates as she ground her bangles hard across her forehead. "Woe be unto me, born a woman in this vast ocean of existence. Untold numbers of other princesses have found suitable husbands by the dictates of fortune. How can I show my face in society bearing such horrible shame? I shall abandon this life by slitting my throat with a knife!" Thus did the king's daughter make clear her intention to commit suicide; and at that very same instant, the crown jewel of *pīrs*, sitting in Mecca, knew of it.

Satya Pīr brooded, "If the young daughter of the king kills herself, then I will never be honored in the kingdom of Vijayanagara again. I must do everything to protect the worldly honor and reputation of this young bride. I will lead this princess from this land to another, where she is not known. When the minister's son finally comes of age, she will return to her homeland and institute my worship." This crown jewel of *pīrs* then disguised himself in a woman's dress to pass as a female playmate and companion of Madanamañjarī.

Using his magic, Satya Pīr—dressed in women's clothes and makeup and looking just like one of Madanamañjarī's friends—miraculously appeared by the side of the distraught princess. Although distracted, Madanamañjarī did notice her new companion almost instantly. In her need, she placed her arms around Satya Pīr's neck and immediately entreated "her" through a veil of tears.[5] "Why have you come to visit me, a luckless, unfortunate woman? I am about to kill myself, to slit my throat. This birth has come to a premature end. We shall not meet again. It is impossible for me to show my face in public under such humiliation. What a wretched disgrace to have to raise your husband on your own lap! When he lies in my lap and demands to suckle my breasts, what consolation can I offer my little lord?"

The Pīr soothed her. "Should you take your own life, all righteousness and good merit will be annihilated and you will head to hell! Heed this sound advice, my princess. Why should you give up this life? While you are unable to stay in the house of your mother and father, you can surely take your husband from this country to another. There you will be able to pass the time," pointed out the Pīr, "until your husband reaches manhood. Whenever you find yourself in any difficulty, you simply remember Satya Nārāyaṇa and call on him. Satya Nārāyaṇa is the Lord of the Kali Age. If you but remember him, all misery will be lifted. You must flee with your husband in the thick of night, and when you return to this land you must institute the formal worship of Satya Pīr with all honor and respect."

The young bride responded, "If Nārāyaṇa really does watch over me, then when I return I promise to establish the worship of Satya Nārāyaṇa." Satya Pīr, who in disguise looked just like one of her regular neighbor women, acknowledged her response, and disappeared as quickly as he had appeared.

Now galvanized, the princess sat right there and immediately began to plan her strategy. "I certainly must leave my parents' house and flee to another country. Only when Nārāyaṇa guides me back to my homeland can I return to live in my paternal house." Then, as the magic worked by the Pīr began to take effect, Madanamañjarī found herself suddenly longing to look at the face of the baby, her husband. Satisfying this urge, she thought carefully through everything her new neighbor had said.

She meticulously removed her wedding dress and stored it for its eventual future use. She gathered up a substantial amount of disposable assets in various forms—coral, rubies, emeralds, pearls, diamonds, and, of course, silver and gold—in the event she needed to pawn them for cash. Then she dressed herself in the rags of an indigent. She carefully strapped her husband to her chest. In her heart of hearts, she paid her most profound respects to her mother and father—but from a distance. She thought, "I must take leave of everyone, no exceptions. What, I wonder, will my parents do? What will my friends say? Still, I must take my husband and leave now."

The flowered bridal chamber then stood empty, desolate and abandoned, for the young woman had already exited through a back door.

Meditating day and night on the wonderful feet of the Pīr, Gayārāma says, "My friend will protect this young beauty."

When the day broke, the servant women awoke and opened the bridal chamber. The room was empty; no one was there. They trembled in a terrible fear. These women helpers debated what to do, and finally went to the queen. Pressing their hands together in deference, they spoke. "The bride and groom are no longer here. The bridal chamber has been left empty."

As soon as she heard these horrible words from her maidservants, Citrāṅginī fell to the ground in shock. Her hair came unbound and her clothing came loose: she was as disheveled as a plaintain tree in a fierce storm. "Where is my darling child? I am in despair. She has left me a wretched, worthless woman. Has she taken her husband and escaped to the forest to avoid public reproach? Or has my little girl left the country altogether? Or thrown herself into the river? She could not bear the agony and humiliation of having a six-month-old husband in her lap. Being the king's only daughter, she is not inured to heartache; she knows nothing of misery. To whose house will she go? Where will she stay? How can she even survive?" Muttering these and similar things the queen rolled on the ground in agony—then the king received the news.

This great lord of the earth was so unsettled that he slipped from his throne and fell to the ground in a dead faint. The ministers gathered around and poured water over the king's head until he finally regained consciousness. The king cried out, "Where is my daughter? Find her and bring her back to me!" And in this condition did the lord of men, overcome with grief, have to break the news to his chief minister. When the minister and his wife heard the story from the king's messenger, the misery they suffered very nearly drove them mad. As soon as the king's command was issued, messengers were dispatched to search the country high and low. When the dragnet produced nothing, they were completely crestfallen, but dutifully informed the king. When the king heard, he withdrew in silence into his private chambers.

With all hopes at the feet of the Pīr, Gayārāma Dasa, steeped in compassion, tells his tale.

Madanamañjarī swept up her husband and took him away from that place. She eventually made her way into the distant kingdom of Rāja Magīndra. When the baby boy cried to be breast-fed, she would secure cow's milk from whatever village was close by and feed him. Locals in the neighborhood inevitably questioned her. "Whose child do you have? Where have you come from? Come on, tell us exactly what is going on. . . ." Madanamañjarī always carefully replied with her well-rehearsed lines, "He is my baby brother. My mother and father have departed this world for that of Yama. My husband has gone mad as the result of some personal defect, and my brother and I have come here to search him out. We have traveled through many lands without finding a trace of him. Finally, at the end of our journeys, we have landed here. Now that I have gotten this far safe and sound, I plan to stay." And then she added, "It would please me immensely should I be able to have a personal audience with the king."

Having declared her intentions, Madanamañjarī left, and soon thereafter made her way into the capital city of King Magendra. Pulling a cloth around her neck in humility, she placed her hands together respectfully and bowed in deep obeisance to the king. The young girl said, "From this day forward I declare you to be my godfather, my father-protector. Please, great lord among men, grant me one tiny plot of land on which to live. There a brother and sister will reside quietly, making it their permanent abode."

The king graciously acknowledged her request, "You are most welcome to take up residence in my kingdom and you may live wherever you so desire." When she received this permission from the king, she pressed her request a little further—of course with great respect, her hands still held in a gesture of humility. "Not far from here, just south of the fort, I should very much like to reside. Please have a small house built for me and when construction is complete, I will pay for it myself."

The king thought to himself, "It appears that this little woman is going mad. Why would she want to live alone in the middle of an open field?" But what the king said was: "Whatever you wish will be done, my child."

When the young girl saw the house that was built, she was thrilled, and moved quickly to inhabit it. She arranged to purchase various furnishings through intermediaries who knew about these things. She bought two milch cows in order to supply the needs of the minister's son, whom she was determined to raise. She likewise purchased a substantial supply of foodstuffs. And there she lived, quite contentedly.

In this simple way did many uneventful days pass. But God had more amusing events in mind.

For the benefit of her husband, the chaste and devoted Madanamañjarī contemplated the name of Satya Nārāyaṇa without cease, by day and by night. Her newfound companion, who had visited her that fateful day in the bridal chamber, had informed her that when she was beset with difficulty, she should call on the Pīr, who was none other than the apostle of God and his messenger, the *paigambar*. So she thought, "I shall call on the Pīr, who is Lord, just this once to test the truth of my new friend's promise. Where are you, Friend of the Abandoned, Lord of the World? Show your mercy to your servant; save her! You once saved and protected the chastity and fidelity of Rambhāvatī Satī, the wife of Jayadatta. Likewise, the beautiful Vallabhā Sundarī once lived in the forest, blind, yet you restored both her sight and her throne. Another time there was a merchant named Vidyādhara and his life you saved when he was in the trap of the dacoits, the famous *phāsarās*. Our own King Magendra had a son named Madhya Gāzī, who, with your help, went out and slew Jāmbuvāna the demon. The life of Prince Śaśīdhara was spared from the clutches of a *rākṣasī* demon, but only through your beneficence. The wife of Jayānanda, Campāvatī by name, you snatched from the hands of the witch. If you still think of me as your lowly servant, then by virtue of your personal qualities, be merciful and protect me!" In this and other ways did Madanamañjarī praise the Pīr.[6] Pleased by her invocation, the Great Helmsman descended from the heavens.

Satya Nārāyaṇa put on his fakir's dress and visited the young woman to show himself. Satya Pīr inquired of her, "What crisis prompted you to call for me, my little mother? Tell me what is your problem so that I can help you through it."

The young girl replied, "Just who are you? I do not recognize you! Please properly introduce yourself to me, O Fakir Gosāin!" The Pīr smiled and said, "Listen my little beauty, I am the Helmsman of Heaven, the Lord of the Kali Age. I was moved to compassion when I heard your humble prayer. Be frank and tell me what afflicts you."

The young girl replied without hesitation, "If you truly are Satya Nārāyaṇa, tell me how I can struggle through these hard times, for I grow weary of the daily demands of raising a child by myself."

The Pīr assured her, "On that count you need not worry yourself. Whatever obstacle besets you, I will see to its removal. Pay close attention to what I say, Madanamañjarī. Tonight, in a single night, I shall have a beautiful mansion constructed for you. It will be magnificent, jewel-encrusted." And no sooner had Pīr Bhagavān promised than Viśvakarma, the celestial architect, and Hanumān, commander and engineer of Rāma's army, were telepathically summoned. The Prophet Pīr greeted them with deep affection, "Please raise a house for this girl, a mansion that is rich with jewels."

Hanumān immediately requisitioned and assembled the materials and supplied Viśvakarma, who labored throughout the night to construct it. This bejeweled palace was neatly enclosed by high walls on all sides, and furnished with everything gold—plates, utensils, pots, etc. To the right they constructed a lake, to the left, a two-story apartment. Feverishly the two men raised the compound to completion, then took their leave. And the Pīr reminded the girl, "If there is the slightest problem, just remember me!"

After Viśvakarma and Hanumān had finished constructing the citadel, they filled it with fabulous wealth. So, when the night gave way to dawn, everyone in the city gathered to gawk, dumbstruck at the sight of the house. They whispered among themselves how just yesterday a young girl had arrived toting a baby on her hip. Somehow, overnight, this house had miraculously appeared, glittering like a mountain of jewels. Everyone had to go and inspect it. The crowd soon surged to a run and headed out into the field to meet the young girl. She, in turn, hosted them with the utmost grace. When they had been sated, cleansing their palates with betel quids, they returned to their own humble dwellings. Each and every one left truly satisfied.

Late that afternoon, when the *mahārāja* came out onto the main road for his constitutional, to breathe a bit of fresh air, he caught sight of the newly constructed building. The king looked hard at his chief minister, and then spoke. "I see it, but I don't believe it! You, my good minister, look and confirm it for me. Yesterday there wasn't even a road to be seen in the middle of this large field of mine—and it has been that way for ages. Where did it come from? Who could have constructed a golden citadel? Do you know anything at all about this, minister?"

The minister, who was totally abashed, could only reply, "My lord, you may recall that yesterday there was a young girl who addressed you as 'Godfather.' In response, you granted her assistance and had a hut built for her. Now, miraculously it would seem, that hut has been turned into a mansion! Clearly this woman is not at all like others. I do not have any idea how she could have constructed such an exquisite building overnight. If it pleases you, let us go there now and we shall get to the bottom of it." The king, as he was wont to do, listened to his minister; and so they went, arriving in no time at the young girl's abode.

The chaste and faithful Madanamañjarī espied the approaching king, lord of the world, and hastened to greet him. She seated him as was only proper. The king's retainers, friends, and counselors alike had found the existence of the mansion impossible to believe. So the king politely inquired. "Yesterday you came to me wearing tattered rags, yet during the course of one night you constructed a mansion. You are clearly blessed. Please tell me just exactly who you are. Are you a goddess or a demoness who has come down to this world of mortals? Or are you a celestial nymph or one of heaven's many attending musicians, a fairy? I am unable to discern so precisely. Tell me truthfully who you are, for in one single night you have raised high a palace!"

Madanamañjarī fell at his feet and said, "You are my godfather, my father-protector. I am neither a demoness nor a fairy, nor a celestial nymph or some siren from the heavens. I am from the ranks of humans, a mere woman. I beg of you, grant me the continued protection of your feet and think of me only as your daughter. Please do not cast me out of your kingdom! Should I be found at fault for my actions, please absolve me of that guilt; that act is certain to redound to your credit on this earth."

When the king listened to her persuasive plea, he was truly delighted—and much relieved! He smiled and spoke to her gently, reassuringly, "From this day forth you shall be my daughter, most blessed in the three worlds. Have no fear, for I shall watch over you." And with this proclamation, the king retired to his own humble abode, but not before providing her with a proper staff of servants, both men and women. The young girl's heart simply shuddered in delight as she and the baby Candrasena took up residence in their new house.

In what seemed like no time at all, the minister's son reached the age of five and the young woman, his wife, began to brood over what should be done. The girl worried herself to death, brooding quietly and alone in a place that was removed from view. She was calculating exactly how she might begin his formal education.

Now the mahārāja, *under whose protection she lived, was a man of great merit. He had for many years maintained a house in the great city of Bombay. In a tiny hut in that great kingdom, the poet Gayārāma Sarkara also lived, in the village of Vāmana Pukkuryā.*

When the minister's son, Candrasena, was five years old, the faithful Madanamañjarī began to plan his future. "In order to educate him properly, I shall enroll him in a school run by a qualified teacher. If he is not formally educated, he will never be truly knowledgeable. . . ." Thinking in just those terms, that daughter of a king spoke sweetly to the minister's boy. "You must go to the king's palace for your education. If you do not study, then you will be known as an illiterate everywhere you go in the world. Your mother and father died when you were but six months old. I have been raising you since then. I am the luckless maidservant of your mother. Listen, my little jewel of virtue, I have assumed the relationship of your sister. Go and study hard at the king's palace and you will earn a fine reputation for your own family lineage."

After informing him of her intention, she summoned the astrologer. When they fixed the auspicious day, he embarked on his formal training. Given a servant to accompany him, the minister's son was sent to the guru to learn. This young boy was handsome without compare—he shamed even the moon. All those who saw him were struck. After he made his formal greeting to the guru, he took his place to learn to write. In the twinkling of an eye he mastered the thirty-four consonants and all of the conjuncts in the alphabet.

At the end of the first day, the minister's son went home, where the princess had arranged for his food and fed him. He ended his meal and rinsed his mouth and hands. Taking some betel to chew, he then stretched out on the bed and Madanamañjarī tucked him in. After he was asleep, the still-radiant Madanamañjarī ate directly from his plate, privately acknowledging that this growing young man was indeed her husband.

This became their routine. She attended him always, but her constant worrying made her body thin. The minister's son carried on each day with his studies: grammar, lexicon, commentary and exegesis, metaphysics, and disciplined speculation. He was constantly poised to do the bidding of his guru, and it was not long until the minister's son had assumed the mantle of the educated. With his schoolmates he laughed and joked, and, of course, played schoolboy pranks, but he just as easily sat in the presence of the king to argue abstruse points of logic.

One day the guru spoke to him. "Listen, Candrasena, I plan to visit your home for the express purpose of fixing my appropriate fee for your education." And so he went there, accompanied by Candrasena. When the guru got a good close look at the mansion in which the boy lived, he was utterly flabbergasted.

This scion of the twice-born took a seat in one of the outer compartments as the young girl, Candrasena's wife, received the news in her interior apartment. She came out and respectfully seated the guru on a stool, elevated to honor his rank. The twice-born could not help but notice that she moved majestically, with the beauty and grace for which elephants are renowned. After getting the brahmin comfortably seated, she returned to the house's interior. The twice-born remarked that he was truly stunned at the opulence he saw all around him. Enjoying his surprise, the twice-born stayed for nearly an hour. Then his fee was ceremonially meted out. He accepted the tribute and returned home.

As he was walking home, the guru kept trying to figure it all out. "Exactly who is that enchanting young young woman I saw? Tomorrow morning I shall find out who she is. I will question Candrasena and get the particulars." By the time he had decided what he would do, the learned brahmin had reached his own home.

The next morning, as was his custom, the minister's son came to study. When he came into the presence of his guru, Candrasena prostrated himself on the ground in reverent salutation before settling in to the day's study. The guru interrupted him, "Candrasena, pay attention to what I am about to say. I want you to respond truthfully and without deception."

Candrasena, somewhat taken aback, responded, "No matter what you ask, I will never tell you anything other than the truth."

Satisfied, the guru pressed on. "Yesterday when I went to your house, whose daughter came out to seat me? Tell me, child, how is she related to you? When I hear I shall dispel the questions that have been forming in my mind."

No sooner had he heard his guru's queries, than Candrasena spoke, while Gayārāma sings of the song of the Pīr's benevolence.

Candrasena, his hands respectfully joined and a cloth wrapped around his neck in humility, stood beside his guru and related the following story.

"Listen, my guru, as my mentor you make my wishes come true. I can never lie to or deceive you. I am not fully aware of all the details, but the young woman about whom you have inquired has been taking care of me since birth. I have no mother, nor do I have a father. I have no brother nor any friends I might call close. We have no relations whatsoever in the house. When I reached the age of five, she explained it all to me like this: 'Listen carefully to what I say. How can I truly explain to you that when you were a mere six months old, your father and mother died. I am your mother's maidservant and I served her faithfully day and night. What I am telling you is a true story. When your mother died, it was I who looked after you. So I became, by way of personal relation, your sister.'

"Since the time that she sent me to be educated, I go home early in the evenings to a routine. I have told you the truth as I know it. Apart from this bit more, Master, I know little else. As soon as I go home each day, she washes my feet and feeds me. Afterward she prepares betel for me. When I have finished eating, she sits at my feet and questions me about my program of study. Everything I am taught at school I have to explain to her in the evening. If I forget some minor point, she immediately supplies the missing information or explanation. At the end of the evening she always comes into my room to sleep."

The guru puzzled over what he heard and then asked Candrasena, "Do you know what kind of education this beautiful young lady has had?"

Candrasena thought for a second and then said, "Most revered Guru and Master, I am not in a position to say."

The guru replied, "Look, my child Candrasena, you do not understand. Being a maidservant is not meet for this woman. I have seen her with my own eyes. One fact you have not discerned: she is most certainly the daughter of some king, a princess. I have now revealed to you the suspicion I have harbored since meeting her. Listen, Candrasena, see if you are able to prove me wrong. You must relay to me whatever you discover. It is for me to determine whether your story holds true or false. Think for a minute. How can a servant be your sister? She must be someone else. Through hints, the little things, I shall ferret out her story."

Candrasena then reassured his guru, "O honorable Guru, I will do only exactly what you tell me to."

The guru then instructed him: "Go home and eat as you normally would, but then go outside the apartment for some fresh air. When she has prepared and delivered your betel, she will slip back inside to sit and eat the leftover food from your plate. You should run back in pretending that you want a drink of water. As you wait, casually drop a speck or two of your burnt tobacco on the plate.[7] Then, tomorrow morning, reveal to me the exact details of what transpired and what she said to you." Candrasena, who had listened attentively, went home and executed his guru's plan.

The poet Gayārāma sings, "Hear me, O Pīr, full of grace. Please do not get upset with your devotees!"

As soon as he heard his guru's instructions, Candrasena returned home. Madanamañjarī, the faithful wife, knew exactly when he arrived. The first thing she did was pick up a pot of water and some herbal massage oil. Within seconds of gathering her things, she met him. After massaging him with the oil, she sent Candrasena to bathe. Then she immediately set up and prepared dinner.

When he finished his bath, Candrasena returned and ate. Then, as planned, the minister's son went outside for a spell. As he chewed the spiced betel quid, he felt strangely contented. Madanamañjarī sat down inside where he had been and began to eat. This daughter of a king was eating with her head bowed when unexpectedly Candrasena reentered the room. He casually flicked some burnt tobacco on his plate. With a surge of embarrassment, he went straight over to lie down on the bed.

This unusal behavior gave the young princess pause. But she decided that now was not the appropriate time to speak to it. "Perhaps," she reasoned, "he threw the tobacco flecks on my plate to tease me—but was it his own doing or at someone else's instigation? If he plays this same game again, I will, after three repeat performances, learn its real origins." So Madanamañjarī said nothing at all and then, hastily ate the remaining food.

Candrasena arose the next morning to go to school, where he related the entire evening's events to his guru. The guru questioned him closely. "This woman said nothing to you whatsoever? I am very surprised. This strikes me as rather unusual. Let us take a different tack. Listen carefully. This time I shall penetrate her façade. After you have finished chewing your betel leaf, discard a portion of that onto your plate. But see to it that when you throw it down, it touches the rice and food that are left on the plate. Observe precisely her response, then come and tell me whether she ate the food or refused to eat it and threw it out."

Candrasena once again listened with care and then headed for home. As he walked he began to experience a certain lightness of heart to which he was unaccustomed—unexpected perhaps, but by no means unpleasant. And so for three straight nights did this minister's son execute to the letter his guru's instructions.

Finally the young lady had had enough and thought to herself, "This is not the boy's idea. He is acting on the express instruction of his guru. It is abundantly clear for he does not possess this kind of mischief; he would have certainly broken into gales of laughter over everything he has done." Thus the princess kept quiet, breathing not a word. After she finished her meal, she kept to the house, maintaining her self-imposed silence.

The following day the minister's son, as usual, went off to study. And again, as usual, he reported to his guru the girl's conduct of the previous night. Once again the guru instructed the minister's son. "Pay close attention, my son. Every morning, before anyone else has arrived or arisen, she single-handedly sweeps up the evening's mess. Follow her. Grab her clothing—rip it from her body if you must—and pull it completely off, stripping her naked. If you can bring yourself to do that, then the truth about this woman will surely be revealed."

This son of a minister acknowledged his guru's instructions, agreeing to carry out to the letter his command. After working out the details with his guru, the boy made his way home that evening as he would any other. That night, after he ate what he wanted of his dinner, he stayed inside the apartment. Recalling each step of his guru's plan, he arose somewhat earlier than usual the next morning. The faithful Madanamañjarī, hearing him stir, bounded out of bed and quickly swept up the place with cow dung. As she was busy about her work, Candrasena discreetly slipped up behind her, grabbed hold of her clothes, and pulled as hard as he could. Off they flew! Suddenly, and of course quite unexpectedly, Madanamañjarī found herself virtually naked. The face of this comely princess registered clearly the extremes of her embarrassment. Momentarily nonplussed, this chaste wife quickly recovered to pull her clothes back up to cover herself. As the clothes ascended, so too did her anger, but not until she fastened her clothes tight did she unleash her emotions.

"Is there no one to whom I can complain about what these awful Fates have inscribed on my forehead? For the very person I sheltered all these long years now rears up to strike me! It is always the case that the snake catches the frog, and from his terrible oppression the frog can only call on Lord Hari. Yet if in his divine plan Lord Hari himself allows that poor frog's death, there is no one I can think of to whom he might appeal. It is final. If a man personally squanders all of his wealth, his personal possessions, then he is simply counted among the ranks of fools everywhere. A husband, especially, will go to any lengths, resort to any device, to protect the honor and purity of his clan by protecting his most important treasure, his wife. When a man, no matter how educated, becomes intoxicated or just infatuated with himself, he is unable to discriminate between those who are his own kin and are dear to him, and outsiders. What could ever have possessed you to rip off my clothes? While it may fall within your right to have done so, you are not yet ready for that. At the appropriate time, when Kṛṣṇa takes residence in your heart, then and only then will you be entitled to look at my body."

Candrasena very carefully noted her reaction and then left. He went straight to his guru's house and entered. His guru said, "Candrasena, now tell me your story. What transpired between you and that young woman today?"

"I did just as you had instructed. This morning I pulled off her clothes and she became furious with me. 'What is this?' she screamed, 'Why have you ripped off my clothes? You are entitled to see anything you may wish. But only after Kṛṣṇa dwells in your boy's body will you be free to look at whatever you want. Why do you, completely unprovoked, harrass me by tearing off my clothes? You are neither ready nor fit to look upon me now!' When she finished her tirade, she went inside the apartment and I left immediately to come to school to study as usual."

As he listened, the guru mulled over the possibilities, and concluded that they were dealing with no ordinary woman. She was too intelligent and learned to be anything but the daughter of a king. And she must have had to seek asylum outside her own land for some strange and unknown reason. No matter how hard he examined this vexing problem, he could find but one solution. Then, with a gentle and loving touch, he spoke to Candrasena. "Listen, my boy, to what I can tell you about her. I am positive that that woman is none other than your very own wife. I can discern enough from various telltale signs to declare her positively to be your wife. But I cannot say that she has revealed it explicitly so that there is no doubt. So, as a final step, tonight you must try somehow to get her to declare the fact."

Embarrassment and confusion seemed to creep over poor Candrasena as he listened. He quickly excused himself and left for home. With his head hanging low, Candrasena went straight to his part of the house. But he seated himself outside in the courtyard, hunched over, brooding. When it was past the day's second watch, well after noon, his faithful wife began to wonder in concern why her husband had not yet returned. She looked outside and spotted him sitting quietly, his normally beaming moonlike face tarnished with a terrible gloom. Madanamañjarī, always the good wife, spoke to him with cheer in her voice. "Hey, why do you sit here with such a long face? Has someone said something to weigh you down? Is that why you sit with that sad look and your head drooping? Come on, get up and take your bath, you will feel better. It breaks my heart to see you so downcast. Tell me, my little precious, did someone say something unpleasant to you? What could make you sit here looking so distraught?"

Candrasena spoke directly to the point. "You must be honest with me. Before I go bathe, tell me exactly who you are. Who am I? Where is my home? Who are my parents? Who was it that bore you? Whose daughter are you really? What is your caste? Where do you come from and why are we here? What is the reason that you have been the one to raise me?"

The young woman attempted to buy some time, saying, "I will explain all of this later, but first I beg of you, go have some food! In all these long days you have never questioned any of this. So tell me now, at whose instigation are you making this sudden inquiry?"

Candrasena calmly replied, "Give me every detail truthfully, otherwise I won't be able to live like this, I shall commit suicide—and you can count on it!"

The young woman relented, realizing she must finally speak her secret. "Listen, then, to some ancient history. It grieves me heart and soul just to talk about it."

Meditating day and night on the sweetness of the Pīr's feet, Gayārāma narrates a portion of this new poem of praise.

The faithful wife Madanamañjarī listened to her husband's ultimatum and offered her account of past events. "Because you have inquired of me directly, I shall reveal everything. Listen, my beloved, to my strange tale. Should I sometimes choke on my words, it is only the sound of my heart breaking in pain, for I was born the most miserable of women.

"There is a king named Vinoda Vihārī, who rules over Vijayanagara. I am his daughter. Listen, my precious, when I reached the age of twelve, the Fates turned away from me. I happened to appear at the place where my mother and my father were talking together privately. The Fates had ordained that my father take a vow when he discovered his own daughter was of marriageable age. 'When I get up in the morning,' he declared, 'I shall betroth my daughter to the very first man I see.' My father made and kept his promise.

"Meanwhile, your first rice-eating ceremony had been fixed for that very same day. Your father is Dharmadhvaja, the chief minister of the king. He sent you with a maidservant to be blessed by the king's audience—a custom in our land. When the king laid eyes on you, he effected his vow and took you to his own breast. We were married later that evening. My father was ever mindful of the sempiternal laws, the *dharma*, and never did anything that was evil or wicked. The ill luck was not his doing, but mine, indelibly etched on my forehead.

"We went to the flowered bridal chamber accompanied by my attendants. There you could only cry, for you needed milk. Hearing your plaintive wails completely unnerved me—I desired only to take my own life. Instead, I began seriously to contemplate alternative action, some scheme to spirit you away. To that end I collected jewelry, gemstones, and other forms of disposable wealth. Rather than tarnish my father's lineage with a suicide, I ran away with you. It was the darkest part of the night of the fourteenth, the blackest night of the lunar cycle. I had no sense of what I should do, what was right and what was wrong, or proper and improper. God alone understood into just what adversity I had fallen.

"In the city I was forced to beg for milk to feed you. It barely saved your life. Because of this series of misfortunes I ended up in this country. Everyone thought I was a lunatic, a crazy woman. Some people spoke ill of me or insulted me. My eyes frequently flowed with tears I could not restrain. I had been born the most wretched of miserable women.

"When I came to this part of the kingdom, I placed all my trust and hopes on your feet and became the godchild of the king. The king, who is meritorious in his action, was gracious toward me and had a small house erected for me. Shortly thereafter the Pīr, that treasure trove of mercy who is the arbiter of destiny itself, granted me the shadow of his feet and acknowledged me as his faithful maidservant. In less than one night he had raised this fabulous mansion for me, a mansion in which I was to take you and raise you, my lord.

"Listen, O son of my father's minister, at the appropriate time I handed you over to the school so that you would be honored and imbued with formal education. The daily sufferings and hardships that I endured, God alone fully comprehends. How can words from my mouth capture their import? I can only plead with the Fates that never again would I be born in this cycle of lives as a woman. To be born a woman is contemptible, a burden on everyone around. Would that such a demeaning birth never again befall me! . . ."

The ever-faithful Madanamañjarī described to her husband his past, filling in each detail. At first Candrasena's eyes grew moist, then they flowed unabashedly, streams of tears eventually soaking his entire body. In a voice choked with emotion and a lifetime of love, he said, "Truly blessed are you on the orb of this earth. You stand out in your king's lineage as dedicated and faithful, a true *satī*, and utterly devoted to your husband, a *pativratā*. There has never been seen the likes of you—the daughter of a king cursed with such misery. Yet through it all, God has vouchsafed your dignity, your honor, and your respect. You had to labor ever so hard just to raise me, yet never did you come to hate me, to hold me in contempt. As long as there is life in my body, I shall carry out your every wish and command. I will never so much as look at another woman. . . ."

Placing all hopes at the feet of the Pīr, Gayārāma the devotee writes about the servant of your most loyal servant. Of all the places possible throughout the length and breadth of this great universe, grant me a tiny spot at your feet, O Pīr, you who counter our aspirations through trials of misery and disaster.

Madanamañjarī finished her story standing directly in front of her husband, her hands respectfully pressed together in obeisance. As he listened, this fine son of a minister reeled from his shock and amazement. "Truly praiseworthy are you, my blessed Madanamañjarī. Blessed too is the man who planted the seed and the woman who carried you in her womb. You struggled to care for me, a six-month-old baby. You, a princess, forced to hide in one place after another. I have heard an old story recorded in the Purāṇas about a faithful wife, a *satī* named Anusūyā, who lived in the country of Atri. In order to test her fidelity, to destroy her chastity if they could, the gods Brahmā, Viṣṇu, and Maheśvara went to her home. Now Anusūyā's fidelity and chastity were renowned throughout the world as exceptionally powerful. As soon as the gods made overtures toward her, she transformed them into baby boys. She had three maidservants care for these three six-month-old babies. They would hold them in their laps and feed them milk from their own breasts. Later, Sāvitrī, Lakṣmī, and Pārvatī, the gods' respective wives, came there looking for their lost husbands. They threw themselves at Anusūyā's feet. Anusūyā said, 'Goddesses, all of you hear well. Identify the baby who is your husband and take him with you.' But none of the three women was able to recognize her husband as long as Anusūyā's maidservants were stationed nearby, such was their devotion. Only by lengthy propitiation of Anusūyā did that famous *satī* allow the three wives to retrieve their husbands. You have looked after and raised me with the same degree of devotion. You are the supreme *satī* and *pativratā* in the triple world. . . ."

In just this way did the couple exchange stories as they declared themselves. And as they did, the son of the minister became uneasy as his newly discovered appetites stirred. The day came to a close and night took its place. Madanamañjarī prepared to quench his desires. First, she cooked. When the minister's son finished his meal, he was momentarily contented and, without pause, walked straight to his golden bed, where he stretched out.

When Madanamañjarī had finished eating, she came and sat on the bed by her husband. The curiosity and anticipation in their hearts grew with each chew of the spiced betel quid. The couple drew great pleasure from indulging in the same kind of affectionate and intimate talk they had just discovered. All the many and fine wedding garments the young woman had so carefully saved, she now brought out to show the minister's son.

"This night, our room will be transformed into our bridal chamber. The Fates have joined us together, making tonight our wedding night. We passed the earlier daylight hours in agonizing bouts of tears, but tonight we will pass happily as we seek pleasure and play."

Mutually agreed, the couple climbed onto a bed of pure bliss. The minister's son passed the night discovering untold physical pleasures. Their lovemaking continued unabated for the duration of the night, until the sun finally climbed into the eastern sky.

The next day, when he had finished those ritual acts that are prescribed for each morning, the minister's son sat outside the living apartments. After finishing her bath, the young bride put on a strikingly colorful sari. Then she cooked at least fifty special dishes: vegetables, fish, and rice. When his meal was completed, Candrasena knew the feeling of real contentment for the first time. Later that afternoon he went to speak with his teacher.

First he stretched himself out fully in obeisance, then stood respectfully to one side and began to retell the adventures of the princess. "Listen, O Guru, who fulfils all wishes. Hers is a strange tale indeed. That beautiful young woman is my own wife. There is one *rājā*, Vinoda Vihārī, in the kingdom of Pampāpura. This Madanamañjarī is his daughter. My name is Candrasena and I am the son of a minister. My father is Dharmadhvaja, and he is famous throughout the world. On the day of my first feeding of solid food, when I was a six-month-old baby, I was taken to the king's palace. Madanamañjarī was a young woman who had just turned twelve, and Rāja Vinoda Vihārī gave her in marriage to me that day. In order to escape the terrible public censure that would follow, this brave young girl spirited me away. She managed to bring me here, completely indifferent to the manifold hardships she suffered. Last evening this woman explained it all to me. I stretch no truth to falsity. I have told you everything, omitting nothing."

The guru, who had listened intently, finally spoke. "This daughter of a king is truly worthy of praise. As a *satī* and *pativratā* she is a Lakṣmī or a Sarasvatī. Go now, my son, to that house that is your own and live in pleasure. In knowledge you are a *paṇḍita* and in virtues you are as vast as the ocean." The guru continued, "The noble keep the company of the noble. Who has ever heard anywhere of the good among the bad and lowly?" Candrasena bowed at his guru's feet and departed.

When she saw him, the princess was filled with a boundless joy. When they finished their dinner, they lay down on the bed seeking pleasure once again. And just as they had previously done, they passed the entire night savoring the joys of erotic play.

Eventually the good news reached the great king and everyone agreed that this *satī pativratā* was indeed blessed and to be admired. There the happy couple lived, experiencing an enviable joy and pleasure.

Gayārāma continues to sing the new lyrics of the Pīr.

Many days passed in the manner just described. But one day God, Khodā, instigated another round of mischief, for thanks to Candrasena, the minister's son, Madanamañjarī completely forgot to perform her daily worship of Satya Nārāyaṇa. This did not go unnoticed by the Helmsman of Heaven. He reflected, "My ritual vow was not undertaken by Madanamañjarī. I shall make her suffer and eventually destroy her. Then she is bound not to forget to perform my worship, my *pūjā*." Talking like this, the Universal Wheel Turner set those wheels in motion and soon, by magic, both Madanamañjarī and Candrasena fell into the great net of illusion called the world.

One afternoon Candrasena was feeling carefree, so he went to the bazaar seeking some entertainment. He walked through the northern and western sections, then to the eastern. Eventually he entered into the Malayā Market in the southern part. There his eye fell upon a wonderful garden, within which lay a lake, its banks neatly hardened and manicured. The flora was of a pleasingly wondrous variety. The Amarāvatī garden of Indra is the first thing that came to his mind. There were mango and jam-fruit trees, sweet coconut, tamarind, jackfruit, date palms, guavas, palmyras, and dark *tamāla* fan palms. He found orange, lime, and citron, along with clove, nutmeg, hog plum, myrobalan, custard apple, and pomegranate. Brilliant *aśoka* trees, guelder rose, small-bud magnolia, and evergreen *vakula* were all blooming, as were a host of others: *gandharāja*, *sephālikā*, *jārula*, and *pārula*. He saw winter-, star-, and white jasmine, screw pine, the glorious *kadamba*, *nāgeśvara*, rose, myrtle, and *ṭagara*. White and red china roses were blooming, as were climbing jasmine, golden *kāñcana*, lily of the valley, *kṛṣṇakeli*, oleander, and ixora. Everywhere he looked he saw whites, reds, blues, yellows in every imaginable shade. And lotuses—red, blue, white—likewise opened their faces.

The fauna was also abundant. Gallinules, moorhens, and wagtails could be seen dancing in pairs. So too paddybirds, openbill storks, black-winged stilts, various geese, and swans. Swarms of bees buzzed the ripe blossoms in search of their founts of nectar. And when mating pairs of cuckoos sang, the effect was nothing less than thrilling.

The spring season had just arrived, and along with it came the god of love, armed with his unerring bow and arrows. When the minister's son saw this paradisical forest grove, his head grew light. And into it blithely he walked, as if drawn inside by powers he could not fathom.

He inspected everything in turn, taking in each and every item, leaving out nothing. While he was so engrossed, a woman called Mālinī—for she was a weaver of garlands—spotted him from afar. It just so happened that this particular *mālinī* was given to playful seduction, and in that she was quite accomplished. Deep in this park, in the middle of a flower garden, sat Mālinī's tiny hut. She lived all alone: she had neither companions nor lovers. Her full name was Surasikā Raṅginī the Mālinī, which means the "She Who Weaves Garlands to Enhance the Play of Love," or Raṅginī, "Erotic Sport," for short. She had been sitting alone in her room, weaving not garlands, but a veil of illusion.

The one named Candrasena had a face that outshone the moon. He wore a fine line of mustache, which filled in his upper lip, a visible signal of his growing maturity. When Candrasena stumbled upon her, Mālinī coyly suggested, "Be pleased, sir, to take a seat here by me. I would very much like to garland you with some special flowers."

Candrasena naïvely asked, "What might be the point of this garland?" To which Mālinī replied, with a twinkle in her eye, "With this garland you will be able to seduce the wives of other men."

Candrasena, being the way he was, protested. "I do not hanker after any other woman. I already have the woman of my dreams! I could never find another woman with such incredible qualities. Perhaps you should wear the garland yourself so that you can seduce the husbands of other women."

Cool and coy Mālinī took careful note of his suggestion and said, "Well, first you should slip this charmed garland around your own neck to empower it." Laughing at her own suggestion, the seductive garland maker then leaned forward and placed the garland around his neck. As she slipped it over his head, she charmed the beautiful blue-and-white *aparājitā* flowers—and they had to be *aparājitā*, for the creeper's name tells that "they cannot be overcome." Instantly Candrasena turned into a parrot, a popinjay, the fabled Indian *totā*! Mālinī picked him up and secured him in a cage.

Before he had even realized what happened, Candrasena was made a prisoner by the inexorable machinery of fate. Everyone must understand that everything that happened, happened because of the magic of the Pīr.

The face of Candrasena, who was now in the form of a bird, was drawn, drained of life, it seemed. As he realized his fate, his voice was so choked with emotion that he could not squeeze out a sound. He perched mute in his cage, his eyes streaming with tears. The thought of Madanamañjarī hit him like a hundred thunderbolts exploding in his head. He could only sigh deeply and wail in his remorse.

"I shall never see her again. There is nothing I can do. Where is my Madanamañjarī, my joy-filled creeper of love? No more in this birth will I meet my faithful wife. She raised me with such selfless care. Now the Fates have dictated that Mālinī make me prisoner!"

As he thought these things, he did so with a mental intensity so great that back at the house, the pure daughter of the king began to grow restless and uneasy. The sun set and the moon rose. The faithful Madanamañjarī was unable to concentrate on anything as her worries grew. "My husband cannot bear to be apart from me for even a second, why then, has he not come home by now?" As she pondered this, a feeling of dread gradually swept over this sensitive woman.

Gayārāma directs his devotion to the feet of the Pīr.

During the night's second watch, the faithful Madanamañjarī wept. She was truly beautiful, even with tears staining her eyes. A battle raged in her mind as she fought to make sense of his absence.

"He just went to wander around the bazaar. But now it has fallen dark. Why has he not returned home where he belongs? Maybe my husband has left me. He has returned to his own home and jettisoned me, this worthless woman, like so much garbage on the side of the road. Granted I have many defects, but what terrible thing have I done to make him abandon his worshipful servant and return to Vijayanagara? Now I think I understand your ways, for a man has no scruples whatsoever. Given the chance, he is determined only to destroy, nay, kill a woman. I abandoned my mother and father in order to protect you. Now, many years later, I receive the reward for that act."

When her thoughts led her to admit this, the sensitive little woman cried out, "Where is the treasure of my life?" And she slumped to the ground in a dead faint. "Be merciful to me this one time. Come back to your miserable wife. I cannot live without you!" The more she thought about it, the more this loving woman wondered at the sense of it all. "Perhaps someone simply abducted my husband when he went to the bazaar," she began to rationalize. "Or," her thoughts tumbling over themselves, "perhaps someone mugged him or even killed him for his money! Or maybe he has been hidden away someplace for ransom! If I do not get him back soon, I shall hurl myself into the sea. Or offer up my pitiful life to the purifying flames."

Round and round her thoughts whirled, the chaste wife giving herself up to an uncontrollable lament, rolling on the ground in paroxysms of grief until she finally passed out. While unconscious, the Lord Bhagavān spoke to her directly, to her heart.

He appeared to her in the garb of a fakir. He called out to her through the mists of her mind. "Listen, faithful woman, to what I have to say. However long you continue to weep, you only prolong your agony. You will eventually retrieve your husband, you can be sure. When your husband was in your arms, you thought only of him and not of me. For that reason and that alone you now suffer."

When he had delivered his pointed message, Pīr Bhagavān disappeared and Madanamañjarī came to her senses.

Madanamañjarī wept bitterly in the agony of separation from her husband. To her the Pīr, Wielder of the Staff of Justice, had offered sage advice. Listen, one and all, to the story of this song, which takes many unexpected turns.

The king who ruled this land was named Magīndra Rājā. He had in his family one unmarried daughter. There was no suitable match for her extraordinary beauty anywhere in the three worlds. The glow of her face was reminiscent of a harvest moon. She was ornamented with glistening lotus-shaped earrings as if flanked by beloved and adoring friends. The high sweep of her eyebrows would have broken the bow of the Limbless One, Anaṅga, the god of love. The red of her lips struck richer than the early morning sun.

This young woman was not yet married, although she was a full sixteen years of age. She regularly worshiped Śiva, her heart swelling with hope for a boon, for a husband. This picture of beauty worshiped Bholanātha every morning without fail, hoping fervently that the Slayer of the Demon Tripura would provide her with a suitable match. Because the woman honored Mṛtuñjaya in all his forms and with great regularity, Raṅginī the garland weaver was hired to keep her supplied with flowers. This princess was born in the late fall, a time that is especially pleasant, and so for this reason bore the name of Hemalatā—the Lovely Creeper of Autumn.

One day the daughter of the king was paying her customary respects to Śiva when Raṅginī the *mālinī* brought her flowers. Smiling with a hint of mischief, Raṅginī handed her the garlands, then giggled. She spoke directly to the young woman, expecting to tantalize her.

"Listen, my dear princess. Do I have some news! I just caught an especially charming and playful little parrot, a popinjay!"

The girl immediately pressed her. "Is the bird a fine specimen? Is it well formed? Please, my dear Mālinī, bring it so that I may examine it for myself."

Mālinī objected. "But if you do not return it, then what, my dear princess, will I be able to do?"

The princess replied, "I have no ulterior motive. I do not need the bird, for I have everything I could want. I just want to see with my own eyes that it is as you say."

Satisfied that she would not lose her pet, Mālinī went home. The next morning she gathered her flowers with a strange and unacustomed happiness. She gathered flowers in an extra large variety that day: *aśoka*, guelder rose, *ṭagara*, and star jasmine. Then she picked rose, golden *kāñcana*, other types of *ṭagara*, and *vakula* for its white, evergreen-scented contrast. And to these she added an assortment of other blooms, creepers, and sprigs of greenery. She strung well her garlands, filled her baskets, and set off. On the way out she grabbed the popinjay parrot, which perched obediently on her left hand.

Mālinī deposited the flowers and the bird directly in front of the princess, who was waiting patiently in her seat. The extraordinary selection of flowers captivated her imagination, and with the mind of one pure, she worshiped Śaṅkara with increased devotion.

At the end of her worship, she prostrated herself in respect. "I beseech you, Bholanātha, Vyomakeśa who has the sky for hair, never to be cross with me! O fair-complexioned Kṛttivāsa, you who wear the skin of a tiger, grant me a boon that by your grace I may find a groom.[8] After making yet another obeisance, this daughter of a king rose and picked up the popinjay parrot that Mālinī had procured.

Hemalatā took the parrot with her into her private inner apartments. Truly this was the special parrot they call the popinjay. She fed the bird clotted cream, milk, and banana,[9] while for his part, the minister's son ate with a distinct pleasure. But as he gazed at the stunning beauty of this princess, all he could think of was his own Madanamañjarī.

"My own young wife in the prime of her youth is truly as beautiful. Yet now I have lost her and through some awful blight on my fortune I am destined to suffer. Mālinī has turned my good fortune to misery, and I have not even seen my wife since that time."

With these and other anguished thoughts, he sat still, depressed, suffering in silence, while right in front of him Hemalatā and Mālinī argued his fate.

"Listen, my dear friend Mālinī, to what I propose. I want you to leave the parrot with me for just one night. Tomorrow you can come and collect the bird. Tonight I just want to fill my eyes with its haunting beauty."

Mālinī had not counted on this and so pleaded futilely in her panic, "But it has become the very heart of my life. I become utterly confounded and bereft of my good sense when the bird is out of sight." But plead though she might, the bird stayed with the princess at her palace, while poor Mālinī had but to return to her empty home empty-handed. She secretly knew that the parrot was lost to her forever, and she berated herself at the irony of it all. "To think that a valuable treasure stolen by one thief is then lifted by yet another."

As they mulled their separate fates, evening approached and then night fell. Hemalatā, the daughter of the king, hurried off to eat an early dinner. She carried the magical popinjay with her to the second floor of her apartment. Then, completely alone, this beautiful young woman entered her bedroom. She went over and lay down on her bed with its golden stand. It had beautifully colored pillows and a finely woven mosquito net, all appropriate for a princess.

Playing with the bird, Hemalatā rubbed her hand across the bird's body and urged it to speak. "Say 'Rādhā Kṛṣṇa!' my fine-feathered parrot. Say the word "Kṛṣṇa," and animals everywhere will be liberated. Look, my pet, it is the horrible Kali Age and the days are fast disappearing. You must speak." And as she was coaxing him to speak, she stroked his body with her hand. Suddenly the bird's head drooped and fell off!

Where there had been a bird moments before, now stood a man. Transformed and dazed he crouched, still gripping the crossbeam of the perch in his hand. Then he stood.

The princess gaped at him, embarrassed. "That coy seductress Mālinī has pulled an incredibly singular feat! It is impossible for a man to be transformed into a bird, yet here he is. He must be a celestial being, a heavenly nymph or musician, possibly even a demigod." She was stupefied, struck dumb in amazement. But, quickly collecting her wits like the king's daughter that she was, she immediately interrogated him about his background and identity. Her questions were polite, but direct, and came in a jumble.

"Who are you? Where is your home? What is your name? How did you come to be in such a wretched state? Tell me everything. How was it that you came to be in the form of a bird in Mālinī's house? Tell me your story and leave out no detail! I will listen very carefully."

At this prompting, the minister's son found his voice and launched into his saga. "Listen, O Princess, to my sad tale. My name is Candrasena and I am the son of a minister. One day, late in the afternoon, I was walking around the bazaar. Quite by chance—or perhaps by divine intervention—I stumbled across Mālinī in her garden. Raṅginī Mālinī was trying to seduce me, and in the process magically transformed me into a bird. She then captured me easily and kept me under lock in a cage. By some crazy turn of fate I became a prisoner in a house of garlands. My lovely wife must be wailing in anguish at this nasty turn of events. You show me great mercy by breaking the secret of my bondage. Please tell me, how can I find my way back to my own home?"

Taking it all in, Hemalatā chose to interpret the events somewhat differently. "Vidhi, the dispenser of fate, has favorably backed me. My most earnest desire has at last been fulfilled. For I have been propitiating Lord Gaṅgādhara, Śiva, to fill it. And after an interminable wait this boon, a groom, has been made my reward. I have been living in the house of my mother and father as a burdensome unmarried daughter. The responsibility of my womanhood now falls to you. During the day you will remain here in my quarters in your parrot form. But by night you will resume your body as a man and we shall pass the time together, a couple making love. When I look at your handsome face and body, my mind is set awhirl. Who knows how much longer it will be before my father manages to arrange a suitable marriage for me. My situation is no different from that of the pure and true Uṣā when she glanced at Aniruddha. She passed all her days and nights intoxicated by the god of love. She had one special maidservant by the name of Citrarekhā. She procured Citrarekhā for Aniruddha and arranged their marriage.[10] Or perhaps it is in the same mold as the wife of Śiva in the house of Hemanta. Day and night, whenever she looked at Śiva, tears flowed from her eyes. So, too, it was with the winsome daughter of Nīladhvaja, whose name was Svahā. Her heart remained in constant agitation for the sake of Agni, the lord of fire. In ways just as these is my heart bewitched to look upon you! May your heart and mine be forever joined as one!"

The more he listened to the princess's declarations, the more the minister's son grew uneasy. But after a while, he considered, "this woman is blessed with a beauty that is truly exquisite. To look at her makes me curse the time lost to blinking. . . ."

And beautiful Hemalatā certainly was. Snow- and star-jasmine highlighted her curly hair in the way lightning plays through rolling masses of dark storm clouds. The beams of her face reminded him of a stainless moon at its full measure. The dart of her eye proved more pleasingly deft than a doe's. The arch of her eyebrows would have broken the flower-bow of the god of love. The redness of her lips was richer than a rising sun. Mesmerizing earrings dangled gracefully from her lobes, while draped around her neck hung the fabled elephant pearls, set in contrast to a string of gemstones. The fullness of her breasts shamed even large earthen waterpots; they were bursting like ripe pomegranates. The splendor of this bewitching woman's beauty exuded pure eroticism. Her arms, like lotus stalks, were more lithe and slender than a serpent's body, while the trim lines of her waist put that of the lion, the king of beasts, to shame. The curve of her hips proved more graceful and enchanting than an elephant's, and the girdle that encircled them shone like the moon. The slope of her thighs was more shapely than a well-grown plaintain, the red of her soles richer than a fully opened red lotus. Bands encircled her arms, anklets her feet, and jangled as she walked. Her gait was a match to the proverbial grace of the elephant or the liquid glide of the swan.

The minister's son was smitten by her breathtaking beauty. With a single vision he stared, like a puppet transfixed on the strings of her charm. The more he looked, the more control of his heart he lost. The caressing words that wafted from her moon-face hit their mark—he listened without protest to what she said.

The minister's son sat on the bed and Hemalatā sat radiantly to his right. It was the season of spring and the sweet breezes blew from the Malaya Mountains. They soon fell prey to not one, but all five arrows of the god of love, who destroys the sense of one lost in love.[11] This young man, full of his youth, took this young beauty, ripe and eager. He pulled her down on the cot and succumbed to the ecstasy of erotic bliss.

The couple passed the entire night in a continuation of this fantasy, but in the morning the princess did not forget to transform him back into a bird. The minister's son found himself to be a bird just as before.

Later that morning, Mālinī returned to the palace. Raṅginī Mālinī wasted no time. "Listen, Hemalatā. Please produce the parrot so that I may take him home."

The young woman lied, "The parrot has flown away. I have been worried sick about it ever since. Here, take some money and go back to your house. Try to catch another one for yourself, and perhaps another to bring to me." And with these slick words she handed her a generous ten rupees while swearing an oath on her own forehead that she was telling the truth. Then she sent Mālinī home.

Mālinī trudged home, devastated. Candrasena, on the other hand, stayed put in the body of a popinjay. The princess brought him mounds of sweets, and Candrasena would eat, sitting there in the second-floor apartment of the princess. Day and night did these lovebirds indulge their erotic fantasies. But—you must understand—it was all done through the magic of the Pīr.

Thus the lovely Hemalatā, in the first flush of her maturing youth, got the man of her dreams and passed her nights with him as her new husband. This is exactly how things continued for quite some time. Gayārāma extols in song the Pīr's clever plan.

Listen, one and all, and concentrate on the glory of the Pīr, who had afforded this young princess her erotic adventures. Listen to this amazing tale.

Hemalatā, the daughter of King Magīndra, became pregnant after not too many days. All of her female companions were secretly alarmed, and finally told everything to the queen. The queen was furious when she heard, so much so that the corner of her sari fell to the ground when Hemalatā arrived, her instant dishevelment signaling her acute consternation.

The queen demanded of Hemalatā, "Tell me the truth. How have you managed to get yourself pregnant? Who has had the audacity to sneak into my house where Indra, the king of the gods, and Yama, lord of death, fear to tread? That you have done such a thing demonstrates you cannot discern right from wrong. How did you build up the courage to do this? You have stained the lineage of your father with an indelible blot of scandal that will make the king hang his head in shame."

Hemalatā stood her ground. "Mother, no human being possesses this kind of power. This man has come from the heavens themselves. How can I describe his beauty? It is a mix of that of Indra and Agni. And he comes to me in a most unusual way. As the night passes into the second watch he magically appears in my room, just as the moon mysteriously rises in the sky. I can hardly contain myself when I gaze at his beauty. He stays with me and we make passionate love."

As the queen listened, her heart filled with despair, but she went straight to the king and said, "Listen, lord of men. Once you could hold high your head, now it will be hung in shame, for your reputation is severely threatened: Your loving daughter Hemalatā is pregnant."

Coming directly from his wife, the news hit him like a bolt of lightning, and he flew into an uncontrollable rage. Anger spewed from the king's eyes as he ordered the chief of police: "Apprehend the criminal immediately. Go and keep watch over all conceivable routes into and out of the inner apartments all through the night, and note every person who comes and goes. If you fail to capture him, then you and your families will be executed and your names destroyed. You will have no refuge anywhere in my kingdom."

As soon as they heard the command, the police fanned out and took up positions to watch Hemalatā's apartments. But the place where the young lady lived was already so tightly restricted that not even an ant could have slipped through, so what was the use of the police? For three days they waited, each one more silent than the last. Still they rousted out no one. The police chief was seething. He stormed up to the second floor and conducted a close search himself. The police chief could only find a popinjay parrot, which out of frustration and fear he produced before his majesty the king.

"Pay heed, my stalwart king. We have had great difficulty in arresting the criminal. Tell me how we should proceed. We searched the second floor, but all we found was the bird. You, I think, should interrogate him. Listen to what the bird says, for it should be able to name everyone who comes and goes in your palace."

The king considered the chief of police's advice and then redirected his questions. "Please speak, my fine-feathered child, for you are the fabled *totā* parrot. Who has entered into my citadel to meet secretly with Hemalatā? Please tell me truthfully whether or not magic was used. . . ." And with these and similar soft words the king coaxed him along. The bird could only think to himself, "My situation has certainly taken an awkward turn."

From the clan of Acyutānanda comes my paternal grandfather, Śambhūcandra. It is I, Gayārāma, his grandson, who sings.

As the king spoke, he gently stroked the bird's body, trying to soothe him. "You, my little bird, are a speaker of truth, so please give your account of what happened." He continued this light massage as he showered him with flattery and praise. "Please tell the truth, parrot, for you are speaking to the king." And so it went: the king simultaneously pleading and stroking.

Suddenly the bird's topknot drooped and fell to the ground. As soon as his crest hit the floor, a man stood before them. Everyone was amazed to have witnessed this spectacle: a bird suddenly transformed into a man.

The king quickly said, "Tell us just what and who you are! From where do you hail? Tell us, who is your father? How is it that you were in the form of a bird in my palace? Please tell us the truth. And speak so that all those present may hear. If you do not, I will have your head cut off. Now!"

The king questioned and threatened him, and as he did, he filled with rage once again. The minister's son addressed him with his palms pressed together in respect.

"I speak the truth, whether you execute me or grant me life. In Vijayanagara there is a king, Rāja Vinoda Vihārī. His chief minister is one Dharmadhvaja, who is renowned throughout the universe, both the animate and inanimate worlds. The king's daughter is named Madanamañjarī. And by the age of twelve, her beauty was legendary, outstripping even Viśvakarma's grandest creation, Tilottamā. In order to honor a vow he had made, the king gave his daughter in marriage to a six-month-old boy. The bride and groom were futilely escorted to the bridal chamber. I was that baby boy. To avoid public humiliation, the young bride secreted me away in the middle of the night. It was to your kingdom that we fled. She took great pains to see that I was properly raised, and I received my formal education within the walls of your own palace. In this way did fourteen years pass. We lived in your land, being very much in love. One day I went to roam about the bazaar. I happened to meet there the coy Raṅginī Mālinī. Being a garland weaver, Raṅginī Mālinī had learned the secrets of herbal magic. The instant she slipped a garland around my neck, she turned me into a bird. I was held captive in Mālinī's house in my bird form. But she, in turn, presented me to your daughter.

"One day the beautiful young woman who is your daughter was rubbing my body with her hand. My topknot fell off and I recovered my male body. Your daughter instantly inquired of my background, and I told her everything from beginning to end, just as it had happened. 'Grant me my freedom,' I pleaded with her, but the young woman turned a deaf ear and claimed me by virtue of her vow. Then she quoted stories from a number of the scriptures to justify it. And that is how she came to keep me in her bedroom as a bird. By day I lived as a bird, by night a man, when I indulged your daughter in endless bouts of erotic play. This, your Majesty, is the entire truth.

"Now I know and understand nothing more than this. Men do not live terribly long lives. I was born and soon I will die. I have no friends or family anywhere here in your kingdom, so there is nothing more for me in this life save death. Raṅginī Mālinī is the one responsible for this wretched turn of events. Through her herbal magic she transformed me into a bird—and that in itself is worthy of recognition. Listen, wielder of the staff of justice. I have but one regret: I will never see Madanamañjarī again. She labored so hard to raise me—I could never find a woman of her fine qualities anywhere on the face of the earth. It grieves me deeply that I cannot see her at the hour of my death. I have violated the sanctity of your home with gross and sinful acts. Yet by my death, inconsequential and deserving though it be, three more will also die. When my wife hears that you have executed me, she will instantly abandon her own life in suicide. Just so your daughter, who lives in the confines of your own palace, for she will not hesitate to follow me in death. But your daughter is also five months pregnant, and my child, which she carries in her womb, will also be put to death. Through the simple deserving death of one, three more undeserving deaths follow. It is no one's fault; it is simply a nasty twist of fate."

As Candrasena filled in the details of his misadventures, the king paid close attention, hanging on every word. The king dropped his gaze as he pondered the situation, but before he could speak, Satya, the crown jewel of Pīrs, took control of his voice.

The *mahārāja* issued his first command to the chief of police. "Fetch Mālinī and bring her to me straightaway!" As soon as he received the command, the chief of police executed it. He immediately arrested Mālinī and produced her in chains.

The king inquired of her, "Where did you learn this secret knowledge? With what motive did you transform this unsuspecting foreign boy into a bird? But it was not enough that you turned the minister's son into a popinjay parrot. Then, you old hag, you acted like a panderer and procured him for my daughter! . . ." Of course the more the king talked, the more shaken with anger he got. But he restrained himself. He publicly disgraced Mālinī in the presence of the entire court. Then he had her head shaved and her cheeks smeared with lime paste and soot to mark her humiliation. Then he drove her out of town.

By this, Magendra avoided the sin of killing a woman. But at Candrasena he continued to look, undecided. Finally the king spoke, "If he is executed, what will be the result? Because of one, several lives will be destroyed. Should he be executed, the ignominy will be doubled; better now to hand my daughter over to him quietly. I will not compromise my position on account of him."

Having made these pronouncements, the king consulted his ministers. They concurred in unison. "Well judged, O King!" Of course no one dared to speak in dissent. Hearing this approval, the king was pleased. He then took Candrasena and escorted him inside the private quarters of the palace.

The king discussed matters with the queen, and they dispatched one of their maidservants to where Madanamañjarī was staying. The maidservant said to her, "Let us go to the king's palace so that you may see the condition of your husband, who is incarcerated there. The king has decreed that he is to be executed. Go quickly so that you may see your husband."

Hearing all of this, Madanamañjarī was sick with grief and rushed to His Majesty the king, crying all the way. The king's wife met Madanamañjarī and received her with due ceremony, profering a seat of honor. Madanamañjarī groveled in obeisance at the feet of the king and queen, contorted from weeping for clemency for her husband. The king consoled her.

"Listen, Mother, to my proposal. There is no need to weep for your husband.

One day a garland weaver named Mālinī cast a spell on Candrasena and he was transformed into a parrot, the fabled *totā*. By chance the parrot fell into my daughter's hands, and as she rubbed his body—poof—a man magically appeared. When I heard about all of the mischief Mālinī had stirred up, I had her brought here and publicly punished. My daughter is now five months pregnant and if the news leaked out, we would have a scandal and become laughingstocks of the land. The chief of police arrested Candrasena and brought him before me, but I chose not to execute him on account of you. If this one man were killed, then three more people would die. I would be crushed by the scandal of it and lose my good reputation in this world. I have forgiven Candrasena all his transgressions and resolved to give him to my daughter. If you give your permission, I will hand over my daughter. It is for this reason that I fetched you to my place."

The king then reiterated: "If you give me the word, I will give my daughter in marriage to your husband."

Madanamañjarī deftly replied. "O Mahārāja, what power have I to countermand any decree you might issue?"

As soon as he heard this, the king sent for the *purohits*, the priests, to fix the auspicious time. At the most auspicious moment on the proper day of the lunar cycle, the king promptly awarded his daughter in marriage. At the conclusion of the wedding ceremonies, the groom headed for the traditional flowered bridal chamber—accompanied by both Hemalatā and Madanamañjarī. The three of them amused themselves with secret delights. And so it continued for several days without break.

Hemalatā, who had been five months pregnant at the wedding, went into labor after ten lunar months and ten days. She delivered a healthy, strapping boy, which Madanamañjarī, good wife that she was, took to her own lap. On the sixth day, they performed the Ṣaṣṭhī *pūjā* to the goddess of children,[12] a special blessing for him, and on the ninth day, the ritual reading of the Veda. The auspicious twenty-first was observed during the first month. At the end of month six, the child was fed his first rice . . . and so he grew.

One day Candrasena had an idea and went to share it with Madanamañjarī. "Listen, my beloved wife and princess. I have a strong yearning to go to visit my ancestral home. Your mother and father are there, as are mine. Let us go home and assuage their grief over our departure many years ago. Think about my proposal, my moon-faced beauty. Tell me if you approve."

Madanamañjarī replied to her husband, "If you have the desire, then let us go to your home."

When he received her support, the minister's son went to the king to take permission to leave. With hands pressed together, Candrasena appeared before the king. He began to speak with courteous words of submission.

"Please listen, O King of kings, to my humble petition. Please grant me permission to visit my ancestral home. If I survive, I will then return here. I shall take my leave, O King, from your illustrious feet."

The king said, "Listen, my child, the son of a minister. I give you my blessings. Go to your own home."

Having taken formal leave of his father-in-law, he touched his head to the feet of his mother-in-law. "Grant your permission, Mother, so that your son can visit his own home. My mother and father are there and they must have been extremely worried all these years."

Then Madanamañjarī and Hemalatā clasped the feet of the latter's mother and father, and wept. Loud wails haunted the inside of the royal apartments. So loud was the expression of grief over their parting that no one could hear what anyone else said after that. They consoled Hemalatā's mother and father with appropriate words and then, on the auspicious thirteenth of the lunar cycle, they undertook their journey. The king supplied them with horses and elephants and treasures of great value, including rubies and other gems and a retinue of male and female attendants. Madanamañjarī, Hemalatā, and Candrasena mounted the elephants.

The procession started for Vijayanagara. They passed by hundreds of petty kingdoms. When Madanamañjarī recognized the kingdom of her father and mother, she spoke to Candrasena, her hands folded in respect.

"Behold the kingdom of my father, son of his minister. Look on the land of your birth." Uttering these words the two bowed deeply. Right before them stood Madanagaḍa, the residence of the minister. And in this fashion did the elephant procession continue.

Locals inquired of them, "Where are you coming from and where are you going? Tell us, please! Who are you and why are you traveling with two wives?"

There on the third floor of the mansion before them, attended by her servants, the wife of the minister sat. The breeze was light and she was enjoying an afternoon repast. Her gaze settled on the two women perched on the elephant. Their complexions and physical charms were those of the golden *campaka* magnolia. And the handsome man with whom they were riding shone in the way the full moon does in a sky filled with bright stars.

"Go quickly, maid," she ordered, "and find out from him who he is, who his father is, and where and when they will visit!"

The maidservant listened to her charge and then departed in haste to the place Madanamañjarī had just reached. The attendant did not recognize the son of the minister, but found herself staring at Madanamañjarī in vague recognition. She was unable to place her directly, for countless days had passed. But she pondered it, bothered by the familiarity. Then it occurred to the maidservant. "I would guess that this princess is Madanamañjarī, the daughter of our own king. And other suspicions are beginning to take shape regarding who these two other people with her really are. I must ask if this is indeed the case." Having reached her conclusion, the maidservant went up to the young woman.

With her hands gesturing respect, she asked, "Tell me truthfully, just exactly whose daughter are you? I seem to recognize you, but I am reluctant to speak out. Yet the princess of our king had exactly the same beauty that you possess. . . ."

Then Madanamañjarī smiled and spoke.

"My father's name is Vinoda Vihārī. This is the son of the minister, whom you carried at the time of his rice-eating ceremony when he was six months old. This other lovely woman is his second wife. And look at the young boy, their son. The Fates have at last brought us back to our homeland. I will honor the feet of my mother- and father-in-law with great joy."

When she heard this, the maidservant rushed inside to report to the minister. "After many long days your son has finally returned! Candrasena has come to see you, bringing his two wives and son. Please go and greet them, O greatest of ministers."

Hearing this, Dharmadhvaja nearly burst with joy. He and his wife rushed out to bring in their lost son. Madanamañjarī watched and pointed them out to her husband. "Look, there are your mother and father, and this is your home."

There the four of them dismounted the elephants. Candrasena came forward, making obeisance at the feet of the minister. He likewise made obeisance to his mother, and then presented his two wives, and his son, whom he carried snuggled against his own chest.

The minister led Candrasena inside to his former apartments. Many of the town's residents rushed out to greet them. When the invocations and formal introductions were properly completed, the minister's household simply swelled with pure joy.

When the king and queen heard, they rushed out to the house of the minister, tears in their eyes. "Where is my daughter, Madanamañjarī?"

Joyous, the king entered the house of his chief minister. The daughter Madanamañjarī, accompanied by Candrasena, bowed at the feet of the king. The great wielder of the staff of justice blessed Candrasena, while his wife, Citrāṅginī, hugged Madanamañjarī.

The king then sat in an impromptu court in his minister's house, whereupon he questioned them about their general weal.

Meditating on his holy feet, Gayārāma composed this new song in praise of the Pīr.

Madanamañjarī pressed her hands together and told her pathetic tale. "Listen, Mother, listen, Father, you who gave me life. My story is one of suffering. To escape public humiliation I slipped away from the bridal chamber carrying my husband with me. During the second watch of the night I followed the back lanes and left my home and emotions behind. Whenever this tiny son of the minister would cry, my heart nearly broke from the pain. I would scour the town begging cow's milk to feed him. I wore the clothes of an indigent woman and roamed aimlessly from place to place. Mean people spoke poorly of me. Here and there I traveled, until I entered the land of King Magendra, where it all came to end.

"I wasted no time and went straight to His Majesty the king and claimed him as my godfather. I made a request of the king, that he construct a house for me, which, when he heard it, pleased him. South of the fort, the king had raised for me a lovely little house. Right after that, however, Lord Nārāyaṇa granted me a vision of himself as the Apostle and the Prophet, the *paigambar*, Satya Pīr. By the power of his mercy, a wondrous mansion was conjured in a single night, and in that house we lived. There I struggled to raise the minister's son.

"After five years, I sent this young minister's son to school to be formally educated. For many long days he studied assiduously, his pursuit of knowledge lasting until he passed his twelfth year.

"One day he came home and sat outside all alone in the courtyard. I saw that he was troubled and I ran out quickly and looked at him directly. He spoke to me and questioned me about the details of our lives from the remote past to the present day. Then I narrated everything that had transpired. When he heard, he was pleased at heart.

"The two of us were then properly joined together at last, consecrating our vows. We lived soaked in the pleasures of young love.

"One day Candrasena went on an ill-fated trip to the local bazaar. A garland weaver, Raṅginī Mālinī, lived there by herself. Listen carefully to her sordid tale. Through the secrets of herbal magic, she gave him a charmed garland, which transformed him into a parrot, a popinjay.

"Although I am but a woman, I went out by myself and searched for him, here, there, and everywhere. The sky had fallen on my head. I got no leads whatsoever. I became mad and desired only to end my miserable life. But the Helmsman of Heaven showed mercy to me and spoke to me, out of the blue. 'Listen to what I say, my princess. To what end do you abandon your life? Not long from now you will recover your husband. I would never mislead you!'

"I listened to his revelation and preserved my feeble life, but suffered there a living death. Meanwhile, Mālinī had taken Candrasena, that jewel of virtue, and given him to Hemalatā. Blessed in beauty and fine qualities, this princess managed to turn him back into a man. By now the minister's son had forgotten all about me thanks to the magical charms of the princess.

"When it was confirmed that Hemalatā was five months pregnant, the king wanted to slay the culprit responsible. Pīr Bhagavān was filled with compassion, so he caused the king to relent. The king then gave his daughter in marriage to Candrasena.

"Now I have come back to my ancestral land, bringing my husband and his son. No other woman has suffered the way I have suffered. How can I describe the depths of my suffering, which only God understands?"

All who heard this admission were stunned. Both the king and queen wept openly. As he wept, the minister spoke: "There is no woman like this in the greater cosmos!"

Gayārāma narrates this tale at the feet of the Pīr, seeking the nectar therein.

The retainers, courtiers, and other court functionaries were stunned to hear what came from the mouth of Madanamañjarī. All praised her, "Blessed, blessed are you, Madanamañjarī. You honor the king's lineage as a *pativratā*, a wife truly devoted to her husband." And in these and other ways everyone expressed his pleasure.

The king then resumed the discussion there in the minister's house. "My daughter and your son—two lost treasures now recovered here in your place. Let us perform the worship of Satya Pīr and rejoice. Send my manservant to the bazaar. We will worship Lord Satya Nārāyaṇa by waving lights. Issue the invitations and bring your friends."

Hearing this royal command thrilled the minister. Then he sent for the artisans. He measured out and provided them with one hundred maunds of gold. The artisans then set to work constructing the ritual abode to house the Pīr. Goldsmiths measured, etched, and inscribed the surface, while blacksmiths efficiently cast the base structure.

All friends and acquaintances accepted the invitation with joyful anticipation. The manservant quickly purchased and organized all the necessary items: mango, jambu, plaintain, pomegranate, coconut, guava, almond, papaya, wood apple, ripe banana, pomelo, date, pineapple, watermelon, muskmelon. Only the finest were brought. Sugary sweets in large quantities—*michari*, *sandeśa*, *bātāsā*, crystallized sugar—and curd, milk, and soured cream were brought and stored. The flower vendors provided untold types of flowers: star-, white-, and multipetaled jasmines, and china roses by the hundreds.

All the guests were brought in and greeted together as a party. In a lighthearted mood, the king personally seated his subjects. The brahmins then performed the worship, the *pūjā,* of Satya Nārāyaṇa. The king and his chief minister sat prominently by, with hands pressed together in respect. Bells clanged, horns blared, and *dundubi* drums thumped. All the women blew conchs and loudly projected the auspicious *hulāhuli* trill. At the completion of the *pūjā*, everyone fell prostrate, fully stretched out in obeisance. The *prasāda* from the *pūjā*—the leftover food offering that becomes ingestible grace—was distributed to everyone present.

Whoever sings of and whoever listens to the Pīr's glory will have all desires fulfilled; wealth, sons, and good fortune will all increase. May everyone let fly the sound of "Hari" and be thrilled.

Gayārāma thus concludes his song of praise. With the feet of Satya Nārāyaṇa filling your minds, repeat the name, "Hari, Hari," and everyone will be happy.

NOTES

Preface

1. See Asim Roy, *The Islamic Syncretistic Tradition in Bengal* (Princeton: Princeton University Press, 1983). The most complete statement of my critique of syncretism can be found in Tony K. Stewart, "In Search of Equivalence: Conceiving Muslim-Hindu Encounter through Translation Theory," *History of Religions* 40, no. 3 (Winter 2001): 261–88. For an alternate way of conceptualizing the works of this literature, see Stewart, "Alternate Structures of Authority: Satya Pīr on the Frontiers of Bengal," in *Beyond Turk and Hindu: Rethinking Religious Identities in Islamicate South Asia*, edited by David Gilmartin and Bruce B. Lawrence (Gainesville: University of Florida Press, 2000), 21–54.

Introduction

1. See Kirin Narayan, *Storytellers, Saints, and Scoundrels: Folk Narrative in Hindu Religious Teachings* (Philadelphia: University of Pennsylvania Press, 1989), which conveys the richness and complexity of these interactions (focusing here on religious instruction), and her more recent *Mondays on the Dark Night of the Moon: Himalayan Foothill Folktales*, in collaboration with Urmila Devi Sood (Oxford: Oxford University Press, 1997), which reconstructs storytelling sessions.

2. Margaret Mills, *Rhetorics and Politics in Afghan Traditional Storytelling* (Philadelphia: University of Pennsylvania Press, 1991).

3. Joyce Burkhalter Flueckiger, *Gender and Genre in the Folklore of Middle India* (Ithaca: Cornell University Press, 1996).

4. It is no longer necessary to expound on the dangers of reading a contemporary or near-contemporary observation (such as the old woman's story that began this essay) into historical reconstructions, for this has been another borrowed plank of the critique of Orientalism. Without rehashing what has now become an all-too-predictable critique with its own excesses of essentializing and unsupported generalizations, it is still useful to survey the full range of arguments as they apply specifically to South Asia; see Ronald B. Inden, *Imagining India* (Oxford: Basil Blackwell, 1990). A distinction should be maintained, however, between historical narrative as argued by Hayden White, and the cultural narratives that operate within the object of study. See especially Hayden White's *Metahistory: The Historical Imagination in Nineteenth-Century Europe* (Baltimore: Johns Hopkins University Press, 1973); *Tropics of Discourse: Essays in Cultural Criticism* (Baltimore: Johns Hopkins University Press, 1978); and *The Content of the Form: Narrative Discourse and Historical Representation* (Baltimore: John Hopkins University Press, 1987).

5. I am indebted to Jonathan Culler's early attempt to formalize what these constraints might be, where to draw the line in reconstructing the discursive space. He isolates logical presuppositions (rules of argument and discourse), pragmatic presuppositions (genre and

other conventions), direct intertextual citation (literary environment), and implied or assumed intertextuality (culturally current but inexplicit textual reference); see Jonathan Culler, "Presupposition and Intertextuality," *Modern Language Notes* 91 (1976): 1380–96.

6. Tony K. Stewart and Edward C. Dimock, Jr., "Kṛttibāsa's Apophatic Critique of Rāma's Kingship," in *Questioning Rāmāyaṇas*, edited by Paula Richman (New Delhi: Oxford University Press, 2000, 243–64; reissued Berkeley: University of California Press, 2001).

7. Saiyad Sultān, "Nabī Vaṃśa" in *Rasul Carita*, edited by Āhmad Śarīph, 2 vols. (Dhaka: Bāṃlā Ekādemī, 1385 BS [1978]).

8. These include poems to Manasā, Caṇḍī, Śītalā, Ṣaṣṭhī, Gaṅgā, Sāradā, and others. For the most comprehensive historical study and recapitulation of stories, see Āśutoṣa Bhaṭṭācārya, *Bāṃlā maṅgalakāvya itihāsa* (Kolkata: E. Mukhārjī1975).

9. Āhmad Śarīph, ed. and comp., *Bāṅlāra sūphī sāhitya: ālocanā o nayakhāni grantha sambalita* (Dhaka: Bāṃlā Ekāḍemī, 1375 BS [1968]).

10. Kavi Āriph (Arif), *Lālamonera kāhini*, edited by Girīndranātha Dāsa (Gokulapur, 24 Parganas: Śrīmati Karuṇāmayī Dāsa, 1984). Two earlier versions were identical save occasional typos; see Kavi Āriph, *Lālamonera kecchā* (Kolkata: Sudhānidhi Yantra, 1274 BS [1867]); and *Lālamonera kecchā* (Kolkata: Viśvambhara Lāha, 1276 BS [1869]). For an extensive analysis of this tale, see Tony K. Stewart, "Surprising Bedfellows: Vaiṣṇava and Shi'i Alliance in Kavi Āripha's 'Tale of Lālamon'," *International Journal of Hindu Studies* 3, no. 3 (1999): 265–98 (reissued New York: Lexington Press of Rowan and Littlefield, forthcoming).

11. Of the many myths of women favored by her retellings, it is perhaps the story of Ahalyā that is most representative of this strain, but there are others. For instance, see Wendy Doniger O'Flaherty, *Women, Androgynes, and Other Mythical Beasts* (Chicago: University of Chicago Press, 1980); *Splitting the Difference: Gender and Myth in Ancient Greece and India* (Chicago: University of Chicago Press, 1999); and *The Bed Trick: Tales of Sex and Masquerade* (Chicago: University of Chicago Press, 2000).

12. *The Ocean of Story* (Somadeva's *Kathāsaritsāgara*), translated by C. H. Tawney, edited with introduction and notes by N. M. Penzer, 10 vols. (1924, reprint Delhi: Motilal Banarsidass, 1968).

13. For a translation of the main story, see Edward C. Dimock, trans., "The *Manasā Maṅgal* of Ketakā-Dāsa: Behulā and Lakhindar," in *The Thief of Love: Bengali Tales from Court and Village* (Chicago: University of Chicago Press, 1963), 195–294. For comprehensive analysis of the many versions of the tale, see W. L. Smith, *The One-Eyed Goddess: A Study of the Manasā Maṅgal*, Acta Universitatis Stockholmiensis 12 (Stockholm: Almqvist and Wiksell International, 1980), and his earlier *The Myth of Manasā: A Study in the Popular Hinduism of Medieval Bengal* (n.p.: the author, 1976). See also the historical analysis by Pradyot Kumar Maity, *Historical Studies in the Cult of the Goddess Manasā* (Calcutta: Punthi Pustak, 1966).

14. Kiṅkara Dāsa, *Rambhāvatī pālā: satyanārāyaṇa pāñcālī*, 4th ed. (Khātai, Midnapur: Madhusūdana Jānā at Nihar Press, 1331 BS [1924]).

15. Gayārāma Dāsa, *Madanamañjari pālā: satyanārāyaṇa pāñcālī* (Khātai, Midnapur: Madhusūdana Jānā at Nihar Press, 1334 BS [1927]).

16. D. C. Sen was the first to attempt a survey and classification of folk literature, although his categories are not altogether clear and he depended on idealized standards of purity that today seem strained at best. He does, however, make important distinctions between fairy tales (*rūpa-kathā*), humorous tales (*kautuka-kathā*), stories of deities (*vrata-kathā*), and narratives interspersed with songs (*gīta-kathā*). See Dinesh Chandra Sen, *The Folk-Literature of Bengal*, with a foreword by W. R. Gourlay (Calcutta: University of Calcutta, 1920).

17. Bruno Bettelheim, *The Uses of Enchantment: The Meaning and Importance of Fairy Tales* (New York: Vintage [Random House], 1988).

18. The earliest edition of *Ṭhākurmār Jhuli* that I have seen dates to 1907, which appears to be the first edition. These and his other tales have been reprinted too many times to enumerate, but are most recently collected in Dakṣinārañjana Mitra Majumdār, *Dakṣiṇārañjana racanāsamagra*, 2 vols. (Kolkata: Mitra o Ghoṣa, 1406 BS [1999]. The preface lists twenty different editions published between 1902 and 1948.

19. Lal Behari Day, *Folk-Tales of Bengal*, illustrated by Warwick Goble (London: Macmillan, 1912 [first ed. 1883]), 61–88, 211–16.

20. F. B. Bradley-Birt, *Bengal Fairy Tales*, with illustrations by Abanindranath Tagore (London: John Lane, Bodley Head, and New York: John Lane, 1920), 179–85.

21. Dvīja Kavibara, *Bāghāmbarer pālā: satyanārāyaṇa pāñcālī*, 10th ed. (Khātai, Midnapur: Nihar Press, 1322 BS [1915]).

22. Kabir Chowdhury, *Folktales of Bangladesh*, vol. 1 (Dacca: Bangla Academy, 1972), 114–24.

23. Kiṅkara Dāsa, *Śaśīdhara pālā: satyanārāyaṇa pāñcālī* (Khātai, Midnapur: Madhusūdana Jānā at Nihar Press, 1322 BS [1915]).

24. See Stith Thompson, *Motif-Index of Folk Literature*, 6 vols. (Bloomington: Indiana University Press, 1955–58). See also Stith Thompson and Jonas Balys, *The Oral Tales of India* (Bloomington: Indiana University Press, 1958), and Stith Thompson and Warren E. Roberts, *Types of Indic Oral Tales: India, Pakistan, and Ceylon*, Folklore Fellows Communications no. 180 (Helsinki: Academia Scientiarium Fennica, 1960).

25. Vladimir Propp, *The Morphology of the Folktale*, translated by Laurence Scott, with an introduction by Svatava Pirkova-Jakobson (Austin: University of Texas Press, 1968).

26. See Frances W. Pritchett, *Marvelous Encounters: Folk Romance in Urdu and Hindi* (New Delhi: Manohar, 1985). The *qissa/qiṣṣah* is paired with the genre of *dāstān*, the distinctions of which can be found in chapter one of Marvelous Encounters, and in Pritchett, *The Romance Tradition in Urdu: Adventures from the Dāstān of Amīr Ḥamzah* (New York: Columbia University Press, 1991), 13–15. No similar studies or translations have to my knowledge been undertaken for the analogous Bangla genres.

27. According to Genette's scheme, this frame would technically qualify as peritext since it is folded into and around the narrative (along with titles, epigraphs, etc., many of which find their way into the printed versions of these tales). See Gerard Genette, *Paratexts: Thresholds of Interpretation*, translated by James E. Lewin (Cambridge: Cambridge University Press, 1977).

28. Todorov makes a distinction between the "fantastic," the "uncanny," and the "marvelous," all of which hinge on expectations (or lack of expectations) of one's acceptance of the violation of an agreed-upon and scientifically verifiable "natural world," which is not of particular concern in the literature at hand. For this reason I have chosen "fabulous" as a more value-free term. See Tzvetan Todorov, *The Fantastic: A Structural Approach to a Literary Genre*, translated by Richard Howard, with a foreword by Robert Scholes (Ithaca: Cornell University Press, 1975).

29. In a study of gender in the sixteenth-century *Caṇḍīmaṅgala* of Mukundrāma, a Bangla text that shares many features of plot and character with the current set of tales, David Curley has argued that gender "roles" are not roles but scalar forms (following Inden following Collingwood) based on transactional relations that overlap depending on context. Many types of activities are shared by men and women, with the lead character (masculine) symbolically assuming activities that dominate the subordinate characters (feminine). Masculine and fem-

inine forms then are determined by who is dominant rather than by gender per se. This approach helps to explain how heroines such as Lālmon can put on armor and fight, and even take a "wife." See David L. Curley, "Marriage, Honor, Agency, and Trials by Ordeal: Women's Gender Roles in *Caṇḍīmaṅgal*," *Modern Asian Studies* 35, no. 2 (2001): 315–48.

30. Judith Butler, *Gender Trouble: Feminism and the Subversion of Identity* (New York : Routledge, 1999), especially 60–71, 171–77.

31. The implications of the census were seen most palpably in the creation of separate electorates and separate domestic law for Muslims and Hindus, but there were other implications. See Kennth W. Jones, "Religious Identity and the Indian Census," in *The Census in British India: New Perspectives*, edited by N. Gerald Barrier (Delhi: Manohar, 1991), 73–101; and Barnard S. Cohn, "The Census, Social Structure and Objectification in South Asia," in *An Anthropologist among the Historians and Other Essays* (Delhi: Oxford University Press, 1990), 224–54.

32. Kinkara Dāsa, *Matilāla pālā: satyanārāyaṇa pāñcālī* (Kā̃hai: Madhusūdana Jānā at Nihar Press, 1322 BS [1915)]), 1. The story is translated below as "The Mother's Son Who Spat up Pearls."

33. For more on *vratas* see Tony K. Stewart, "The Goddess Ṣaṣṭhī Protects Children," in *The Religions of India in Practice*, edited by Donald S. Lopez, Jr. (Princeton: Princeton University Press, 1995), 352–66. See also Sudhir Ranjan Das, *Folk Religion in Bengal: A Study of Vrata Rites* (Calcutta: S. C. Kar, 1953); and Eva Maria Gupta, *Brata und Ālpanā in Bengalen*, Beiträge zur Südasien Institut, Universität Heidelberg 80 (Wiesbaden: Franz Steiner, 1983).

34. By the late nineteenth century, the worship was subject to elaboration in a manner akin to well-known processes of Sanskritization, and by the mid to late twentieth century, the simple offering of *śirṇi* required multiple priests and elaborate instructions, evidence of its incorporation into mainstream traditions, in this case Hindu. For instance, a publication that first appeared in 1898–99, the *Satyanārāyaṇa o śubhacaranīra kathā*, edited by Śyāmācaraṇa Kaviratna, 2d ed. (Kolkata: the editor through Gurudāsa Caṭṭopādhyāya at Bengal Medical Library, 1315 BS [1908]) gives seven pages of detailed instruction for making and offering *śirṇi*, which is made up of some twenty-eight ingredients. In the same year another small publication, the *Satyanārāyaṇa vratakathā*, edited with Bengali translation by Rāsavihārisāṃkhyatīrtha (Murshidabad: Rāmadeva Miśra for Haribhaktipradayinīsabhā of Baharamapura at Rādhāramaṇa Press, 1315 BS [1908]) provides twelve pages of instructions. A decade later, Rāmagopāla Rāya's edition of *Satyamaṅgala bā satyanārāyaṇa devera vratakathā o pūjāpaddhati* (Kolkata: Jayakṛṣṇa Caudhurī, 1835 Śaka [1913]) includes twenty-two pages of instruction.

35. Carl Ernst distinguishes between the historical *malfuẓat*, composed by a disciple and believed to contain the authentic words of the master, and the later hagiographies that eulogize but do not carry the same force of authority. See Carl W. Ernst, *Eternal Gardens: Mysticism, History, and Politics at a South Asian Sufi Center* (Albany: State University of New York Press, 1992), 62–84. For more on the distinction between *malfuẓat and taẓkirah* genres of Sufi hagiography, see Bruce B. Lawrence, *Notes from a Distant Flute: Sufi Literature in Pre-Mughal India* (Tehran: Imperial Iranian Academy of Philosophy, 1978). It is not clear how a mythical *pīr* such as Satya Pīr would fit into this scheme. For the best survey of the Bengali *pīr* literature and the relationship of mythical to historical figures, see Girīndranātha Dāsa, *Bāṃla pīr sāhityera kathā*, 2d ed. (Kolkata: Suvarṇarekha, 1998).

36. Kṛṣṇahari Dāsa, *Baḍa satya pīr o sandhyāvatī kaṇyāra punthi* (Kolkata: Nurūddin Ahmād at Gāosiya Lāibreri, n.d.). I am indebted to Professor A.K.M. Zachariah of Dhaka, who allowed me to copy from his private library the only known manuscript of this book and the source of the printed edition.

37. Śaṅkarācārya and Rāmeśvara, *Śrīśrīsatyanārāyaṇera pāñcālī: līlāvatī kalāvatī daridra brāhmaṇera upākhyāna* (Kolkata: Tārācāñda Dāsa and Sons, n.d.); Śaṅkarācārya and Rāmeśvara, *Śrīśrīsatyanārāyaṇera pāñcālī: līlāvatī kalāvatī daridra brāhmaṇera upākhyāna (pūjādravya pūjāvidhi, dhyāna o praṇāma sambalita)*, compiled and edited by Avināśacandra Mukhopādhyāya, revised by Surendranātha Bhaṭṭācārya, 3d ed. (Calcutta: Calcutta Town Library by Kārttika Candra Dhara, 1360 BS [1953]); and Śaṅkarācārya and Rāmeśvara, *Śrīśrīsatyanārāyaṇera pāñcālī: līlāvatī kalāvatī daridra brāhmaṇera kāhinī (pūjādravādi o pūjāvidhi sambalita)*, edited by Gaurāṅgasundara Bhaṭṭācārya (Kolkata: Rajendra Library, n.d.). A sample of the cycle can be found translated by the current author; see Tony K. Stewart, "Satya Pīr: Muslim Holy Man or Hindu God," in Lopez, ed., *Religions of India in Practice*, 578–97. For more on the strategy of accommodation and the divisions of literature, see Tony K. Stewart, "Alternate Structures of Authority: Satya Pīr on the Frontiers of Bengal," in *Beyond Turk and Hindu: Rethinking Religious Identities in Islamicate South Asia*, edited by David Gilmartin and Bruce B. Lawrence (Gainesville: University of Florida Press, 2000), 21–54.

38. Farina Mir has argued persuasively that the *qissa* literature in the Punjab functions in much the same way, creating a space for moral and social order that is not sectarian first. See Farina Mir, "The Social Space of Language: Punjabi Popular Narratives in Colonial India, c. 1850–1900" (Ph.D. dissertation, Columbia University, 2002).

39. Perhaps the most striking example is Lālā Jayanārāyaṇa Sena, *Harilīlā*, edited by Dīneśacandra Sena and Basantarañjana Rāya (Calcutta: Calcutta University, 1928).

40. One of the most interesting versions of this tale can be found in the previously noted work (*supra* n. 34), edited by Rāsavihārisāṃkhyatīrtha, who refers to its as the *Tuṅgadhvaja gopa saṃvāda*; see also the *Satyanārāyaṇa vratakathā*, compiled by Meghanātha Bhaṭṭācārya (Kolkata: Saṃskṛta Press Depository, 1306 BS [1899]), who calls it the *Vaṃśadhvaja gopa saṃvada*.

41. Gayārāma, *Madanamañjari pālā*, translated below as "The Unwilting Garland of Faithfulness."

42. Pierre Macherey, *A Theory of Literary Production*, translated by Geoffrey Wall (London: Routledge, 1978), 44.

43. Ibid., 45.

44. Ibid., 59.

45. D. C. Sen provides an entertaining synopsis of the story by Wazed Ali; see his *The Folk-Literature of Bengal*, 103–13.

46. Kavivallabha, *Satyanārāyaṇa puthi*, edited by Munsī Abdul Karim, Sāhitya Pariṣad Granthāvalī no. 49 (Kolkata: Baṅgīya Sāhitya Pariṣat by Rāmakamala Siṃha, 1322 BS [1913]).

47. Munśī Oyājed (Wazed) Āli Sāheb, *Satya pīrer pūthi: madana sundara pālā* (Dhaka: Mohāmmad Solemān, n.d.).

48. Karṇa, *Madana sundara pālā* (Cuttuck: H. M. Dutta at Dutta Press, n.d.). The same tale somewhat emended with paraphrase translation can be found in *Pālās of Śrī Kavi Karṇa*, edited and translated by Bishnupada Panda, Kalāmūlaśāstra Series, vols. 4–7 (New Delhi: Indira Gandhi National Centre for the Arts and Motilal Banarsidass, 1991), 4:144–233.

49. Karṇa, *Madana sundara pālā*, 1–2; Panda, *Pālās of Śrī Kavi Karṇa*, 4:144–46.

50. Munśī Oyājed (Wazed) Āli Sāheb, *Satya pīrer pūthi: madana sundara pālā*, 1.

51. Anonymous, *Manohara phāsarāra pālā: satyanārāyaṇa pāñcālī*, 10th ed. (Kāthai, Midnapur: Nihar Press, 1313 BS [1906]), translated here as "The Erstwhile Bride and Her Flying Horse." This text is essentially the same as Rasamaya, *Galakāṭā phāsyarāra pālā*, Bengali manuscript no. 214, Dhaka University Library (17 folios; complete; dated 1264 BS [1857]).

52. The translation here follows the sole mansucript of the text written by Kavi Kaṇva [=Karṇa]; *Satyanārāyaṇa kathā* of Kavi Kaṇva, Bengali manuscript no. 59b, Dhaka University Library (14 folios, complete, dated 1273 BS [1866]). Bishnupada Panda worked from the same manuscript, but with considerable disagreement in readings; see *Kavikarṇera pālā*, 4:2–93. The well-known poet Rāmeśvara also produced a version of the text that is essentially the same story with only relatively minor digressions; see Rāmeśvara, *Ākhoṭi pālā: Satyanārāyaṇa pañcālī*, 3d ed. (Khātāi, Midnapur: Madhusūdana Jānā at Nihar Press, 1924), and the more critically edited version titled "Ākhoṭi pālā" in *Rāmeśvara racanāvalī*, edited by Pañcānana Cakravartī (Kolkata: Baṅgīya Sāhitya Pariṣat, 536–49).

The Wazir's Daughter Who Married a Sacrificial Goat

This tale is translated from two early versions that are identical save occasional typos; see Kavi Āriph (Arif), *Lālamonera kecchā* (Kolkata: Sudhānidhi Yantra, 1274 BS [1867]); and *Lālamonera kecchā* (Kolkata: Viśvambhara Lāha, 1276 BS [1869]). A more recent edition, with no significant changes, has appeared as Kavi Āriph (Arif), *Lālamonera kāhini*, edited by Girīndranātha Dāsa (Gokulapura, 24 Parganas: Śrīmati Karuṇāmayī Dāsa, 1984).

1. The *Bismillah* is an invocation to God to oversee whatever task is being undertaken, and is always recited at the beginning of any kind of work or undertaking; it appears prominently appears at the opening of every chapter of the Qur'ān save the 9th: *Bismillah al-Raḥmān al-Raḥim*, which translates as "In the name of the merciful Lord of Mercy."

2. Eating betel is an act of intimacy between those who have shared a nuptial bed or its equivalent in romantic assignation.

3. Games of dice are played with very high stakes on the wedding night, in a "winner-take-all" competition designed to heighten the anticipation of love play and of course to break the ice. The obvious meaning of having taken her chance with him also holds.

The Unwilting Garland of Faithfulness

This tale was translated from Kiṅkara Dāsa, *Rambhāvatī pālā: satyanārāyaṇa pāñcālī*, 4th ed. (Khātai, Midnapur: Madhusūdana Jānā at Nihar Press, 1331 BS [1924]).

1. Sītā, Rāmā's wife, is the Indic epitome of wifely virtue, having retained her honor when captured by the demonic Rāvaṇa. Mandodarī, Rāvaṇa's wife, turned to Rāvana's brother, Vibhīṣaṇa, for aid after the capture of Sītā. Known for his sense of righteousness, Vibhīṣaṇa alone counseled Rāvaṇa to return Sītā; eventually Vibhīṣaṇa changed allegiance to Rāma.

2. *Kāhana* or *kāhaṇa* is an old measure worth 16 *paṇa*s or 1280 cowries, a measure difficult to estimate now except that it was a princely sum for food and would have provided a feast for large numbers.

3. The "eye of silver" was to "bring the boat to life" so that it would be dedicated to the men it carried; a bimini is a canopy stretched across the cockpit to provide shelter from the sun.

4. Apart from the obvious comparison of Rāmbhāvatī to her servant, it is a common expression to say that someone eats whey when they have been put to shame.

5. The *bimba* fruit is a brilliant red-orange cucurbit of the gourd family.

6. Symbolically, the wife would be seated on the left, so she has tricked him, as will become apparent.

7. A maund is currently one hundred pounds troy weight or 82.20 pounds avoirdupois; but it is also a traditional unit of measure that would fill a large basket called a maund.

The Fabled *Beṅgamā* Bird and the Stupid Prince

The translation here follows the sole mansucript of the text written by Kavi Kaṇva [=Karṇa]; *Satyanārāyaṇa kathā* of Kavi Kaṇva, Bengali manuscript no. 59b, Dhaka University Library (14 folios, complete, dated 1273 BS [1866]). Bishnupada Panda worked from the same manuscript, but with considerable disagreement in readings; see *Kavikarṇera pālā*, 4:2–93. The well-known poet Rāmeśvara also produced a version of the text that is essentially the same story with only relatively minor digressions; see Rāmeśvara, *Ākhoṭi pālā: satyanārāyaṇa pañcālī*, 3d ed. (Khātāi, Midnapur: Madhusūdana Jānā at Nihar Press, 1331 BS [1924]) and the more critically edited version titled *Ākhoṭi pālā* in *Rāmeśvara racanāvalī*, edited by Pañcānana Cakravartī (Kolkata: Baṅgīya Sāhitya Pariṣat, 1371 BS [1964), 536–49.

1. Viṣṇu disguised himself as a dwarf and then asked the arrogant King Bali for the boon of all the land he could cover in three steps. Against the advice of his minister, Bali granted the boon, whereupon Viṣṇu assumed his cosmic form and covered the three regions of the universe.

2. The text here reads "banyan," but the word is often generic for "big tree"; later the author identifies the tree as an *aśoka*, a more precise designation.

3. The *beṅgamā*, alternate *behaṅgamā*, is a fabled bird that, in addition to being able to speak with a human voice, is often credited with being able to tell the future, such that what it says comes to pass—a handy oracle indeed. It is likewise believed to carry a precious gem embedded in its head or throat.

4. *Pakṣirāja* means "king" (*rājā*) of "birds" (*pakṣi*, literally "winged ones"), but it also refers to winged horses, and that suggests something of the size of this particular bird. A secondary epithet equates *pakṣirāja* with Viṣṇu's gigantic bird-mount Garuḍa. In the story of "The Erstwhile Bride and Her Winged Horse," *pakṣirāja* is in fact a winged horse.

5. This and the other episodes of Kṛṣṇa to which the the author, Kavi Kaṇva, routinely alludes can be found in the *Bhāgavata Purāṇa*, unless otherwise noted. The most well-known will not be cited. There are likewise numerous general references to Rāma and his companions in the *Rāmāyaṇa* epic, which will not be noted unless the passage would otherwise remain obscure.

6. It would appear that one or two couplets have dropped out of the manuscript at this point, otherwise Takṣaka would be bribing the *muni* who levied the curse not to see it undone. The story stages a test between the two, with Takṣaka destroying a massive tree with his poison and Kaśyapa easily restoring it to its pristine form. Then he bargains with him. The tale is from the *Devī Bhāgavata*, *skandhas* 9–12. An earlier version in the *Mahābhārata*, *ādi parva*, chapter 20, and *Bhāgavata Purāṇa*, *skandha* 2, names the brahmin Kaśyapa in place of Dhanvantari.

7. The manuscript is only partially decipherable for the first verse of this couplet, but the gist is clear enough.

8. Uṣā was provoked to this lustful act after witnessing Śiva and Pārvatī making love, and wishing for the same. Pārvatī advised her to watch her dreams, and within three days she would see the man she could captivate. Her companion, Citralekhā, drew pictures of famous princes and kings until she landed on Aniruddha, and Uṣā reached for the picture. Citralekhā then conjured Aniruddha while he was asleep by means of a powerful *mantra*. It was shortly after the great commotion of his arrival that King Bāṇa imprisoned him in the snake ropes. The story is from *Bhāgavata Purāṇa, skandha* 10, chapters 61–63.

9. The scribe appears to have dropped one or two couplets here.

10. Baka had assumed the form of a giant bird, and lay in the road with his beak open.

Kṛṣṇa innocently entered the bird's stomach, and then in a whirlwind ripped up his stomach, causing the bird to vomit out Kṛṣṇa along with his own guts.

11. Brahmā kept the stolen cows—and the cowherd boys—for a year, but when he returned to the banks of the river, he discovered all the cowherd boys and their herds as usual. Then they began to transform into the miraculous image of the celestial Nārāyaṇa, which humbled Brahmā, who, scared, returned the cows and boys.

12. Vṛndāvana, Kṛṣṇa's childhood home in north central India, not far from the city of Agra, is about eight hundred miles from the setting of this story.

13. Among Vaiṣṇavas in Bengal, the traditional signs of true devotion are called the *sāttvika bhāvas*, and include fainting, shaking, sweating, crawling gooseflesh, shouting, rolling on the ground, and torpor. The signs are very similar to those of epilepsy.

14. In a conflict with his father, Hiraṇyakaśipu, over the worship of Viṣṇu, Prahlāda endured endless tortures, including serpent bites, trampling by wild elephants, having spikes rammed through his body, being buried under a mountain, and being thrown into the bottom of the sea. In the end, Viṣṇu descends as the *avatāra* Narasiṃha, half-man and half-lion, to slay Hiraṇya. This popular story is found in the *Bhagavata Purāṇa, skandha* 7 and the *Viṣṇu Purāṇa, aṃśa* 1, chapter 20, with references in the *Vāmana Purāṇa* and *Agni Purāṇa.*

15. Dhruva was the son of Utthānapāda's second wife, Suniti; when he was a child, he was denied the opportunity to sit in his father's lap because he was not first in line. After being insulted by the first wife, Suruci, Dhruva vowed to exceed his father's position based on his own accomplishments, and retreated to the forest to meditate. His great meditation resulted not only in a personal visit by Mahāviṣṇu but also in the attainment of great powers, and eventually ruline over the kingdom of his father; see *Viṣṇu Purāṇa, amśa* 1, chapters 11–12. Dhruva attained a permanent place in the heavens, where he sits in eternal meditation in the Viṣṇupāda, the highest point of heaven, where the Gaṅgā flows into the mundane egg; today that place is called Dhruvamaṇḍala; see *Devī Bhāgavata, skandha* 8.

16. According to the *Mahābhārata, ādi parva* 29–34, Garuḍa was incensed that his mother, Vinatā, had been enslaved by the *nāgas* in what amounted to a battle of pride with Kadru, mother of a thousand *nāgas.* To secure her release, he agreed to bring the *nāgas* the nectar of immortality from *devaloka*, high in the mountains of the Himalayas, even though the *nāgas* were his mortal enemies. There seems to be an ambiguous message here, because ultimately Garuḍa colluded with Indra to steal the nectar, which allowed Garuḍa to keep his promise in the letter but not the spirit.

17. That the text calls a Hindu Vaiṣṇava a Muslim fakir suggests that the image of the holy man is interchangeable. Vaiṣṇava ascetics are generally called *vairāgīs* or generically *saṃnyāsīs*, and Sufi ascetics *fakirs*. The mixed image parallels that of Satya Pīr himself.

18. This is the name of a mythical mouse in Bengal that is credited with bringing about floods; the mice do this by chewing through the wood of dams, causing them to give way, releasing the waters.

19. This folk tradition is observed to help childless couples have children. Cowries are small shells that serve as cash.

20. Qādir is Bangla *kādir*, meaning a fakir of the Qādirīyah school of al Jilānī in Baghdad.

21. *Rathayātrā* is the term usually reserved for the Car Festival of Jagannātha in the city of Puri in Orissa. The festival falls between mid-June and mid-July at the beginning of the monsoon. Puri is not specifically named. Unlike other tales of Satya Pīr, which give detailed accounts of trading routes that can still be located today, this one is vague about direction and locale. But in this case, the Car Festival appears to be a more local phenomenon, perhaps the king's annual formal tour of the city or the processional of a local deity.

22. This dance is common among Vaiṣṇavas who, in group singing of the stories and names of Kṛṣṇa, will often dance in this unique style. It was, tradition has it, originated by the great god-man Kṛṣṇa Caitanya (1486–1533).

The Disconsolate Yogī Who Turned the Merchant's Wife into a Dog

The translation comes from Dvīja Kavibara, *Bāghāmbarer pālā: satyanārāyaṇa pāñcālī*, 10th ed. (Khātai, Midnapur: Nihar Press, 1322 BS [1915]).

1. "Regiment" is *bāhinī*, which is a traditional unit with 81 elephant riders, 81 charioteers, 243 cavalry, and 405 infantry. These numbers are derived from multiples of primes (so $81 = 3^4$, $243 = 3^5$, $405 = 3^4 \times 5$) and therefore auspicious, perfect, or complementary.

2. Kṛṣṇa Caitanya (1486–1533) was a historical figure believed by his followers to be Kṛṣṇa, and so his departure from his wife, Viṣṇupriyā, at renunciation has always been compared to Kṛṣṇa's abandoning Rādhā when he left for Mathurā.

3. See "The Fabled *Beṅgamā* Bird and the Stupid Prince," note 1.

4. Each of these figures is filled with the arrogance of his own might and eventually destroyed by Nārāyaṇa or Kṛṣṇa and his kin, as told in the Purāṇas and epics.

5. *Jalāñjalī* is the final offering of water after cremation.

6. The *Tantrasāra* is perhaps the best-known *tantrika* digest in Bengal, compiled by the great scholar Kṛṣṇānanda Āgamaviśa.

7. Nimāi is the childhood nickname of Kṛṣṇa Caitanya, mentioned above.

8. Agha, the *asura* brother of Bakāsura and Pūtanā and servant of King Kaṃsa, took the form of a serpent, lay on the road where Kṛṣṇa and the other boys were playing, and opened his mouth like a cave. They entered, and all save Balarāma and Kṛṣṇa were overcome with the noxious fumes of his poisons. The two brothers then expanded their size and went about the business of slaying the *asura*; see *Bhāgavata Purāṇa*, *skandha* 10, chapter12.

9. Kīcaka was born of an *asura* as son of Kekaya, king of the Sūtas. When the Pāṇḍavas were in hiding in Viraṭa kingdom, he attempted to force himself upon Draupadī, wife of the five Pāṇḍavas, who was disguised as a servant girl Mālinī. She was forced into assignation, which she informed Bhīma, who showed up to slay the hapless general; see *Mahābhārata*, *viraṭa parva*. The comparison is a singular admission of guilt on the part of the yogī.

10. King Satrājit possessed the famous gem Syamantaka, and one day his brother Prasena went hunting while wearing the gem. A lion killed Prasena, but Jāmbavān came along and killed the lion. Kṛṣṇa retrieved the gem and returned it to Satrājit, but not without scandal about the means of its procurement.

11. Jarāsandha was the cruel ruler of Magadha. He fought with Kṛṣṇa and Balarāma, but just as he was about to die, a voice intervened from the heavens and proclaimed that now was not the time; he was released. Later Kṛṣṇa, Balarāma, and Bhīma visited the king in disguise, and challenged him to fight one of them; he chose Bhīma, who then killed him; see *Mahābhārata, sabhā parva*.

The Mother's Son Who Spat up Pearls

This tale is translated from Kiṅkara Dāsa, *Matilālera pālā*: *satyanārāyaṇa pāñcālī* (Khātai, Midnapur: Nihar Press, 1322 BS [1915]).

1. One of the literary conceits used to describe the moon with its dark blotches, more commonly noted in Indian letters as the rabbit in the moon.

2. Because Satya Pīr is sitting in Mecca, one might be inclined to envision him surveying

all of the Indian subcontinent or even a larger world, but in fact, as will become clear, he is speaking exclusively of Bengal.

3. Kṛṣṇa Caitanya's mother, Śacī Ṭhākurāṇi, is an object of great sympathy in Bengali literature because of the way her son abandoned her to become an ascetic; her lament is the standard of motherly grief.

4. The eight ornaments (*aṣṭa-ābharaṇa*) include those for a woman's hair, neck, arms and wrists, waist, and ankles; silk saris, luxurious or at least comfortable housing, and fine foods. David Curley indicates that in the text of the *Caṇḍimaṅgala*, arms and wrists are separate, and so the list does not include waist ornaments; see Curley, "Marriage, Honor, Agency, and Trials by Ordeal: Women's Gender Roles in *Caṇḍīmaṅgala*," *Modern Asian Studies* 35, no. 2 (2001): 326–27.

5. Dakṣiṇa (southern) Triveṇī is Bengal's version of the more famous confluence of Yamunā, Gaṅgā, and underground Sarasvatī rivers. In this literature it is variously located in southern Bengal.

6. The *makara* is a fabled water creature that resembles half crocodile and half fish; significantly, here it is the emblem of Kāmadeva, the god of love, and is equated in European astrology to the constellation of Capricorn.

7. A *daṇḍa* is 24 minutes, so between 288 and 312 minutes into the night. It is not clear from the context which form of reckoning time is being used, but clearly this period falls well after midnight.

8. *Gorocanā* is a yellow orpiment produced from the processing of cow's livers, highly prized for ritual.

9. Gaura is the "golden one," Kṛṣṇa Caitanya, who has the coloration and personality of Rādhā; here Nityānanda, his ascetic companion, is likened to Kṛṣṇa.

10. The text here has "brother," which makes no sense.

11. See "The Disconsolate Yogī Who Turned the Merchant's Wife into a Dog," note 2.

12. A *bāṅgāliṇī* literally means a women indigenous to East Bengal, but coming from the pen of someone not from the area the term is derogatory, indicating an uncouth, untutored, poor villager or even aboriginal, generally credited with being a ne'er-do-well and potential troublemaker.

13. What follows is an epitome of the *Rāmāyaṇa* epic as told in Bengal.

14. As in many cultures, only virtuous and high-ranking women will give birth to beautiful children.

15. There is a pun here, for *lālā* means "saliva" or "spittle," and *lāl* means "reddish" or "ruddy," the color of the pinkish pearls he spits up; *mohana* means "enchantment" or "fascination." He is alternately called Motilāl, the name of the pearl he spits.

16. An oath taken on the head of someone puts that person's life at stake. There are many cautionary tales about swearing on the head of your children or some other loved one; it is a powerful statement of intention to swear on your own head.

17. See "The Fabled *Beṅgamā* Bird and the Stupid Prince," note 1.

The Erstwhile Bride and Her Winged Horse

This translation is made from the anonymous *Manohara phāsarāra pālā: satyanārāyaṇa pāñcālī*, 10th ed. (Kāthai, Midnapur: Nihar Press, 1313 BS [1906]). The text is very close to Rasamaya's *Galakāṭā phāsyarāra pālā*, Bengali manuscript no. 214, Dhaka University (17 folios; complete; dated 1264 BS [1857]), a likely source for the heavily edited print edition.

1. Kaikeyī had received two boons, one of which she used to place her own son Bhārata on the throne and to exile Rāma for fourteen years.

2. See "The Fabled *Beṅgamā* Bird and the Stupid Prince," note 15.

3. See "The Fabled *Beṅgamā* Bird and the Stupid Prince," note 8.

4. There is a pun on the phrase *kāli karāli*, referring both to the goddesss Kālī, who is bloodthirsty, black, and fanged, and to the stain, *kāli,* on his lineage.

5. Dhanvantari was a celestial *deva* who was preceptor in the Ayurveda medical treatises. He had several encounters with serpents, most notably Takṣaka and those sent by Manasā to slay him and his followers, but he always revived his students and vanquished the snakes with his superior knowledge of poisons and their antidotes.

6. The old man insultingly addresses the merchant with *tui*, the inferior second-person pronoun "you," generally reserved for servants, dogs, and the most intimate settings, such as with God or a lover.

7. Kṛṣṇa and Balarāma met the hunchback Trivakrā, attendant to King Kaṃsa. Out of love for Kṛṣṇa she gave him the special unguents she was carrying for the king. In return, Kṛṣṇa raised her up by the chin and straightened her back.

8. It should be noted that Bangla does not mark gender in its pronouns, so the ambiguity of this charade is easily executed in the language, whereas in English we are forced to choose he or she, making the text less subtle.

9. The following speech bears an affected lexicon, grammar, and syntax that produces a pidgin Urdu, an attempt to disguise the origins of the speaker, who pretends to be from the northwest portion of the subcontinent, a land famed for its warriors.

10. The *Mahābhārata*, *vana parva*, chapters 52–79, recounts the tale of Nala and Damayantī, the former of whom was separated from his wife and then turned into a hideous form by the serpent Karkoṭaka, whom he had saved from a fire in a forest where he had been cursed to remain until Nala freed him. He bit Nala with poison to kill Kali, who was possessing Nala at the time, with poison, which eventually forced Kali from Nala's body. The curse here is Nala's forgetfulness of his identity while under the possession of Kali.

11. This is the famous scene in which Uddhāva brings news of Kṛṣṇa to the women of Vraja, and tries to convince them that Kṛṣṇa is really with them at all times; they roundly chastise him for his stupidity, since Kṛṣṇa is there in Mathurā while they are stuck in Vṛndāvana.

The Bloodthirsty Ogress Who Would Be Queen

This translation is made from Kiṅkara Dāsa, *Śaśīdhara pāla: satyanārāyaṇa pāñcālī* (Khātai, Midnapur: Madhusūdhana Jānā at Nihar Press, 1322 BS [1915]).

1. These are the three great departures represented in Bengali literature, the first two in the well-known epics, the third that of the religious figure Kṛṣṇa Caitanya or Gaurāṅga, "the Golden Limbed One," who left his wife, Viṣṇupriyā, and mother, Śacī, to renounce the world.

2. The Gaṅgā, the Yamunā, and the mythical Sarasvatī, which joins the other two from underground.

3. See "The Fabled *Beṅgamā* Bird and the Stupid Prince," note 8.

4. The first book of the *Devī Bhāgavata* tells the story of Śukadeva, who was the son of the sage Vyāsa, and was born by a celestial nymph or *apsaras* named Ghṛtācī. Ghṛtācī happened along when the ascetic was completing one hundred years of austerities or *tapasya*, and feared his advances, so turned her herself into a parrot, which because of its celestial beauty, incited

by its flight just as much eroticism as her regular form. Vyāsa cast his seed on a stick, which he then used to prepare his fire, the smoke of which impregnated the parrot. Because Vyāsa had done austerities for the sake of a son replete with all accomplishments, composed of the perfection of the five elements, Śukadeva was cognizant while still in the womb.

5. Śikhidhvaja and Mayūrdhvaja are synonyms, and epithets of Kārttikeya, a Hindu god of war. Because Śikhidhvaja is a synonym of his father's name, the connection allows the prince to speak truthfully, though in a manner somewhat veiled.

6. The gem was the fabled Syamantaka, retrieved by Kṛṣṇa after he had been falsely accused of stealing it, then refused when Śatrājit attempted to place it in his daughter Satyābhāma's dowry when she wedded Kṛṣṇa.

7. Because there is no distinction in the pronunciation of these sibilants, there is a pun on the name of the cucumber (*śasā*) and its taking (*dhāra*) in the name of the hero Śaśīdhara.

The Princess Who Nursed Her Own Husband

This translation is made from Gayārāma Dāsa, *Madanamañjari pālā: satyanārāyaṇa pāñcālī* (Khātai, Midnapur: Madhusūdhana Jānā at Nihar Press, 1334 BS [1927]).

1. Ṣaṣṭhī, "the Sixth," is worshiped for the welfare of children on the sixth day after birth, on the sixth of each month in the household women's ritual cycle, and at other auspicious moments, as here. See also Introduction, note 33.

2. *Darśana* is a term used to describe the auspicious act of beholding one's Lord, whether God or the Goddess in the form of an icon, or an important or famous person, such as the king. When the object of attention returns the gaze, the individual is blessed.

3. A "division" is an *akṣauhiṇī*, composed of 109,350 infantry, 65,610 cavalry, 21,870 elephant mounts, and 21,870 charioteers.

4. According to the *Kathāsaritsāgara*, Rati prayed to Śiva to restore Kāma's life after he had been incinerated by Śiva in his wrath. Śiva granted her request, but with the proviso that she would raise him herself. And so, with the name of Māyāvatī, she became kitchen maid to the *asura* Śambhara, who held the boon that he would live until Kāma was reborn. Meanwhile Kṛṣṇa, having received a boon from Śiva, had a son with Rukmiṇī, which upon inquiry Śambhara stole and threw into the sea. A giant bottom-scavenging fish swallowed the child, but was soon caught, and by the workings of fate, given to Śambhara, who cut it open and found the child. He gave the child over to Rati, who cared for it with special zeal when she was told by the peripetetic Nārada that the child was none other than Kāma himself, and so the latter was raised at the hands of his mother.

5. See "The Erstwhile Bride and Her Winged Horse," note 8.

6. The enumeration of these tales appears to be a not-so-subtle advertisement for Nihar Press publications, all of which are among their catalog. The tales of Rāmbhāvatī, Vidyādhara, Śaśīdhara, and Campāvatī have been translated for this volume. The inclusion likewise suggests that the story was committed to print later than the rest, or at least redacted by an enterprising editor.

7. Charred tobacco was occasionally used as a dentifrice and gum stimulant after meals in Bengal during this time, probably the late eighteenth or early nineteenth century.

8. Appropriately enough, the word *vara* means both "groom" and "boon."

9. This concoction is actually a simple form of *śirṇi*, which is the preferred offering to Satya Pīr.

10. See "The Fabled *Beṅgamā* Bird and the Stupid Prince," note 8.

11. There is a mistake in the text here, having Smarahara, the "Destroyer or Enemy of Smara," (i.e., Śiva)—Smara is the god of love—shooting Kāma's own arrows. I have rendered *smarahara* as the "destruction of memory or sense" equivalent to the English "lost in love."

12. See note 1.

GLOSSARY

adharma violating the standards and norms of society (*dharma*).

Āgama a sacred text that in popular Bengali terms contains esoteric knowledge associated with the manipulation of spells and incantations; often paired with Nigama (q.v.).

akṣauhiṇī a military "division" composed of 109,350 infantry, 65,610 cavalry, 21,870 elephant mounts, and 21,870 charioteers.

apsaras a celestial nymph of exceptional beauty and grace, skilled in music and dance.

āstānā a small pedestal or dais that serves as the focal point for the aniconic worship of Satya Pīr, and made of gold for more elaborate forms of worship.

asura a demonic celestial who is in perpetual conflict with the gods and the forces of good; not to be confused, but often paired with, *rākṣāsa* (q.v.).

avatāra literally a "descent" of god to earth, usually affiliated with Nārāyaṇa or Viṣṇu, in whole or in part, to restore the proper order of the world (*dharma*); in popular usage it can refer to any extraordinary individual who is believed to be divine or divinely inspired.

badshāh overlord or king, usually a designation for a king who has lesser kings under his rule.

bāhini a military "regiment" composed of 81 elephant riders, 81 charioteers, 243 cavalry, and 405 infantry; these numbers are derived from multiples of primes (so $81 = 3^4$, $243 = 3^5$, $405 = 3^4 \times 5$) and are therefore auspicious, perfect, or complete.

bālī, bālī piṇḍa offerings of riceballs to feed the ancestors for seven generations in both directions (past and future), ensuring salutary transmigration.

bāṅgāliṇī a perpetually poor and destitute woman encountered in the rural parts of eastern Bengal.

bel wood apple, *aegle mamelos*; sometimes referred in English literature as the Bengal quince, but technically a different fruit.

beṅgamā, beṅgamī fabled birds inhabiting the deepest forest, who have priceless gems embedded in their heads or throats, and who are famous for their ability to speak and reason.

Bhagavad Gītā eighteen chapters from the *Mahābhārata* epic in which Lord Kṛṣṇa explains to Arjuna the necessity of fighting the war with his cousins; often the touchstone for popular notions of *avatāra* and the role of god in human affairs.

Bhāgavata Purāṇa foundational text of worshipers of Nārāyaṇa Viṣṇu, the tenth book of which is especially prominent for detailing the exploits of Lord Kṛṣṇa.

bhajana worship by singing the praises of the deity.

bhaṇitā signature line in which the poet comments on, or enters into, the action of the narrative.

Bhāṣya name of Patañjali's commentary on Pāṇini's *Sūtras*, the key to Sanskrit grammar for any student; also the shorthand name of Śaṅkara's commentary on Bādarāyana's *Vedānta Sūtras*.

Bidhātā the celestial figure who writes an individual's fate on the forehead.

bimba a brilliant red-orange cucurbit of the gourd family; this fruit is frequently invoked to describe the fullness and redness of a woman's lips.

Bismillah an invocation to God to oversee whatever task is being undertaken, always recited at the beginning of any kind of work; and it appears prominently at the opening of every chapter of the Qur'ān save the 9th: *Bismillah al-Raḥmān al-Raḥim*, i.e., "In the name of the merciful Lord of Mercy."

brahmācārī a celebate student or, more generally, a practicing *paṇḍita* or scholar who observes strictly the brahminical regulations.

Brāhmaṇa ritual text explicating the Veda.

campā, campaka an especially beautiful and fragrant magnolia blossom, used in garlands and offerings to gods and holy people.

crore millions, ten million; an indefinitely large number.

dacoit a highwayman or robber, usually roaming in gangs of five or more, the word originating in Bengal, where it entered the British penal code.

ḍākinī witch, female goblin.

daṇḍa rod, staff; metonym for punishment and law; a unit of time equivalent to twenty-four minutes.

daṇḍapati literally "lord of the staff," enforcer of law and justice; a king.

darśana a view or vision; the act of beholding the icon of a deity or someone important as a way of showing respect and receiving blessings.

dāstān a genre of folk tales extolling the virtues and exploits of figures in early Islamic history.

deva (m), devī (f) deity.

devaloka heaven.

dharma moral and cosmic order; proper behavior; personal duty.

Dharma Śāstras texts that lay out and adjudicate the intricacies of *dharma* and the law.

dhoti a traditional man's garment, consisting of approximately two to three meters of cloth wrapped around the waist and between the legs.

dundubī a small double-ended drum with a small ball on the end of a string that hits one end and then the other with a flick of the wrist.

durbār royal court; the holding of court.

durbbā a sacred grass that is generally spread for the celestials gathered at a sacrifice or other ritual, or for honored guests.

fakir a Muslim Sufi holy man.

gajamati the fabled "elephant pearl," an exceptionally large, perfectly round, unmottled, and flawless pearl.

gandharva heavenly musician.

gāzi warrior saints who defend Islam.

ghat landing steps on the banks of rivers, ponds, or tanks that allow easy entry to the water.

gopī cowherd girls and women, generally associated with the pastoral idyll of Kṛṣṇa, the cowherd boy, who romances the village girls; *gopī*s figure prominent in the tenth book of the *Bhāgavata Purāṇa*.

gorocanā a yellow orpiment made from the liver of cows, highly prized for use in brahminical ritual.

haṃsarājā literally the "lord among swans or geese" or "the king of birds;" in mythic terms the bird capable of carrying humans or deities.

hulāhuli a high-pitched trill made generally by women at auspicious moments.

jalāñjalī offerings of water in a display of reverence and respect.

kāhana, kāhaṇa an old measure worth 16 *paṇa*s or 1280 cowries, now difficult to estimate, but substantial.

kāhini story or tale, synonym for *qissa*.

kalimā the creed of Muslims, "There is no God but God, and Muhammad is the Apostle of God."

kautuka-kathā humorous tales.

karamāt the wonder-working power of a Sufi saint, often demonstrated to unbelievers.

kecchā, kissā Bangla terms for the genre of *qissa* (q.v.).

kokil cuckoo, fabled for its songs appropriate to romance.

kṣatra a generic social designator of a class of rulers, warriors, and administrators; *kṣatriya* caste.

lakh 100,000; an impressively large number.

madhyadeśa the "middle land," a domesticated area of habitation constituting the upper Gangetic plain of the subcontinent, whose limits are defined in the east by the course of the Gāṅgā River; anything lying outside that (here the eastern portions of the Bangla-speaking region, primarily today Bangladesh) constituted a kind of frontier or wasteland unsuitable for habitation by proper brahmins.

Mahābhārata the great epic of the Bhārata civil war that pitted the five Pāṇḍavas against their cousins, the Kauravas, both sides cousins of Kṛṣṇa. The *Bhagavad Gītā* (q.v.) is found in the *bhiṣma parva* of this text.

mahārāja a king or great king, often designating relative rather than absolute rank.

makara a mythical beast, half crocodile, half fish, emblematic of Kāmadeva, the god of love.

malfuẓat a class of Sufi biography generally containing the discourses of the master.

mālinī (f) a garland weaver or flower vendor, who is generally associated with the creation and manipulation of potions and ensorcelling charms and spells for things as benign as capturing the heart of a lover, or as malevolent as enslaving people; hence the secondary meaning of "witch."

maṅgala kāvya semi-epic poems in early Bangla literature dedicated to the promotion of a local goddess or occasionally a god, whose recitation incites auspiciousness (*maṅgala*).

mantra an utterance of one or more syllables understood to harbor mystical power to increase the efficacy of action or to be used as a weapon of others' destruction, or a prophylactic device against others' attacks; popularly used to signify the power of magic.

maund currently one hundred pounds troy weight or 82.20 pounds avoirdupois; but also a traditional unit of measure that would fill a large basket called a *maund*.

mohara a gold coin or sovereign of considerable value.

motilāl a pearl common to Bengal that is pink in luster.

muktab traditional primary school for Muslims, often associated with courts.

mulmul an exceptionally fine, lightweight muslin cloth, woven so delicately that a bolt can be pulled through a finger ring.

muni seer or sage.

murśid a spiritual teacher or guide.

nāga serpent, cobra; lords of the region beneath the surface of the earth, who often function to signify lordship or divinity by spreading their protective hoods over the individual.

Nātha member of a religious sect who utilizes yoga to reach a state of immortality; generally a worshiper of Lord Śiva, and who is often affiliated with the workings of magic.

Nigama a text explicating the Veda, often paired with Āgama (q.v.) in popular lore, signifying an esoteric knowledge affiliated with the workings of the sciences of astrology and necromancy, and other forms of black magic.

ojhā a professional snake handler and master of antidotes.

paigambar a north Indian word that encompasses the meanings of both the Arabic *nabi* (prophet) and *rasul* (apostle).

pakṣirāja literally "king" (*rājā*) of "birds" (*pakṣi*, literally "winged ones"), but it also refers to winged horses capable of carrying humans through the skies; a secondary epithet equates *pakṣirāja* with Viṣṇu's gigantic bird-mount Garuḍa.

pālā, pālāgāna story or tale, often set to music and sung (*gāna*); an episode within a larger cycle of tales, such as the Satya Pīr cycle.

pāñcālī a folk narrative genre of a distinctive meter, often interchanged with *pālā* (q.v.).

paṇḍita a learned brahmin who can teach, advise, or conduct rituals for a fee; a pandit.

pativratā an ideal, chaste, and devoted wife who sacrifices everything for her husband and honor.

payār the most common Bangla metrical form, generally a couplet of fourteen syllables per verse with caesura after the sixth and eighth syllables.

phāsarā a highwayman or cuthroat, popularly called a dacoit in Bengal.

piṇḍa, piṇḍadāna the ritual offering of riceballs to the manes or departed ancestors.

pīr a Muslim holy man and guide, considered to wield enormous powers.

piśāca (m), *piśācī* (f) a type of demon that feasts on flesh.

pitṛloka ancestral manes.

prasāda the leftover food offerings to a deity or divine figure, eaten by the devotee as a form of ingestible grace.

pūjā the ritual demonstration of honor and respect for a deity or holy figure; worship.

Purāṇa a class of texts from which much of the classical Hindu mythology is derived.

purohit, kulin purohit a proper and respected brahmin ritual officiant of impeccable breeding, training, and culture.

qazi a local judge who rules on civil, communal, and personal issues in a village or town.

qissa genre of tale that migrated from Persian into north Indian vernaculars via Urdu and Punjabi.

rājā king.

rākṣasa (m), *rākṣasī* (f), *rākṣasakā* (f) a class of anthropophagous demon, cannibal.

Rāmadān the fast observed by Muslims to celebrate the month during which the Qur'ān was first revealed to Muhammad.

Rāmāyaṇa one of the two great epics of India, whose hero, Lord Rāma, avenges the kidnapping of his wife, Sītā, by the demon Rāvaṇa, and restores moral order in his vast kingdoms.

rāsa-dance, *rāsa-līlā* the famous circle dance described in the tenth book of the *Bhāgavata Purāṇa* in which Kṛṣṇa multiplies himself so that every *gopī* (q.v.) imagines herself to be dancing alone with him.

rūpa-kathā fairy tales.

sādha the insatiable cravings for often difficult-to-obtain foods that pregnant women have, and which are often addressed through special rituals.

sādhu (m), *sādhvī* (f) holy or pure, often indicating an idealized condition; in a religious context, the masculine reference is to holy men; in the femine to the ideal wife; *sādhu* is also a word for merchant in old Bangla.

Śākta followers of *śakti*, the feminine power permeating the universe, personified as the Goddess, Śakti.

saṃnyāsī a holy man who has formally renounced the world in pursuit of religious goals and who is often renowned for the practice of yoga.

sandeśa popular Bengali milk-based sweets that are considered delicacies.

saśa a long cucumber that grows on climbing creepers and can often be found entwined around a tree or running along the roof of a house; the form in which the souls or life forces of demonic figures are contained.

śāstra ancient religious texts that serve as the source of Hindu authority.

satī a woman who is pure, chaste, and totally devoted to her husband, so much so that in extreme cases she immolates herself on his pyre, and is believed to ignite the flames with the power of her own purity.

satītva the quality of being *satī*.

sāttvika-bhāvas the physical signs of the presence pure love for the divine, including such manifestations as incessant crying, loud expostulations, fainting, the display of goose-flesh, stupor, catalepsis, and so forth; in Vaiṣṇava theology it indexes the quality of devotional experience.

sayyid a Muslim who claims descent from Muhammad through his daughter Fātima and her husband ʻAlī.

seer a unit of weight that was nonstandard; generally reckoned about 2 or 2-½ pounds Troy weight making forty seers to the maund (q.v.).

siddha a perfected one, one who through yoga has attained certain extraordinary powers (*siddhi*).

śirṇi (alternate *śirṇī*, *śīriṇī*, *śinni*, *śinnī*) a concoction of rice flower, banana, sugar, milk, and spices, prepared as offering to Satya Pīr.

śloka a traditional Sanskrit couplet composed of sixteen syllables per line, with caesura after the eighth and sixteenth syllable.

śrāddha obsequies; the funerary rites performed by the eldest son after the death of his father, usually observed at a famous pilgrimage center such as Gayā in current-day Bihar.

tabasheer lit. "the sugar of bamboo," this substance is on occasion found in the joints of bamboo and prized for its medicinal qualities and rarity.

taitala an astrological conjunction of stars and planets considered very powerful and auspicious.

Tantra a class of ritual texts, originally paired with the *sūtras* as the woof and warp, respectively, of Vedic exegesis; popularly, a class of texts connoting bizarre ritual action, often including magical rites, resuscitation of the dead, and so forth.

Tantrasāra a famous treatise or digest of *tantrika* ritual in Bengal.

tantrika pertaining to the texts called Tantras or the practice of Tāntra.

Tāntrika practitioner of Tāntra.

tapasya religious austerities through the practice of yoga, which generate heat and other powers as byproducts.

tarpaṇa oblations of water to the manes; a more generalized form of ritual appeasement of departed ancestors that supplements the *piṇḍadāna* (q.v.) or, when the latter is not possible, substitutes for it.

ṭīkā a specialized verse-by-verse commentary on an important religious text.

tilaka the mark on the forehead indicating sectarian affiliation, occasionally social rank, or among women simply cosmetic ornament.

ṭippaṇī a commentary that often glosses words or phrases in an important religious text or further elaborates the more formal *ṭīkā* (q.v.) commentary.

totā the popinjay or parrot, famous for its ability to imitate human speech; in mythical terms a parrot who actually talks and reasons.

tripadi a three-footed meter in old Bangla that generally observes symmetrical patterns of two short followed by one long verse (e.g., six, six, and eight-syllable lines); a meter often employed to explore deep emotional experience, positive or negative, and often used to describe the nature and effects of love.

Tritantra a *tantrika* text of unclear provenance.

vairāgī a Vaiṣṇava ascetic who lives a disciplined life, similar to a *saṃnyāsī* (q.v.); in general terms, someone who is indifferent to the world.

Veda the ancient poetry texts of India, sources of moral and ritual order; the standard against which all other orders are measured.

vedi technically the hourglass-shaped fire pit of Vedic ritual; in more general terms, the fire pit or even altar of any ritual.

vīṇā a classical stringed instrument of ancient India, with gourds on both ends that serve as sounding boards.

vrata a promise or a vow to honor or cherish a deity or holy figure in exchange for some gain or the general weal; *vrata*s tend to be the primary domain of women in the domestic setting, but can, in the case of Satya Pīr, be observed by anyone.

vrata-kathā the story that is told to accompany the *vrata*.

wazir (m), *wazirāṇī* (f) the primary minister in a state ruled by Muslims, who, by virtue of the king's reliance on his judgment, wields a power that rivals that of the most important generals and other state functionaries; the feminine refers to the wazir's wife, not to a female advisor.

yavana foreigner, literally "Ionian," but later applied in Bangla primarily to Muslims who ruled or were present in traditional Hindu realms.

yoga a highly disciplined mode of meditation in which the practitioner gains superhuman powers in the quest for immortality.

yogī (m), *yogiṇī* (f) a practitioner of yoga who gains extraordinary powers; the feminine form connotes a woman who has gained nefarious powers and is, then, a witch.

FURTHER READINGS

The Fabulous Tales of Satya Pīr: Bengali Sources Used in This Translation

Anonymous. *Manohara phāsarāra pālā: satyanārāyaṇa pāñcālī.* 10th ed. Kãtai, Midnapur: Nihar Press, 1313 BS [1906].

Dvīja Kavibara. *Bāghāmbarer pālā: satyanārāyaṇa pāñcālī.* 10th ed. Khãtai, Midnapur: Nihar Press, 1322 BS [1915].

Gayārāma Dāsa. *Madanamañjari pālā: satyanārāyaṇa pāñcālī.* Khãtai: Madhusūdhana Jānā at Nihar Press, 1334 BS [1927].

Kavi Āriph (Arif). *Lālamonera kāhini.* Edited by Girīndranātha Dāsa. Gokulapur, 24 Parganas: Śrīmati Karuṇāmayī Dāsa, 1984.

———. *Lālamonera kecchā.* Kolkata: Sudhānidhi Yantra, 1274 BS [1867].

———. *Lālamonera kecchā.* Kolkata: Viśvambhara Lāha, 1276 BS [1869].

Kavi Kaṇva [=Karṇa]. *Satyanārāyaṇa kathā.* Manuscript no. 59b. Dhaka University Library. 14 folios, complete, dated. 1273 BS [1866].

Kavi Karṇa. *Ākhoṭi pālā.* In *Pālās of Śrī Kavi Karṇa*, compiled and edited by Bishnupada Panda. Kalāmūlaśāstra Granthamālā, vols. 4–7. New Delhi: Indira Gandhi National Centre for the Arts and Motilal Banarsidass, 1991, 4: 1–93.

Kiṅkara Dāsa. *Matilāla pālā: satyanārāyaṇa pāñcālī.* Khãtai, Midnapur: Nihar Press, 1322 BS [1915].

———. *Rambhāvatī pālā: satyanārāyaṇa pāñcālī.* 4th ed. Khãtai, Midnapur: Madhusūdhana Jānā at Nihar Press, 1331 BS [1924].

———. *Śaśīdhara pālā: satyanārāyaṇa pāñcālī.* Khãtai, Midnapur: Madhusūdhana Jānā at Nihar Press, 1322 BS [1915].

Rāmeśvara. *Ākhoṭi pālā.* In *Rāmeśvara racanāvalī*, edited by Pañcānana Cakravartī. Kolkata: Baṅgīya Sāhitya Pariṣat, 1371 BS [1964], 536–49.

———. *Ākhoṭi pālā: satyanārāyaṇa pañcālī.* 3d ed. Khãtāi, Midnapur: Madhusūdhana Jānā at Nihar Press, 1924.

Rasamaya. *Galakāṭā phāsyarāra pālā.* Bengali manuscript no. 214. Dhaka University Library. 17 folios; complete; dated: 1264 BS [1857].

A Select Bibliography of Bengali Folk Narratives in Translation

Banerjee, Kasindranath. *Popular Tales of Bengal.* Calcutta, 1905.

Bradley-Birt, F. B. *Bengal Fairy Tales.* Illustrated by Abanindranath Tagore. London: John Lane, Bodley Head, and New York: John Lane, 1920.

Chakravarty, Padmaja. *Folk Tales from Bengal.* New York: HarperCollins, 1996.

Chowdhury, Kabir. *Folktales of Bangladesh.* Vol. 1. Dacca: Bangla Academy, 1972.

Dasgupta, Sayantani, and Shamita Das Dasgupta. *The Demon Slayers and Other Stories*. New York: Interlink Books, 1995.

Day, Lal Behari. *Folk-Tales of Bengal*. Illustrated by Warwick Goble. London: Macmillan, 1912 [first ed. 1883].

Devi, Shovana. *The Orient Pearls*. London: Macmillan, 1915.

Dimock, Edward C. *The Thief of Love: Bengali Tales from Court and Village*. Chicago: University of Chicago Press, 1963.

Majumdar, Geeta. *Folktales of Bengal*. New Delhi: Sterling, 1971.

McCulloch, William. *Bengali Household Tales*. London: Hodder and Stoughton, 1912.

Mode, Heinz, and Arun Ray, eds. *Bengalische Märchen*. Frankfurt: Insel Verlag, 1969.

Panda, Bishnupada, comp., ed., and trans. *Pālās of Śrī Kavi Karṇa*. 4 vols. Kalāmūlaśāstra Series, nos. 4–7, edited by Kapila Vatsyayan. New Delhi: Indira Gandhi National Centre for the Arts and Motilal Banarsidass, 1991.

Sen, Dinesh Chandra. *The Folk-Literature of Bengal*. Calcutta: University of Calcutta, 1920.

A Select Bibliography of South Asia Folk Narratives in Translation

Birla, L. N. *Popular Tales of Rajasthan*. Bombay: Bharatiya Vidya Bhavan, 1967.

Bompas, Cecil Henry. *Folklore of the Santal Parganas*. London: David Nutt, 1909.

Dracott, Alice Elizabeth. *Simla Village Tales, or Folk Tales from the Himalayas*. London: John Murray, 1914.

Edgerton, Franklin. *Vikrama's Adventures: Or the Thirty-Two Tales of the Throne*. Harvard Oriental Series, no. 26. Cambridge: Harvard University Press, 1926.

Jacobs, Joseph. *Indian Fairy Tales*. New York: A. L. Burt, n.d.

Knowles, James Hinton. *Folktales of Kashmir*. London: Kegan Paul, Trench, Trubner, 1893.

Munshi, K. M., and R. R. Diwakar, eds. *Stories of Vikramaditya (Simhasana Dwatrimsika)*. Bombay: Bharatiya Vidya Bhavan, 1960.

Narayan, Kirin, in collaboration with Urmila Devi Sood. *Mondays on the Dark Night of the Moon: Himalayan Foothill Folktales*. Oxford: Oxford University Press, 1997.

Parker, Henry. *Village Folktales of Ceylon*. 3 vols. Dehiwala, Sri Lanka: Tisara Prakasakayo, 1971.

Penzer, N. M., ed. *The Ocean of Story, being C. H. Tawney's Translation of Somadeva's Kathā Sarit Sagara*. 10 vols. London: Charles J. Sawyer, 1924; reprint Delhi: Motilat Banarsidass, 1968.

Pritchett, Frances W. *The Romance Tradition in Urdu: Adventures from the Dāstān of Amīr Ḥamzah*. New York: Columbia University Press, 1991.

Ramanujan, A. K. *Folktales from India: A Selection of Oral Tales from Twenty-Two Languages*. The Pantheon Fairy Tale and Folktale Library. New York: Pantheon, 1991.

Steel, Flora Annie. *Tales of the Punjab*. London: Macmillan, 1894.

Swynnerton, Charles. *Romantic Tales from the Punjab with Indian Nights' Entertainment*. London: Archibald Constable, 1908.

Index

Printed in the United States
By Bookmasters